Guidance for Healthcare Ethics Committees

Second edition

Guidance for Healthcare Ethics Committees

***

Second edition

Edited by
D. Micah Hester
University of Arkansas for Medical Sciences, College of Medicine

Toby L. Schonfeld
US Department of Veterans Affairs

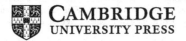

CAMBRIDGE
UNIVERSITY PRESS

University Printing House, Cambridge CB2 8BS, United Kingdom

One Liberty Plaza, 20th Floor, New York, NY 10006, USA

477 Williamstown Road, Port Melbourne, VIC 3207, Australia

314–321, 3rd Floor, Plot 3, Splendor Forum, Jasola District Centre,
New Delhi – 110025, India

103 Penang Road, #05–06/07, Visioncrest Commercial, Singapore 238467

Cambridge University Press is part of the University of Cambridge.

It furthers the University's mission by disseminating knowledge in the pursuit
of education, learning, and research at the highest international levels
of excellence.

www.cambridge.org
Information on this title: www.cambridge.org/9781108791014
DOI: 10.1017/9781108788250

© Cambridge University Press 2012, 2022

First published 2012
Second edition 2022

A catalogue record for this publication is available from the British Library.

Library of Congress Cataloging-in-Publication Data
Names: Hester, D. Micah, editor. | Schonfeld, Toby, editor.
Title: Guidance for healthcare ethics committees / edited by
    D. Micah Hester, Toby L. Schonfeld.
Description: Second edition. | Cambridge, United Kingdom ; New York, NY :
    Cambridge University Press, 2021. | Includes bibliographical references
    and index.
Identifiers: LCCN 2021029075 (print) | LCCN 2021029076 (ebook) | ISBN
    9781108791014 (paperback) | ISBN 9781108788250 (epub)
Subjects: MESH: Ethics Committees, Clinical | Hospital Administration–ethics |
    Ethics, Clinical | Delivery of Health Care–ethics | Practice Guidelines as Topic |
    BISAC: MEDICAL / General
Classification: LCC R724 (print) | LCC R724 (ebook) | NLM WX 150.1 | DDC
    174.2–dc23
LC record available at https://lccn.loc.gov/2021029075
LC ebook record available at https://lccn.loc.gov/2021029076

ISBN 978-1-108-79101-4 Paperback

In memory of J. David Hester:
"We can be Heroes, just for one day"
– David Bowie/Brian Eno

Contents

Contributors

Peter Angelos
MacLean Center for Clinical Medical Ethics, University of Chicago

Jessica Berg
Case Western Reserve University

Georgina D. Campelia
University of Washington School of Medicine

Felicia Cohn
Kaiser Permanente Southern California

Jana Craig
Kaiser Permanente Northern California

Thomas V. Cunningham
Kaiser Permanente Southern California

Sabrina F. Derrington
Center for Pediatric Bioethics, Children's Hospital Los Angeles

Arthur R. Derse
Center for Bioethics and Medical Humanities, Medical College of Wisconsin

Douglas S. Diekema
University of Washington School of Medicine

Denise M. Dudzinski
University of Washington School of Medicine

Claretta Y. Dupree
Captain, US Navy, Retired

Kelly East
HudsonAlpha Institute for Biotechnology

Joseph J. Fins
Weill Cornell Medical College
Yale Law School

Paul J. Ford
Cleveland Clinic

Cynthia M. A. Geppert
National Center for Ethics in Healthcare, US Department of Veterans Affairs

Kenneth W. Goodman
University of Miami Miller School of Medicine Institute for Bioethics and Health Policy

D. Micah Hester
University of Arkansas for Medical Sciences, College of Medicine

Nancy S. Jecker
University of Washington School of Medicine

Whitley Kelley
HudsonAlpha Institute for Biotechnology

Nancy M. P. King
Wake Forest School of Medicine

Kathy Kinlaw
Center for Ethics, Emory University

John D. Lantos
Children's Mercy Hospital Bioethics Center

Stephen Latham
Yale University

Anne Drapkin Lyerly
University of North Carolina at Chapel Hill

Thomas May
Washington State University, Elson S. Floyd College of Medicine

Jennifer L. McCurdy
Michigan State University
The Center for Bioethics and Social Justice

Margaret Moon
Johns Hopkins University School of Medicine

John C. Moskop
Wake Forest School of Medicine

Thaddeus Mason Pope
Mitchell Hamline School of Law

Toby L. Schonfeld
US Department of Veterans Affairs

Darryl Schuitevoerder
University of Chicago

Wayne Shelton
AMBI
Albany Medical College

Alissa Hurwitz Swota
Wolfson Children's Hospital/Baptist
Health System

Katherine Wasson
Neiswanger Institute of Bioethics,
Loyola University Chicago

Mark R. Wicclair
Center for Bioethics and Health Law,
University of Pittsburgh

Lucia Wocial
John J Lynch, MD Center for Ethics
MedStar Washington Hospital Center

Preface

In 1992 The Joint Commission on Hospital Accreditation (The Joint Commission) began requiring every accredited hospital to have a mechanism to handle ethical concerns within its institution. In response to this (and other cultural forces in medicine), hospitals across America have come to satisfy the requirement by constituting an institutional healthcare ethics committee (HEC).[1] Physicians, nurses, administrators, social workers, chaplains, community volunteers, and, others populate these committees. Yet by their own admission, many of these individuals, while well intentioned and personally invested, have neither training in ethics nor the tools at their disposal to aid in their ethical considerations. Even more basically, not many members of an HEC, not to mention a healthcare institution writ large, are comfortable explaining what constitutes an ethical consideration. So, while these individuals are the people both medical professionals and patients turn to for ethical insight into the complexities of medical decision-making, they themselves recognize that they are often underprepared to handle the depth and complexity of many moral problems raised by health care.[2]

It is within this context that we offer this book. The purpose of this text is to serve as a primer for members of HECs regarding the three main roles that comprise the function of an HEC: consultation, policy, and education. The book provides material to aid in elucidating and educating about these functions for the many different persons who find themselves confronted with ethically challenging medical situations by virtue of being members of some HECs.

While we, the editors, have worked for decades in this field, we know our limitations, and thus, to facilitate attaining this goal, we have invited leaders in the field of ethics to author chapters in their areas of expertise. Chapters are directed at educated individuals who are members of HECs, whether they are new to the committee or they simply seek to solidify their knowledge on particular topics. The chapters herein try to cover each topic in such a way as to inform and support the work of HECs specifically. For example, the chapter on Advance Care Planning does not go into detail about forms, conversation partners, and other features of Advance Directives (these can vary by state and there are many other sources to find and describe those specifically). Instead, the authors describe the ways in which HEC members may encounter ethical concerns about Advance Directives and end-of-life planning, as well as how HEC members can engage productively with the issues presented.

Further, in order to make the material as accessible as possible, we have oriented each chapter around a consistent format. Every chapter opens with a set of objectives, then proceeds to a case or series of cases, followed by key content, and concludes with questions for discussion. We would like to take a moment to explain each of these features:

---

[1] Some writings call these "hospital ethics committees," some call them "institutional ethics committees", or "clinical ethics committees." We have chosen the term "healthcare ethics committee," and will use that term throughout this volume.

[2] In this text, we use the terms "ethics" and "morals"/"morality" as well as "ethical" and "moral" interchangeably.

(1) **Objectives:** Objectives for each chapter were negotiated between the editors and the chapter authors. When possible, we used objectives suggested in the *Education Guide for Improving Competencies in Clinical Ethics Consultation* (2009) published by the Clinical Ethics Education Task Force of the American Society for Bioethics and Humanities (ASBH). However, since this guide is directed exclusively at ethics *consultation*, many objectives were altered or authored with a broader committee charge in mind. Nevertheless, the connection to the ASBH Task Force helps to standardize, where possible, the topics and approaches contained herein.

(2) **Cases:** All chapters begin with at least one case. Many chapters include multiple cases, or iterations of the same case, throughout the work. The purpose of such cases in this work is twofold. For one, cases give a concrete demonstration of the way the individual chapter topics may present themselves to members of HECs. Note that such demonstrations are not meant to be representative or categorical; rather, they are meant to be illustrations of the kinds of things to which an HEC must attend. Second, when taken as a whole, the cases in the text demonstrate how individual personal, professional, institutional, social, cultural, or religious values can affect the emergence of and response to ethical issues in a clinical setting. These conflicts of value are important motivators of ethics cases, and it behooves members of HECs to consider the ways in which these conflicts broadly construed may affect both the form and function of their committee.

(3) **Content:** We felt it was important to have scholars recognized in specific fields to write the chapters for which they have particular expertise. This experience not only lends expert, knowledgeable insight to the text but also enables HEC members to be introduced to the individuals who help shape scholarship in this arena. However, because the chapters are all independently authored, they may vary a bit in terms of tone and style. We have ensured consistency of format whenever we could, but as editors we felt it was important for each chapter author to present material in their own voice.

(4) **Questions for Discussion:** Each chapter ends with three kinds of questions to prompt thought and discussion within the HEC: Conceptual questions focused on broad considerations of values and norms; Pragmatic questions designed to look at practical considerations; and Strategic questions that look to issues of implementation and action. However, partly because of the diversity of authorship described above, the orientation of the questions at the end of the chapters will vary as well. Some authors chose to ask summary or reading comprehension sorts of questions to ensure that readers understood the main points of the chapter. Others use the questions to further the conversation on the topic and to challenge the reader to think beyond the text contained in the chapter. Regardless, we think that the questions at the end of each chapter may be useful tools for beginning a dialogue within the HEC about each topic at hand.

This volume is organized into three main sections: introduction/preliminaries, consultation, and a final section capturing policy development, organizational issues, and education. Among these sections, the bulk of the chapters focus on consultation, as this often presents the most significant challenges to committee members and clinical topics are wide and varied. While conceived of as a comprehensive volume, each chapter of this text is capable of standing alone as a teaching module through which an ethics committee can work together or members can work individually.

* * *

This text is now in its second edition, and we have been motivated by the feedback from previous readers and reviewers while updating this volume. We began by rethinking the chapters included in the volume, and then eliminated some chapters from the previous edition (typically by marrying with another chapter) and added chapters on topics that were not in the previous volume. We also decided to loosen the word count restriction for a few chapters where the topics were such that they needed a little more space in the volume than others (though, to be sure, we believe in tight, digestible chapters; thus, no chapter is more than 5 000 words). Also, every chapter that was kept from the previous edition has been updated/rewritten by its author.

The other major shift that occurred well into the writing of this edition is the SARS-CoV-2 pandemic. To say that this has transformed the way we think about health care is by no means an understatement. Global health really has become local health as the mobile nature of contemporary society ensured that few areas were spared the need to consider carefully how to both care for those infected and protect those who were not. Indeed, this is one of the times in health care when the work that we do in ethics – namely, identify core values and help to adjudicate values conflicts – took center stage. Healthcare leaders at all levels collaborated with their ethics staff to ensure they were able to allocate scarce resources in a way that was fair, consistent, transparent, and inclusive.

Yet despite ethicists' considerable expertise in these areas, it was by no means an easy activity in which we engaged. There was much debate in the professional ethics community about the best way to allocate scarce resources; to identify, prioritize, and communicate public health ethics principles as compared with more traditional individually focused healthcare ethics principles; and how to address the clear inequities in care that the pandemic illuminated. Early data demonstrated that there were clear differences in approach by different ethicists at different institutions, and only time will tell if greater unanimity emerged with the broad sharing of information that characterized the response to pandemic planning.

We can only imagine how those engaged in ethics at smaller institutions, without the benefit of a professionally trained ethicist, fared during these difficult times. To the extent that state health departments collaborated with professional ethicists and the resulting material was widely available, ethics committees ought to have been able to avail themselves of both the ethical justifications and practice standards enumerated therein. But for those states that were slower to publish such documents, or those institutions without good access to ethical resources, we suspect that ethics committees may have been relied upon to an extent not previously witnessed in their organization. And it is those individuals, and those committees, to whom this volume is directed. We can only hope that the background and thought processes demonstrated in these chapters will help to form the foundation for those called upon to respond to both local and global challenges in healthcare ethics.

* * *

Large projects like this are never done by one or two persons, and we want to express our gratitude to many others (and our apologies for anyone we might miss). First, we appreciate the work of the chapter authors; both previous and new authors put in a great deal of time with already busy schedules. Further, we thank those who, over the past decade, used the previous editions and then gave us their insights and support for a new edition. This leads us to Cambridge University Press for readily supporting the publication of this book. To Nick Dunton, who was of invaluable help in making this second edition happen, we wish fair winds and following seas on your retirement. We also appreciate the work of Jessica Papworth and Olivia Boult who stepped in and continued the effortless partnership with the Press.

As we noted in the first edition, the idea for this book was generated from the time we have both spent serving on HECs at a variety of institutions. We are grateful for the insights that have been gleaned from these experiences, especially in recognizing the challenges of educating a group of diverse, time-constrained, dedicated healthcare professionals. We continue to have these HECs in mind as we assembled this text and hope that our efforts have proved fruitful.

Finally, we are grateful to our institutions and our families for their support of this work. Toby has had important support from the Center for Ethics at Emory University during the first edition and Prime Review Board and the National Center for Ethics in Health Care at the US Department of Veterans Affairs during the development of the second. For Micah, the Department of Medical Humanities & Bioethics, and its parent unit, the College of Medicine at University of Arkansas for Medical Sciences has allowed the time and provided the resources necessary to produce this work. We are, however, most indebted to our families: James (for Toby) and Kelly, Emily, Joshua, and Matthew (for Micah), without whom nothing good in our lives is possible.

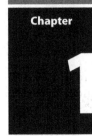

Chapter

Introduction

D. Micah Hester and Toby L. Schonfeld

Objectives

Upon reading and considering the content of this chapter, the reader should be able to:

1. Explain how the concept and function of ethics committees have developed in of modern health care.
2. Define the relationship between clinical ethics consultation and the ethics committee.
3. Describe the roles, constitution, and authority of ethics committees in institutions.

Ethics in the Hospital: A Brief History

Case

Conrad is a 68-year-old former parole officer. He has been in the hospital for the past week on the oncology service. He has a sarcoma in his shoulder that the physicians are saying is inoperable, and that they believe he will ultimately die from complications of this cancer. When talking about this with Conrad and his family, however, the physicians become frustrated because Conrad, while aware of others in the room, does not seem to understand anything that is going on, and the family dynamics are challenging.

Conrad's family consists of three children and his girlfriend of 30 years with whom he lives. One of the children is from this relationship while the other two are from his former wife. The oldest, a son named Artemis, is constantly at the bedside, and he refuses to acknowledge the others in the family. The team, out of confusion and expediency, treats Artemis as the primary decision maker, and when he instructs the nursing staff to keep the other children and the girlfriend away, the staff feel obligated to do so. Meanwhile, the rest of the family are confused and frustrated by the lack of information since they cannot even call in because Artemis keeps changing the call-in password to give to the hospital.

Meanwhile, Conrad lies in the hospital getting intensive medical treatments, insisted upon by Artemis, that the team does not believe will make any long-term difference to Conrad's eventual demise. On the few opportunities that the other children have been able to talk with the team, they do not think their dad should continue on intensive treatments but should be transitioned to home hospice.

Conrad's case is sadly frustrating for most everyone involved, and all the while he lies in a kind of medical limbo that might stretch on for months. While everyone believes they are doing what is in Conrad's interests, the complex family dynamics, the tragic state of Conrad's disease, and the team's inability to navigate all this successfully make knowing whether or not Conrad is getting the care he wants and deserves hard to determine. In addition, there are some important value conflicts that are reflected in the family's approaches to decision-making: quality versus quantity of life, authority and resources for decision-making, and fundamental existential values may all be under debate in Conrad's case. The atmosphere surrounding this case is charged with emotion and frustration, both for the family and the healthcare providers.

Cases like Conrad's often benefit from review by a group that is not directly involved in the care of the patient but is familiar with cases like this one. Such a group might be able to diffuse tensions, clarify the meaning of terms like "medical futility" and "comfort care," and suggest a way to reconcile conflicting obligations. Further, they could create educational programs to prepare the staff for similar situations in the future, and even develop policies that would help resolve future conflicts that appear intractable. Such a group is a healthcare ethics committee (HEC), whose purpose is to improve the quality and delivery of health care through the identification, analysis, and resolution of ethical questions or concerns.

While now ubiquitous in hospitals in the USA (though less so in other parts of the world) (McLean, 2007; Hajibabaee et al., 2016), the presence of an institutional *committee* to address ethical problems is a relatively recent one. The origins of HECs can be traced to the allocation decision committees of the 1960s (sometimes known as "God Squads"), the end-of-life committees recommended by the Quinlan ruling (1976) and the President's Commission (1983), and the neonatal review requirements of the Baby Doe Regulations (1984). Particularly since the President's Commission's promotion of and outline for HECs, a number of influential organizations have subsequently endorsed the concept of HECs, including the American Hospital Association (1986) and the American Medical Association (1985; see Ethical and Judicial Council, 1985). However, in the USA, the most influential stimulus for the creation and proliferation of ethics committee is The Joint Commission on the Accreditation of Healthcare Organizations (The Joint Commission), which began in 1992 to require some kind of formal "mechanism" to assure that ethical issues in patient care were addressed effectively (The Joint Commission, 1992). It is worth noting that The Joint Commission language has changed over the decades, moving away from "mechanism" to "framework" and "process," but still much of the responsibility for implementing that framework or process falls to an HEC.

As we come into the second decade of the 2000s, most US, Canadian, and European hospitals have an HEC, with the percentages lower but still existent in Asian Pacific and Middle Eastern countries (Hajibabaee et al., 2016). Looking at the USA, specifically, a conservative estimate would be that 30,000 people (and probably double that) in the United States currently serve in some manner on an HEC.[1] Even while the American Society for Bioethics and Humanities (ASBH) – the dominant professional organization in US bioethics with approximately 2 000 members – has begun certifying clinical ethics consultants (ASBH, 2020), the vast majority of HEC members would not consider themselves professional clinical ethicists. Thus, most of them may find themselves uncomfortable in the role as a "go-to" person for ethical concerns in the hospital. The present volume aims at reducing that discomfort by helping prepare HEC members for the challenges they are likely to face in this role.

---

[1] These numbers, while rough estimates, are supported by surveys by Fox et al. (2007, 2021).

Three Functions of HECs

As developed by the President's Commission, there has come to be a traditional threefold mission of an HEC. The most visible and often controversial role is to provide case review or, as it is often referenced, to consult on difficult clinical decisions. Equally important, though sometimes forgotten, are the other two functions: formulating institutional policies (consistent with the organization's function and mission) to guide the professional staff in making ethical decisions, and educating hospital personnel about these policies and about healthcare ethics in general. The case of Conrad at the beginning of this chapter presses on all three functions: the HEC might be called in to consult with the staff and family, it might be asked to develop a policy for conflict resolution or patient access, and it might be asked to provide staff with further education about the ethical and legal considerations of family and other involved persons. We have devoted a section of this book to each of these topics, and, thus, will only briefly discuss them here.

Function 1: Case Consultation

Ethics is a specialty discipline with its own domain of inquiry. It leads to the development of moral norms and a deliberation of values in light of those norms. Thus, when an acute *ethical* problem arises in clinical care, turning to individuals with special education and/or experience to address it is akin to consulting a cardiologist when the patient has heart-related medical concerns. This explains the need for the ethical case consultation. The consultative role of the HEC may vary both in terms of the goal of the process and the model of consultation. Goals for the process may include clarifying the situation and/or providing recommendations, ensuring effective communication and/or mediating among diverse groups, empowering clinical staff to assess and address ethical issues themselves, and recognizing patterns of consultation that may result in broader educational or policy implications (see Chapter 7 for more on this). Regardless, several different models are effective ways of achieving these ends; brief descriptions of the three most common models follow below (Smith et al., 2004).

1. **Individual Consultant:** Available in many large institutions or health systems with deep resources, individuals with trained expertise (and now, even certification) can serve as the primary ethics consultant. The individual's training typically consists of education in healthcare ethics (formally or informally) often supplemented with demonstrated competence in an academic discipline that informs the field (such as philosophy or religion), as well as familiarity with the clinical setting. In addition to the training, the individual consulting model has the benefit of expediency and flexibility, with a single person who is able to respond quickly to a request for help and meet with key individuals in an efficient manner.

2. **Multidisciplinary (aka "Whole" HEC) Committee:** An older model that remains common in smaller hospitals is that of a multidisciplinary committee that conducts consultations. A multidisciplinary committee ensures a variety of ethical and professional perspectives and gathers partial expertise from a larger number of individuals. This approach mitigates the lack of strong expertise in ethics through the use of multiple perspectives, values, and voices. An important detriment to the use of committees for review is that they can be cumbersome to assemble on short notice to respond to a pressing ethical consultation. Additionally, patients and/or families may be overwhelmed by the presence of an entire committee during the consultation process.

3. **Consultation Subcommittee (aka "Team-Based" Approach):** The third, quite popular, approach across a wide range of hospitals involves the appointment of select members of an HEC onto a consultation subcommittee. Members of the group are chosen for their special abilities and training in ethics and agree to be available to provide help when consults arise. This model attempts to incorporate some of the best features of both the individual consultant and the whole committee models. Like the individual consultant, a small group that is "on call" is able to respond quickly to an urgent need, can be flexible in meeting with involved parties in various locations in the hospital, and is less intimidating to patients and families. Additionally, as an interdisciplinary group, it would be expected to contain different ethical perspectives as well as differing sets of skills and experience.

Choosing from among these models involves matching the needs, resources, and scope of the HEC to the institution or organization more broadly. An HEC should consider carefully which model best suits the institution and provide specific support for the chosen model in order to help it succeed.

As noted above, ASBH has developed a credentialing process, the Healthcare Ethics Consultant-Certified Program, as a way of professionalizing the practice of providing clinical ethics consults. This program requires individuals to get hundreds of hours of ethics-related experiences in the healthcare setting and then pass an exam. Earning the credential (an HEC-C) reflects endorsement of a minimum knowledge of key concepts and skills in healthcare ethics (ASBH, 2020). Because it only reflects basic competency, many people with certification would do well to work in teams and on ethics committees, rather than as solo consultants. This volume can provide some useful education for certification, but more importantly, it should help all members of an HEC be better prepared in the face of ethical challenges in the hospital.

Function 2: Policy Development, Review, and Implementation

Of the vast number of policies that each hospital creates, many policies deal with ethical concerns. Some have obvious ethical content, such as policies that govern advance directives. Others that are not overtly ethical in content may still have ethical dimensions – for example, policies concerning admission, discharge, and transfer of patients. When done well, writing or revising policies provides HEC members with an opportunity to engage in meaningful interdisciplinary work with clinical departments likely affected by the (proposed) policy. Policy work is some of the most important work undertaken by HECs: The very character of the hospital is expressed, in part, through its policies, and thus, the ethical climate of any institution is determined in large part by the policies it adopts. This is particularly true when considering policies that govern the organization. Per The Joint Commission, every institution must address "organizational ethics," but it remains an open question how much responsibility the HEC should take on regarding these issues. Yet ethics committees clearly have a role in addressing the organization's mission by offering reasonably clear guidelines for difficult situations: Good policies help individuals make good decisions and thus prevent some ethical problems from arising. They may also help to shape the institution's policies on workplace conduct, hiring practices, and the allocation of resources broadly construed.

Function 3: Education

Last but not least, the educational role of an HEC is twofold: looking internally at the HEC membership and externally at the institution's staff. As we have noted, the great majority of HEC members likely have little academic training or other formal background in healthcare ethics; some training, then, is necessary for this new role. But in addition to this, an HEC should also provide education to the entire hospital community. This becomes particularly important when policy is adopted or revised that has ethical dimensions, when a specific ethical concern comes to the committee repeatedly or for some other reason seems to gain traction in the institution, or simply to address perennial issues in healthcare ethics – like surrogate decision-making or the allocation of scarce resources. Such initiatives can forestall problems that arise from lack of awareness and can enhance the visibility and credibility of the committee.

HEC Constitution and Authority

While some states and countries do have laws regarding some aspects of HEC work, most HECs do not operate under required legal or regulatory standards. Similarly, The Joint Commission fails to articulate expectations of an HEC (or even the processes by which ethics is addressed in the hospital). Thus, we can offer no definitive and authoritative guidelines about how the committee should be developed: its administrative location in the organizational structure of the institution, its charge, and its membership. However, we can provide some guidance based on considerations of the benefits a committee might bring to its institution.

Location and Accountability

All institutional committees are established by a particular administrative unit. They are given a purpose or charge and are responsible for reporting on their activities to the parent unit. There is no one single "home" for HECs. HECs have been created by the medical staff, by the hospital administration, and even some by the hospital's board of directors. Although it may not be a crucial decision, the location of the HEC in the institution's administrative structure can have some practical consequences, since guidelines for constituting and operating the committee may vary according to the group to which it reports.

In some hospitals, for example, medical staff committees must be chaired by physicians, thus restricting the options for filling this important position. On the other hand, developing the HEC as a medical staff committee intent on quality improvement, it may be easier to shield proceedings of the HEC from any potential legal scrutiny. Where the organized medical staff has yet to embrace fully the concept of an ethics committee, it might be advisable to establish the HEC as a unit of the hospital administration. If it is an administrative committee, however, its purpose must not be perceived as making the hospital run smoothly. The third possibility, board committee status, can carry both positive and negative messages. On the one hand, the HEC is answerable only to the highest authority, which gives it significant status. On the other, this may carry the implication that its purpose is to oversee and perhaps report on medical and administrative decisions, creating distance from the very people it is intended to help. Given all these potential benefits and detriments placement of the HEC within the organizational structure requires careful thought. Determining the best place for an HEC to be "housed" within the organization will involve many subtle factors that vary from place to place and may change over time in any given institution.

Leadership

Committees are rarely effective if they do not have good leadership. Thus, the chair of an HEC is always a critical position to fill. The chair(s) often will become the de facto face of the committee and should be someone who enjoys respect and credibility among the many professions in the institution. The most important quality, however, is commitment to the idea of an HEC. The chair must believe in the mission of the committee and consider the position an important part of their job. Meetings will be perfunctory and unproductive unless the chair takes care to construct a meaningful agenda.

Where should one look for a suitable chair? There are good reasons to support a physician as chair of an HEC. A physician chair tends to have more immediate credibility with physician-colleagues, perhaps making it easier for them to call on the committee for help. As we have noted, in some institutions, the committee is under the auspices of the medical staff, and only a physician is allowed to function as chair. However, in other hospitals, no such rules exist, so there may be a diversity of leaders. A professional ethicist may chair the committee in these instances, which lends credibility to the work of the group given the professional training and general expertise of the leader. This will work only in cases where the committee and the chair are well-respected members of the organizational community, and where the chair has clear partners with other key stakeholders. Nurses, social workers, and other healthcare professionals may serve well as chairs, too. Consider a co-chair model, as well; co-chairs can help gain credibility from different constituencies in the hospital, and they can share the workload in order to keep the committee moving forward, not getting stale. Regardless, there are no hard-and-fast rules; committee founders need to assess the available resources and the pragmatics of the institution to determine who should chair the HEC.

Membership and Structure

Importantly, an ethics committee allows for an array of knowledge and perspectives to be brought to bear on consultation, education, and policy issues; otherwise, the hospital might as well be served by one or two individuals. Thus, the committee should be multidisciplinary, composed of members with a variety of professional perspectives and disciplines on clinical care (physicians, nurses, allied health professionals) and on broader social issues (for example, social workers, chaplains, and ethicists). Second, a committee allows for a variety of expertise. Since general familiarity with ethical issues in health care is clearly desirable, particular physicians and nurses with training or deep interest in ethical issues are obvious targets for membership. At the same time, policies or cases tend to cluster in or overly affect certain units. Thus, it might be important to have, say, a critical care specialist on the committee, as cases from acute care units are often fraught with ethical concern.

While special knowledge is desirable on the committee, some areas of expertise deserve special note. For example, some committees include a member of the hospital's risk management or legal team, and some include members of hospital administration.

In these particular roles, conflicts of interest are the primary concern. While ethics committees are *institutional* committees, they are charged to be "objective" in their deliberations, looking out for what is the best solution to a difficult case or complicated policy from a dispassionate perspective. As a result, the outcome of deliberation may not be an action that is in the best interests of the institution more generally. Thus, to the extent that the risk manager or hospital administrator also has a responsibility to protect the institution, this conflict of interest may raise tensions given their roles. On the other hand, having a representative from hospital administration or risk management could prove quite beneficial to the committee; this is particularly true when the committee considers organization-level decisions (like policies on resource allocation) or when there are real questions about how a state statute may apply in a particular case. In addition, having a member of hospital administration on the committee may lend it legitimacy, and may enable resources to be allocated to the committee for education or other purposes that might otherwise be devoted elsewhere. It may be desirable to create ex officio (without voting privileges) positions for such roles, but regardless, these are issues about which an HEC should be thoughtful when deciding on its composition.

Another unique category of membership is that of the "community" member. While not a requirement, many HECs, perhaps following the President's Commission's recommendations or structuring themselves after the institutional review board model, employ community members – that is, persons not directly associated with the institution. The purpose of the role is to provide a kind of corrective should the institutional members of the committee become insulated from public perceptions or too interested in institutional protection. This is a daunting role to perform. It may be difficult to identify persons to fill the role. In fact, the person filling the role often has some relationship with the institution (e.g., ex-patient, former employee, member of a hospital advisory council, etc.), raising questions whether that individual can adequately fulfill the intended role of the community member. Nevertheless, some committees may find it useful to have a community member, even two, on the committee, especially if the committee is particularly involved with issues that impact the community directly.

In addition to their knowledge and positions in the institution, a number of personal qualities of its members are critical to the success of an HEC. While about a quarter of HECs require references and interviews to become a member, some have an expectation that members will also demonstrate character traits like integrity and honesty (Prince et al., 2017). Further, members must demonstrate a sincere belief in the importance of the committee's work and be willing to devote significant time and energy to it. They should also try to take advantage of opportunities for self-education. Moreover, for an HEC to function smoothly and effectively, members must respect one another and the various perspectives they represent; egalitarianism should pervade the committee's work. Differences of status within the organization should be left at the committee room door: It is intent to do good and right with cogency of reasoning that should matter, not position in the institution. Members should be respectful but not deferential to one another, and anyone who expects deference should be dropped from the committee.

Bylaws

Like any other working committee, an HEC needs a set of bylaws or a detailed committee charge to give it structure and allow for necessary changes in an orderly manner. In addition to leadership and categories of membership, the by-laws should address size of the committee, terms of membership, frequency of meetings, and the scope of the three roles of consultation, policy review, and education.

HECs vary in size. One survey showed that larger hospitals (550 or more beds) can have over 30 members on the HEC, while smaller hospitals may have memberships as small as 10 persons. Further, length of service on the committee varies as well. About half of the HECs in the country have unlimited terms, while others have restricted terms as short as 1 year (Prince et al., 2017). Short terms and a rapidly rotating membership will result in instability and inexperience, whereas indefinite or permanent membership may burden a committee with uninterested and unproductive members. The reasonable solution to the extremes is probably a compromise, such as staggered, fixed terms of several years with the possibility of reappointment. Uninvolved members can easily be dropped and committed ones retained as long as they contribute to the group.

Frequency of meetings is another item the bylaws should address. Regular mandated meetings are expected. While it is easy for overburdened professionals to slip into the "only when necessary" mode, which in effect means only when there is a consult to conduct, without regular meetings the "preventive" work of the committee – education and policy review – will suffer. Self-education and self-assessment will also falter, affecting the quality of the consults, and the committee will lose a sense of its continuing importance to the life of the hospital. Quarterly meetings are the minimum to retain a sense of continuity, with more frequent meetings highly desirable.

Ultimately, committee members should be encouraged to own each function of an HEC, and as such, the bylaws should define as clearly as possible the role that the HEC is to play in all three of its primary activities. The educational function will probably be left entirely to the committee, to design and implement programs that it can offer on its own or through departmental meetings (having a budget for this purpose is highly desirable). Further, the bylaws might specify a base level of ethics education that committee members themselves should have.

With respect to policy review, the HEC should be charged to recommend changes up through the administration or to the medical board. In this it is similar to every other committee in the institution, as committees are generally created to make recommendations rather than final decisions about policy matters. If there are particular policies the committee is to "own" or review regularly, they should be specified in the bylaws, or a list should be kept as part of the HEC's standard processes and operations documents. And in other situations, the HEC may initiate the creation of a policy based on a series of clinical consultations; members should consult institutional procedures for performing such an action.

The most important function to clarify in the committee's bylaws is case consultation, both in terms of what role it plays and outcomes to expect. An HEC may take on the consulting task itself or may provide oversight of a consulting service that is established separately from the committee itself. Further, although committees are typically charged only to make recommendations to others, some are in fact constituted (often through a specific policy) to make binding decisions about particular cases. Nevertheless, there is sometimes considerable apprehension about the ethics committee "taking control" of a case when called to consult. Committee bylaws should specify that the committee is advisory only and does not make decisions about patient care. Some committees build this into their name (e.g., "Medical Ethics Advisory Committee") to make clear the limit to their authority. There may be a small subset of cases that the committee is given explicit authority to decide; if so, these should be spelled out carefully in the committee bylaws.

Conclusion

The healthcare ethics committee is a firm and ubiquitous fixture in American hospitals, yet, like any complex institution, it is still defining itself. The concept has been scrutinized in the scholarly and professional literature for some 50 years, including several books and countless articles focused on the consultative function of an HEC. There are ethics committee networks in many states and regions of the country (Fausett et al., 2016). There is no lack of resources to aid an institution in organizing, educating, or revivifying a moribund committee. In the end, however, the general idea of an HEC must be adapted to the particular structure, mission, and size of the institution, and just as important, to its professional and community resources. This book can help by presenting current thinking about major issues to be considered, indicating resources for further information, and suggesting ways to tailor an HEC to fit local conditions.

Questions for Discussion

1. Conceptual: How is the HEC viewed by staff, patients, and families in your institution? What challenging barriers and attitudes shape this view?
2. Pragmatic: Which of the three functions of an HEC present the greatest challenge to your institution, and what can you do to overcome these challenges?
3. Strategic: How ought the bylaws and membership of your own HEC be constituted, given the needs of your organization and the expertise of your personnel?

References

American Hospital Association. (1986). Guidelines: Hospital committees on biomedical ethics. In Ross JW, ed., *Handbook for Hospital Ethics Committees.* Chicago: American Hospital Publishing, 57, 110–111.

American Society for Bioethics and Humanities (ASBH). (2020). Healthcare Ethics Consultant-Certified (HEC-C) program. https://asbh.org/certification/hcec-certification

Ethical and Judicial Council. (1985). Guidelines for ethics committees in health care institutions: Ethical and Judicial Council. *JAMA*, 253(18): 2698–2699.

Fausett JK, Gilmore-Szott E, Hester DM (2016). Networking ethics: A survey of bioethics networks across the US. *HEC Forum*, 28(2): 153–167.

Fox E, Myers S, Pearlman RA (2007). Ethics consultation in United States hospitals: A national survey. *American Journal of Bioethics*, 7: 13–25.

Fox E, Danis M, Tarzian AJ, Duke CC (2021). Ethics consultation in U.S. hospitals: A national follow-up study. *American Journal of Bioethics*, March 26.

Hajibabaee F, Joolaee S, Cheraghi M, Salari P, Rodney P. (2016). Hospital/clinical ethics committees' notion: An overview. *Journal of Medical Ethics and History of Medicine*, 9: 17.

McLean SAM (2007). What and who are clinical ethics committees for? *Journal of Medical Ethics*, 33(2): 497–500.

Prince AER, Cadigan RJ, Whipple W, Davis AM (2017). Membership recruitment and training in health care ethics committees: Results from a national pilot study. *AJOB Empirical Bioethics*, 8(3): 161–169.

Smith ML, Bisanz AK, Kempfer AJ, Adams B, Candelari TG, Blackburn RK (2004). Criteria for determining appropriate method for an ethics consultation. *HEC Forum*, 16(2): 95–113.

The Joint Commission on Accreditation of Healthcare Organizations. (1992). *Accreditation Manual for Hospitals.* Oakbrook Terrace, IL: The Joint Commission on Accreditation of Healthcare Organizations.

Brief Introduction to Ethics and Ethical Theory

Toby L. Schonfeld and D. Micah Hester

Objectives

Upon reading and considering the content of this chapter, the reader should be able to:

1. Explain the family of related concepts to which the terms 'ethics' and 'morality' refer.
2. Identify a variety of common sources of moral guidance and authority.
3. Describe several approaches to ethics and explain the difference between ethical discourse (a systematic approach to ethics) and related areas such as etiquette or custom.
4. Use an ethical theory and its associated methods to help identify, clarify, and analyze clinical ethics issues.

Case

Janet S. is a 65-year-old stage 4 breast cancer patient whose third round of chemotherapy has failed. She knows her status well, as she suffers from significant pain from bone metastases. In a thoughtful conversation with her oncologist, she asks for help in hastening her death. She states clearly that she finds her life insufferable and that dying quickly while she still has some "dignity" is of utmost importance to her. She has made peace with her friends and family and states that she is ready to die. The oncologist calls the healthcare ethics committee (HEC) for guidance.

The Meaning of "Ethics"

The term "ethics" originated with the Greek term *ethikos* meaning habit or custom; similarly, our word "moral" arose from the Latin *mos*, also meaning "custom." But ethics (which we will not distinguish from "morality") has certainly not come to mean the description of our "accustomed habits." In fact, ethics is what we call a "normative" endeavor, meaning that ethics is not simply descriptive but prescriptive. While there are a variety of approaches to ethics that have been offered up over the centuries, all of them attempt to speak not to how we *do* live and act but to how we *should* live and act. Given the myriad uses and conceptions of what ethics is, though, it may help to discuss several of them in order to clarify better the purpose and work of a healthcare *ethics* committee.

In everyday usage, ethics concerns how each individual deals with "right" and "wrong," "good" and "bad" as part of our living in the world. We talk about things like our "personal ethics," and in this light most, if not all, of us believe we are "good people" who make the right choices most of the time. In this sense, then, ethics is tied closely to *values* and *character*.

In addition, though, we also play different *roles* in our communities and in society that reflect a different understanding of ethics. For example, as members of professions we might be governed by "ethics." This governing is often manifest in codes of ethics or other lists of expected professional behavior, but it also resides in our sense of what our roles or being a professional are all about: the responsibilities and obligations that come along with the actions we perform in our roles as healthcare professionals. This sense of ethics is often associated with judgments of what actions or behaviors are *right* and *wrong*.

Finally, we carry with us our values and interests, and it is easy to recognize that others have their own interests as well. Further, the roles we play, not only as professionals but as family members, friends, citizens, and members of multiple communities each carry corresponding obligations. Often, between personal interests, cultural values, and professional and relational obligations, it is not uncommon to find ourselves in conflict with others, with institutions, even with the many aspects of ourselves. Since it can be hard if not impossible to fulfill all these competing interests and obligations, our interpersonal conflicts often lead to questions concerning ends we really should pursue and what means are appropriate in those pursuits. This sense of ethics can be characterized as weighing *outcomes* as *good* and *bad*, *better* and *worse*.

No one of these three senses of "ethics" should be ignored, nor is any one of them always dominant. It is worth noting that each of us is a "values carrier," whether as a product of biology, nurturing, education, or some other means. Further, we do, in fact, find ourselves in relation to others – familial, professional, and so forth – and those relationships commit us to others and to expectations for which we are held accountable. At the same time, in a finite universe of limited abilities and resources, with a plurality of individual and communal interests, we are confronted often by concerns for what we should do, and why.

Ethics, then, concerns each of these aspects of moral living – values (character), duties (roles), and goods (ends). We might say, then, the "field" of ethics – that is, the territory of and inquiry into values and interests covered by moral considerations – comprises those *evaluations* of human (and some other animal) conduct, both arising from and affecting character, which result in appraisals of "good" and "bad," "right" and "wrong."

Value-Conflicts in Health Care

Ethics is part and parcel of human living, as it is nearly impossible to move in the world without either being held accountable or holding others accountable for their choices and actions. And yet a reasonable question remains: Why *study* ethics? This question is brought into even greater focus if we limit ourselves specifically to health care as a profession. We see that, in fact, each of us has a set of personal values that has helped shape us into the kinds of people who pursued the "healing professions." Also, professions have codes of ethics or other standardized lists of acceptable behaviors. This might seem to be enough. What role does a rigorous focus on ethics, medical ethics, or even just ethics committees play?

To answer this question, consider Janet's case from the beginning of this chapter. Simply relying on the fact that you are a "good" person and that you recognize professional obligations may not be enough to settle the moral issue for you. These features may help you begin to think about the issue, but they may in fact *produce* the value tension here: You may have personal or religious commitments that prevent you from supporting hastening someone's death, but also have professional commitments to alleviate suffering to the best of your ability. How are you to *know* which values should have priority in this situation? Holding values is not enough, especially when values conflict with each other.

Thus, no matter how "ethically equipped" we seem to be, challenges to how or whether to act on our values will arise in health care. Frankly, resolving ethical conflict is not always an easy task, and this makes ethical reflection all the more important. At the same time, ethical reflection is incapable of stopping at the "borders" of the particular conflict in front of us. Each consideration raises issues of "principle" rather than just expediency or prudence; thus, reconsideration of our professional obligations as well as our individual values is implicated in our ethical decision-making. Furthermore, while it is also the case that our values and professional obligations are the products of past experiences, this still may not help. On the one hand, it is impossible to guarantee clear applicability of these experiences to any new situation, and, on the other hand, we often generalize these experiences to such an extent that what "applicability" even means comes into question.

In addition, everyone's character and the practices of every profession are subject to continual (if not cataclysmic) change; this, then, requires a certain routine vigilance with respect to reflecting on who we want to become, what we are willing and able to do, and how we should interact with those around us. What will help us in responding to Janet's request is having some systematic way of approaching questions of value tension in a way that respects the perspectives of the various stakeholders but also enables professionals to act with personal and professional integrity.

Ethical Reflection

The history of moral theory is a history of attempting to develop the kinds of systematic responses to moral considerations desired in Janet's, and most any other, case. Whether the values in question are situational, culturally specific, or more universal, our response to conflicts in values is strengthened by careful attention to what makes our reasons for one moral judgment or another acceptable. In what follows, we look at three broad approaches that have been taken to systematize ethical reflection. These three approaches correspond roughly to the three "meanings" of ethics discussed above. There are a number of ways to approach ethical reflection, and we do not suggest that what follows is in any way exhaustive. However, since some version of these three meanings of "ethics" often manifests itself during our ethical considerations, a basic sketch of these three approaches may assist an HEC in its work.

Virtue Theory

Though our conduct is often where moral evaluation comes into stark relief, our beliefs and actions both demonstrate and affect who we are; that is, they arise from and impact character. As such, one important moral question we often ask ourselves is: What kind of person do I want to be? This question prompts individuals to consider in what ways they should live their lives in order to find meaning and cohesion and will likely involve considerations about appropriate interactions with others and with the environments in which they reside. This process of self-reflection and adapting of oneself to a particular conception of the moral life takes ethics to be, in part, a matter of virtue and integrity (cf. Aristotle, 1999).

Proposed long ago by such philosophical luminaries as Plato and Aristotle and carried on more recently by theorists such as Alasdair MacIntyre and Martha Nussbaum, the idea behind virtue theory is that the moral life consists of aiming to live a good life, and such a life is best achieved by developing one's character through traits and habits that will guide a moral agent in knowing how to act in a variety of situations. Of course, these character traits will necessarily be broad and general; courage, kindness, temperance are some examples. Traits and habits do not arise from performing any one action. Rather, virtue theorists champion careful attention to the collection of a person's activities, practices, and routines. They often encourage individuals to seek out positive role models of moral action and to learn from and through these moral exemplars how one ought to respond in a variety of situations. Though not reducible to this approach, virtue theory asks, at least in part, that one be a moral apprentice to others who are acknowledged as typically "getting it right." Most often, we look to our parents, teachers, coaches, and other "role models" to learn about appropriate behavior in this way. Note well, though, that role models may be both positive and negative. Determining what makes a role model one or the other is challenging, but both kinds can be helpful in assisting someone to know how to conduct one's life, since even if we determine that someone is a negative role model, we judge their conduct as *not* worthy of replicating.

Bioethicists such as Edmund Pellegrino and Daniel Sulmasy have championed the importance of virtue-development in their works. In the context of health care, the process of moral development goes beyond personal virtues to those that are central to the professions. For example, virtues of honesty and trustworthiness may achieve greater importance in the clinical context than they do in other arenas. As such, healthcare professionals are encouraged to focus on responding openly and consistently, fighting against urges to mere self-preservation or expediency. It is worth noting that much of the training experiences of healthcare professionals relies on a "mentorship" model, and so while there are multiple ways to identify and nurture healthcare virtues, surely in health care, as in other cases, one might look to those whose actions one admires professionally, and subsequently approach their own professional practice guided by similar features.

Consider how a focus on virtue and character may affect considerations in Janet's case. Such a focus may help a provider consider the broader implications of acceding to Janet's request. Those who act from the virtue of compassion and who strive to be physicians whose goal is to alleviate suffering may look differently at Janet's situation than those who herald the virtue of "never giving up." Those who highly value life over death may take it as a matter of personal integrity to decline to act on Janet's request, while others who highly value personal self-determination may see it as a weakness of moral courage not to be able to help Janet fulfill this wish. Whether you lean more to one approach over another, the point here is that acting from virtue requires the identification of a set of values and then performing those actions that best accord with the virtues so identified. But still further, we want to note that whichever actions are taken, one's character is reflected in those actions. Thus, some attention to the moral importance of virtues, character, and integrity is not merely warranted but important.

Duty-Based or Intention-Based Approaches

Following our values and interests, often we are motivated to act in particular ways. For example, in stopping a child from running into the street, I may act with the intention of wanting to protect the child from potential harm. However, others might perform the same action for different reasons. For example, depending on one's character, psychology, and other issues, another person may think that rambunctious children could damage their car or property when running in the street, or they may simply believe that the street looks better when it is free of people running around on it. Surely, though, we would morally judge someone motivated to protect a child from harm differently from someone whose intent is to maintain an aesthetically pleasing street. That is, while clearly related to one's character, it is different, and not unimportant, that we appraise the morality of one's *intentions*. In fact, some moral theorists take intentions and motivations to be the central feature of any ethical judgment (cf. Kant, 1983).

Even more narrowly, we might argue that only particular kinds of motivation can survive ethical scrutiny. So, a store clerk knocking down a robber in the store and thus thwarting theft can look from the outside as a courageous moral act and outcome. But suppose that the clerk simply tripped or was pushed by someone else; in this case, are their actions still morally praiseworthy? Philosophers such as Immanuel Kant and Thomas Scanlon are unconvinced and, thus, have argued that only those decisions that intend to fulfill our moral duties (e.g., respect others' self-determination) and follow moral rules (e.g., do not harm the innocent) should be judged as ethically acceptable. Because of their emphasis on "duty," such theories have been labeled "deontologies" (from the Greek word *deontos*, meaning "duty").

Similarly, some bioethicists argue that rather than focusing on the characteristics of a good physician, nurse, respiratory therapist, etc., ethical action requires instead the professional to consider carefully their duty to the patient and the family. It is this duty that specifies right action, and as a result the agent's motive or intention is of primary importance: Actions are right to the extent that they derive from a good-faith effort to do one's duty, and wrong to the extent that the duty has been somehow misinterpreted or ignored.

However, sometimes this duty is not so clear. In Janet's case, for example, the duty to care for her and to alleviate suffering may suggest one action, but the professional duty to preserve life may prescribe a different action. So, saying that we ought to act from our professional duty may not resolve tension.

As a way of addressing this tension, some people appeal to rules or principles as guides for appropriate action. Famously, Bernard Gert, K. Danner Clouser, and Charles Culver have argued that there are ten basic rules of common morality (e.g., do not kill, do not lie) that must guide our actions for those actions to be considered morally acceptable. Others, such as H. Tristram Engelhardt, focus on principles of permission and beneficence, among other guiding concepts. Regardless, deontological approaches to ethical reflection consider duties, principles, and rules as ways of determining right action.

Consequentialism

The moral life is messy. We may intend to do good things, and yet nothing but bad consequences follow our actions. For instance, I may take a new, better-paying job, motivated by a moral obligation to support my family, and yet the family falls into disarray because the move created too much stress, left children without friends, required persistent travel, and more. Of course, we might rightly say that we cannot control, and thus should not be blamed for, all the effects of our actions. Yet it seems as though it matters morally when our actions produce bad results (cf. Mill and Bentham, 1973).

The final type of theory we will examine, then, is one where the results of our actions are of primary moral importance. Supporters of this approach to morality address ethical dilemmas by focusing primarily on the outcomes of action; they attempt to produce the best possible consequences in a given situation. While utilitarianism (à la Jeremy Bentham and J. S. Mill – actions are morally good that produce "the greatest good for the greatest number of people") is the most famous version of a theory that prioritizes consequences, any approach that looks primarily at producing optimal outcomes, even if it violates a moral rule, can be categorized in this class.

Because consequences are of central concern in these theories, motive and intent are reduced in importance, even to the point of irrelevancy in some theories. Thus, some versions of consequentialism allow for the possibility that an agent could do the right thing (i.e., produce the best possible outcome) for the "wrong" reasons (i.e., to bring fame and fortune to himself), but as long as the action produced an optimal outcome, then the intent does not matter. Such theories are a kind of extreme, however. Many consequentialist theories, from those of G. E. Moore to P. Singer to D. Parfit, evaluate the effects of our actions to determine morally good acts, but reserve moral praise or blame for moral agents based on whether the actions arise from careful reflection rather than from mere intuition or whim.

Janet's situation illustrates that the *best* possible outcome in a case may still be a grim or tragic one. Janet is dying, and in that context she describes a wish to take control of the dying process as a way of maintaining her dignity and autonomy. Those who consider motive important, as with deontology, may focus on the fact that the medical professional's duty is to heal, not to kill, and therefore Janet's request is both anathema and an impossibility. Yet no amount of aggressive care will restore Janet to prior form or function, and no therapeutic intervention will likely prevent her inevitable demise. In this case, a "good" outcome may consist simply in dying on one's own terms rather than the course dictated by the pathogen coursing through her body. A consequentialist, if convinced that this is the best possible outcome, will work to achieve this goal, despite the fact that successful action will result in Janet's death and may conflict with other professionals' sense of moral duty.

In sum, ethical theories attempt to put together an acceptable story of the moral life and provide a coherent basis for moral reflection, evaluation, and judgment. We, here, have only noted three constellations of theoretical approaches, and in so doing only account for select aspects of each grouping of theories. The point, in part, is to show how the multiple meanings of "ethics" noted at the beginning of the chapter map to carefully considered moral theories. Further, we want to emphasize the importance of the work that moral theory does while also noting that the complexity of moral considerations may not easily lend itself to be encapsulated by any one theory or theoretical approach. Finally, by recognizing the way in which moral reasoning often occurs, one is better equipped to hear why others reason and act as they do, thus avoiding the significant problem of talking past each other while reflecting on ethics. As such, the better HEC members understand moral philosophy, the better they will be able to analyze and discuss the many features of morally challenging situations in health care.

Bioethical Theory and Methodology

Given the difficulties of "applying," not to mention merely understanding, ethical theory, the brief history of bioethics itself has focused much more on reflective methodologies and moral rubrics than the theories that ground those methods. Most famous among these are the four "mid-level" principles developed by Tom Beauchamp and James Childress (Beauchamp and Childress, 2019): respect for autonomy, beneficence, non-maleficence, and justice. According to Beauchamp and Childress, the principles themselves arise out of common morality and medical practice and are not directly beholden to any particular ethical theory. The function of the principles is to guide bioethical reflection by setting forth important considerations of patient self-determination, of beneficial treatment, of avoiding harm to patients, and of treating all individuals fairly in our systems of health care. The principles are, for Beauchamp and Childress, both deontological (requiring adherence to moral obligations) and consequential (aiming at good outcomes). Ultimately, however, the principles themselves provide no framework for how to weigh, for example, issues that pit self-determined choices against fair distribution of resources. For the HEC, then, these (and others, like fidelity and caring) principles best serve the purpose of developing important questions to be asked and considerations to keep firmly in mind.

Of course, "principles" are but one of the many bioethical methods and tools developed in the last few decades. Some have pointed out that more fundamental than principles are rules of conduct. Whereas principles tell us to respect others, rules specify that harming others and coercion are wrong. And yet, these more particular rules themselves admit of a need for specification in certain contexts (Gert et al., 2006). At the same time, of at least equal importance are narrative considerations that put the patient's context at the center of ethical reflection. In a narrative approach to bioethics, how a person's life story is shaped in and through medicine is as important as the ethical principles at play (Hester, 2001). Such a view might emphasize the meaning and importance of a person's roles and relationships, not just rules of conduct.

We could multiply these considerations significantly. The point here is simply that while the history of moral philosophy has given us many ethical theories and methods – Aristotle's virtue ethics, Kant's deontology, Mill's utilitarianism, Gilligan's ethics of care, casuistry, narrative ethics, pragmatism, and so forth – and the much briefer history of bioethics has a variety of reflective methodologies, short of a full-blown course in (bio) ethical theory and method, no one can be expected to have a firm handle on these. However, this does not mean that theory and method are, therefore, unimportant or that anything goes. As stated earlier, each of our actions is not performed in isolation, nor are policies written in a vacuum. *Reasons and justifications are necessary* components of ethical determinations, whether concerning particular situations or institutional policies. Further, consistency of considerations is not unimportant either. Consistent reasoning stems from justified principled positions, and those arise from long processes of inquiry into the moral life itself. It is not good enough simply to care about the consequences of our actions for some issues and about our dutiful obligations toward others depending on our mood. We must be able to account for the legitimacy of our use of methods and theories that underlie the deliberations we perform and decisions we make.

Closer to home, we might also say that there is a "kind of progress possible through reflection in ethics" (Buermeyer et al., 1923, 323) that may be noted in four types: First, ethical reflection can bring our own values to light, "values which we might otherwise overlook" (323). Second, reflection aids in clarifying our aims and desires. Third, ethical reflection allows us to separate wheat from chaff, helping "us see what problems really are most vital, and thus bring[ing] us nearer to actual solutions" (324). And fourth, reflection leads us to own our actions, making "our conduct more fully our own, more voluntary and less of a blind obedience to custom" (324). For more detailed information about how this works, please see Chapter 8, "A Method of Consultation."

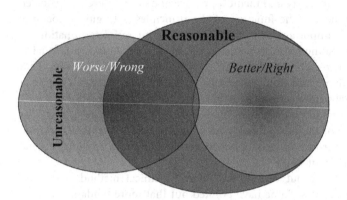

Figure 2.1 The scope of reasonable moral arguments

Relationship of "Reasonable" to "Right"/ "Unreasonable" to "Wrong"

A final note: It is often said that there are no "right" or "wrong" answers in ethics. This is misleading, at best. In fact, it is very important to understand that ethical quandaries do admit of better and worse responses. How we determine "better" and "worse" is what the entire process of ethical reflection is all about.

But while we may aim at "right" responses to ethical concerns and since we can only guarantee "better" ones, different ethical conclusions may be reached through a plurality of reasonable considerations. And all *reasonable* positions deserve consideration, though they may not always be determinative. What this means is that some people can hold *reasonable* ethical positions and *still not win the argument* (see Figure 2.1). Just because someone disagrees with you or their position is not considered to be as strong as yours does not mean they are unreasonable or irrational (though, they *may* be, of course). Also, just because you hold a position grounded on reasons does not mean it is the best position to hold in the given situation. So, keep an open mind when pursuing ethical outcomes.

Questions for Discussion

1. Conceptual: Discuss the ways in which the membership generally approaches ethical questions (character-based, rule-based, or consequence-based), how this affects the choices made, and why one or another approach predominates. Can those approaches be defended – for example, if one member argued for a harms–benefit analysis (consequentialist) and another member disagreed with that approach?

2. Pragmatic: How might someone use any one of the theories or methods to respond to Janet's case? Which approach is the "best" choice here, and why?
3. Strategic: Identify the members of your HEC who typically champion one approach to ethics (consequentialist, character-based, etc.). How might this knowledge enable more robust approaches to ethical questions?

References

Aristotle. (1999). *Nicomachean Ethics*, 2nd ed. (Irwin T, trans.). Indianapolis, IN: Hackett.

Beauchamp T, Childress J (2019). *The Principles of Biomedical Ethics*, 8th ed. New York: Oxford University Press.

Buermeyer L, Cooley W, Coss J, et al. (1923). *An Introduction to Reflective Thinking.* Boston: Houghton Mifflin.

Gert B, Culver CM, Clouser KD (2006). *Bioethics*, 2nd ed. New York: Oxford University Press.

Hester DM (2001). *Community as Healing.* Latham, MD: Rowman & Littlefield.

Kant I (1983). *Ethical Philosophy* (Ellington JW, trans.). Indianapolis, IN: Hackett.

Mill JS, Bentham J (1973). *The Utilitarians.* Garden City, NY: Anchor Books.

Chapter

3

Healthcare Ethics Committees and the Law

Stephen Latham

Objectives

Upon reading and considering the content of this chapter, the reader should be able to:

1. Explain legal mandates for and uses of healthcare ethics committees (HECs) in certain situations.
2. Describe legal parameters that affect the actions and deliberations of HECs.
3. Identify the importance of becoming familiar with your own state's law.

Case

Tina is an 11-year-old female with HIV. She acquired her HIV at birth, from her infected mother, Barbara. (Barbara had not sought medical care during her pregnancy.) Barbara and Tina moved into the community shortly after Tina's birth, and since then Barbara has been bringing Tina to the hospital's outpatient pediatrics clinic for HIV treatment and drugs. (Barbara sees a different physician.) Tina's viral load is well controlled. Because Tina has been visiting the clinic since before she can remember, she regards her trips there as a normal part of life, and has never questioned them. The clinical team has asked for an ethics consult because Barbara has never told Tina the nature of her illness, and has forbidden the team from informing her, either. Tina's physicians are concerned that Tina may soon become sexually active; they want her to understand about her HIV status and the risks of transmission. They also point out that Tina is approaching the age at which she could consent on her own to simple medical treatments; they argue that she ought to know her HIV status in order to be able to communicate it to caregivers. Barbara is vehemently opposed to informing Tina about her HIV status. She is worried that if Tina knows she is HIV+, she will let that fact slip to her peers, and will become stigmatized. She also argues that Tina will not become sexually active for many years – and by that time, she says, God will have cured Tina. She therefore sees no need to trouble Tina with knowledge of her illness. One of the nurses on the medical team thinks that Barbara may also have another motive for not telling Tina: Barbara is afraid that her new boyfriend will find out that Tina is HIV+, and will then deduce that Barbara is, too. Barbara has not disclosed her HIV status to her new boyfriend. She says she is "being careful" and "waiting for the right moment."

Introduction: Surrounded by Law

This chapter is designed to give ethics committee members a basic introduction to laws (particularly in the USA) affecting the committee's work. These include:

- a small number of federal cases and statutes
- a small number of state laws directed at ethics committees themselves and
- a large body of state-law rules governing medical treatment

Every ethics committee member needs to know something about the laws that shape and govern the clinical encounter. This is not because the law will typically determine the answers to the questions faced by the committee – far from it! Most of the problems faced by HECs aren't answered by any statute, regulation, or judicial holding. But that doesn't mean that law is irrelevant to the work of ethics committees. In some cases, law may define the terms in which a particular problem is discussed: "She needs to get his informed consent." In others, law may rule some possibilities out: "We can't just turn her out into the street." In still others, law may authorize or even require the committee's deliberation: "We can't avoid making this decision." In sum, law works mostly not to solve ethics committees' problems, but to shape them.

The case of Tina and Barbara illustrates the pervasiveness of law in medicine. Obviously, the case raises a number of ethical issues: When is it appropriate to tell a child about the nature of a serious illness like HIV? How much control should a parent have over that timing? Is it fair for the medical team to make judgments about the quality of this mother's reasoning, that is, that she is naïve about the possibility that her daughter will soon be sexually active, or that her religious conviction that Tina will be cured is incorrect, or that her "real" motives are self-interested? What responsibility, if any, does the team have regarding Barbara's relationship to her boyfriend? And so on. But for present purposes it's important to notice that the entire case is couched in a network of laws, and that some of the ethical problems will be better answered if the ethics committee has some legal knowledge.

For example, the committee should be aware that as a matter of law, in pediatric cases the medical team is bound to pursue the best interests of the child, not simply the parents' view of those best interests. This principle will help the committee evaluate Barbara's claims. The committee should have some knowledge of their state's standards regarding children's ability, at different ages, to consent to medical care; this will help them estimate how likely it is that Tina will soon be making her own medical choices. (Most states have a sliding-scale standard, permitting children to consent to simpler procedures early, and requiring parental consent for more complex or dangerous treatments.) And they should understand, or have access to, their state's laws regarding HIV. Some states have criminalized the act of knowingly exposing an unconsenting party to the risk of HIV infection; others have mandatory reporting laws that might or might not apply to Barbara. Note that while the law really does not supply knock-down, final, unassailable answers to any of the ethical questions raised by the case, knowledge of the law nonetheless permits better ethical analysis.

We turn now to look at some particular laws with which your committee should become familiar as a matter of course.

A Little Federal Law

The USA has a strong tradition of leaving medical matters to be regulated by states, rather than by the federal government. State governments are better equipped to judge local needs, and there are important variations among the states with regard to their healthcare resources, the numbers and training of their healthcare providers, and the public health problems they face. Most of the core areas of medical law are still centered on the states, for example, licensure of medical personnel and facilities, medical malpractice, public health. Although there are a few federal cases and statutes of which ethics committees should be aware, most of their work will be framed by state law.

Even the relatively few US Supreme Court decisions that relate to clinical ethics end up directing ethics committees toward state law. For example,

- *Cruzan* v. *Director, Missouri Department of Health*, 497 US 261 (1990). In this important bioethics case, the Supreme Court announced a constitutional right of competent patients to refuse life-sustaining medical treatment, and further that this right could be exercised on behalf of patients by their duly-authorized surrogates. But though it is a constitutional holding, *Cruzan* leaves some very important matters for the states to determine, such as: Who is authorized to serve as a surrogate? How much and what kind of evidence do surrogates need in order to prove that they are making the same decision the patient would have made?

- *Roe* v. *Wade*, 410 US 113 (1973), *Webster* v. *Reproductive Health Services*, 492 US 490 (1989), *Planned Parenthood* v. *Casey*, 505 U.S. 833 (1992). These US Supreme Court decisions underpin a constitutional right to early-term abortion. But these and subsequent decisions have left states largely free to determine whether any of their state resources or facilities will be used in connection with abortions, and, crucially, to determine the scope of regulation of both pre- and postviability abortions, and to determine whether postviability abortions will be permitted at all (if the mother's life is not at stake).

- *Washington* v. *Glucksberg*, 521 US 702 (1997) and *Vacco* v. *Quill*, 521 US 793 (1997). These cases determined that there is no US Constitutional right to physician aid-in-dying. The upshot of the two cases is to leave states free to decide whether and in what manner physicians or others may assist terminally ill patients who wish to die.

There are also many federal laws relating to health care: the laws establishing and implementing the Medicare and Medicaid programs; the Affordable Care Act, which expanded access to Medicaid in many states, and changed the way private insurance is regulated and marketed; federal regulations governing research on human subjects; Food and Drug Administration standards for prescription drugs and medical devices; the Genetic Information Nondiscrimination Act, and more. However, relatively few of these have much effect on the work of a clinical ethics committee. Among these few are:

- **The Health Insurance Portability and Accountability Act (HIPAA):** This act establishes privacy standards for healthcare professionals and institutions to use in connection with patients' identifiable health information. In fact, HIPAA does very little to interfere with ordinary, common-sense communication among healthcare professionals, ethics committee members, patients, families and friends (see US Department of Health and Human Services, Office of Civil Rights, 2017).

- **The Emergency Medical Transfer and Active Labor Act (EMTALA):** This law obliges hospitals to screen any patient who comes to the emergency department requesting examination or treatment, and to stabilize or transfer anyone suffering from an emergency medical condition. Most questions arising under EMTALA have to be resolved before there is time for an ethics committee consultation, but ethics committees sometimes consider EMTALA-related policy.

- **The Americans with Disabilities Act (ADA):** This law acts to prevent hospitals and healthcare workers from discriminating against persons with disabilities. Many provisions of the law (e.g., those governing physical accessibility of facilities) are outside the ethics committee's purview, but ethics committees may sometimes be called upon to assist physicians and others in understanding and complying with provisions such as those involving communication with the deaf, healthcare access by people with mobility problems, and toleration for service animals such as seeing-eye dogs.[1]
- **The Patient Self-Determination Act:** This act requires hospitals and other healthcare institutions to provide patients, upon admission, with information about patients' rights and the use of advance directives. Ethics committee members may periodically be called upon to review or assist in their hospital's implementation of the act's requirements.

The vast, vast majority of law touching on the actions of ethics committees is therefore state law. We may divide that law into two basic kinds: first, the relatively rare state laws that affect the formation and functioning of ethics committees themselves; and second, the much larger universe of state laws that will inform the committee's deliberations about clinical matters.

Law Relating to the Committee Itself

Committee members should of course have a basic understanding of any law relating to the existence and function of the ethics committee itself; but there is little such law. No federal requirements govern clinical ethics committees. The private Joint Commission does mandate that hospitals establish and follow a process allowing staff, patients, and families to address ethical issues. Ethics committees can satisfy that mandate. Joint Commission accreditation is required for hospitals to accept Medicare and Medicaid patients and, in some states, for licensure.[2]

Only about a half-dozen states have law mandating the creation of ethics committees. Maryland, New Jersey, Colorado, and New York have general "ethics committee" statutes; Texas law requires ethics committees in some state-funded facilities; Massachusetts law requires committees to consider a subset of complex issues arising in neonatal intensive care. Some of these laws recommend or require specific membership structures for such committees, and some basic practice standards, for example, written recordkeeping, notice to family members of committee deliberations, etc.

Ethics committee recommendations are usually purely advisory in nature, but a few state laws empower committees to make some binding decisions. Hawaii law laconically lists the making of ethical decisions as one of the functions of an ethics committee. Other states (Alabama, Arkansas, Georgia, Tennessee, Iowa, and, with regard to certain patients

---

[1] Detailed guidance on these and other ADA requirements is available at the US Department of Justice ADA website, www.ada.gov.

[2] This and the following three paragraphs draw extensively from Pope (2011), which contains specific citations to state statutes. In general, the "Legal Briefing" column in the *Journal of Clinical Ethics* is an excellent source of general information about laws governing clinical ethics consultation. But any given column may be out of date, so it is always best to consult on legal issues with a health-law attorney from your state.

in long-term care, California) have more specific laws permitting ethics committees to make or contribute to decisions for patients lacking surrogates. Massachusetts requires committee approval before life support can be withdrawn from any child under the supervision of the state department of children and families. New York law empowers ethics committees to approve surrogates' decisions about withholding and withdrawing life support and nutrition/hydration, and to approve the life-support decisions of emancipated minors. Maryland and Delaware law requires ethics committees to adjudicate disputes between surrogates and insulate physicians from liability if they follow the committee's recommendations. A controversial Texas law empowers ethics committees in certain circumstances to make binding determinations that particular treatments are futile and may be withdrawn.

Ethics committee members may be forgiven for having particular interest in laws that protect them from liability. New York, Ohio, Texas, and Maryland have laws protecting the confidentiality of ethics committee deliberations and preventing committee deliberations from being introduced in court cases. Alabama, Florida, Georgia, Hawaii, Maryland, Massachusetts, Montana, and New York all have specific statutes shielding ethics committee members from liability; and some states' general laws governing medical quality review committees may also act to shield ethics committees.

Ethics committees and their individual members have been sued when patients or their families were dissatisfied with their decisions. Such suits have been rare, but there will be more. Committees should therefore verify that all of their members – including those who, like community representatives, are not hospital employees – are covered by the hospital's institutional liability insurance. In addition, scholars have suggested recently that some kinds of decisions by ethics committees may amount to practicing law without a license (Prince and Davis, 2016). It is very unlikely that any lawyer would bring a complaint against an ethics committee on these grounds. However, to minimize risk, committees should avoid making decisions about what laws mean (leaving those to licensed attorneys!), and instead concentrate on making ethical decisions within the bounds of the law as attorneys have described it to them.

Law Relating to the Work of the Committee

We turn now to consider some of the laws that will frame the committee's deliberations and decisions about clinical matters. Here we face some serious expository difficulties posed by the fact that it is state, and not federal, laws that we are attempting to consider. First, the relevant laws may differ substantively from one state to another; physician-assisted suicide, for example, is permissible in Oregon, but criminal in Connecticut. Second, and more subtly, the laws in different states may have been created in different ways, using different legal mechanisms. Rules that were enacted as statutes by a legislature in one state may have been set out in health department regulations in another and may have been worked out gradually through a series of court decisions in a third. The following discussion of state law will therefore necessarily be a mere overview of the areas of law with which ethics committee members ought to make themselves familiar.

Ethics committees can use a number of strategies to get themselves educated in their state's law. In some states there are handy guides to medical law published by professional associations; these could be used by the committee for group study. But by far the best approach is to invite an experienced health-law attorney (perhaps the hospital's general counsel, or a local health-law professor) to meet with the committee a few times and lay out the state's basic medico-legal standards. It is vitally important that the committee get its education in law (whether in the form of training materials or lectures) not from nonlawyers, and not even from general-practice lawyers, but from experienced health lawyers.

Here, then, are the most important areas of law for ethics committee members:

- **Informed Consent:** Generally, state laws require that physicians obtain patients' informed consent prior to performing any procedure on them. Physicians are required to inform their patients of their diagnosis; their prognosis; the recommended course of treatment and its risks and benefits; and the risks and benefits of available alternatives, including nontreatment. But there is significant variance among states on the narrower question of exactly which risks it is important to disclose. There are two major camps: states that require physicians to inform patients about risks that any reasonable patient would like to hear about ("patient-standard" states) and states that require physicians to inform patients about risks that physicians customarily disclose ("physician-standard" states). In addition, some states have special consent laws addressing particular procedures – notably abortion, but also sterilization, fertility treatment, and others. And some have, or are entertaining, consent laws requiring disclosure of the particular physician's personal experience with the procedure in question, or of financial conflicts of interest.

  The legal situation with children is importantly different. Most states legally recognize a sort of "sliding scale" of children's competence to make their own medical decisions. A mature 15-year-old may be competent to make their own medical decisions, even about some fairly serious matters, while a 5-year-old may not. The child's intelligence, maturity, and previous experience with medical care are all variables that feed into the judgment whether that child is competent to consent to a given medical treatment; and, of course, the more risks and uncertainties attend the treatment, the more intelligence, maturity, and experience will be required for competence. If the child is not competent to consent, then the child's parents or guardians must decide. But, unlike competent adult patients, parents cannot just make any decision they want to. They are required to make their medical decisions in the best interest of the child. Sometimes it is not clear exactly what decision is in the child's best interest; in these cases, which may involve difficult weighting of risks or competing value-systems, physicians often defer to parental judgment. But if the medical team or the ethics committee are convinced that the parents are not deciding in the child's best interest, they are obligated to override the parents' decision, and may seek a court order to do so.

- **Refusal and Withdrawal of Treatments:** Every state recognizes a competent patient's right to refuse medical treatment of any kind, including life-sustaining medical treatment. State laws start to differ when the patient has become incompetent. In general, state laws require the medical team to obey, first, the wishes of a competent patient, their duly appointed guardian, or someone with their durable power of attorney for health care; and next the wishes expressed in a valid living will. Where there is no living will, or the living will is inapplicable or unclear, most states shift to a "substituted judgment" standard, requiring surrogates to make decisions as the patient would have made them. If there is not enough evidence to establish the patient's wishes, the surrogate must decide in the patient's best interest. The move from substituted judgment to "best interest" is extremely significant, since courts have been reluctant to hold that it is ever in anyone's best interest to die. Thus, where there is insufficient evidence to establish the patient's wishes, the default state-law position has been to "do everything" to save the patient. The problem is that state standards regarding how much evidence is sufficient to establish the patient's wishes are quite variable. In some states, recalled casual conversations about "not wanting to live hooked up to machinery" can be enough to justify a surrogate's substituted judgment in favor of treatment withdrawal. Other states demand powerful evidence such as signed writings, or testimony from an attorney about a serious advance planning conversation.

- **Advance Directives:** Committee members should be familiar with the basic state law governing the use of advanced directives, including living wills in which patients express their wishes about medical care and durable powers of attorney through which patients formally appoint surrogate healthcare decision makers. Some states separate regular healthcare powers of attorney from powers related to end-of-life decision-making. Some states also limit the ability of patient directives to halt the provision of nutrition and hydration, whether orally or through medical means. In many states, adherence to a patient's advance directive is not mandatory; instead, following the directive normally shields the medical team from liability. But a growing number of cases have found liability for physicians who have not followed advance directives, particularly in egregious circumstances (see Pope, 2017).

- **Surrogate Decision-Making:** In some cases, it will be clear to both the treatment team and the ethics committee who is legally authorized to make medical decisions in a given case. Of course, the competent patient makes their own decisions. An incompetent patient may have appointed a healthcare proxy, or the hospital or a state agency may have had a court appoint a guardian for the patient. Where there is no clearly authorized surrogate decision maker, though, the committee will need to make reference to state law. Luckily, a large majority of states have passed statutes that help determine who should serve as a patient's surrogate medical decision maker if the patient or a court has not designated one.[3] Commonly, the patient's spouse is first in line, followed by an adult child, and then by other family members. Some states permit even "close friends" to serve as surrogates, and a few (as we have seen above) permit ethics committees to sign off on treatments for patients with no other option. Incredibly, however, some states have no law on the question. In those states, both the treatment team and the ethics committee simply have to use their best judgment as to which of a given patient's relatives is the appropriate surrogate with whom to consult.

- **"Do Not Resuscitate" and Similar Orders:** Committee members should understand the variety of physicians' orders recognized in their state (and in their institution). Some state laws authorize patients and their physicians to cooperate in framing advance Physician Orders on Life Sustaining Treatment (POLST, also sometimes

---

[3] The ABA (American Bar Association) Commission on Law and Aging maintains a summary of state surrogate consent statutes at www.americanbar.org/groups/law_aging/publications/bifocal/vol_36/issue_1_october2014/default_surrogate_consent_statutes/.

called Medical Orders on Life Sustaining Treatment or MOLST). These are binding on all caregivers. But most other special orders relating to end-of-life care (Do Not Resuscitate, Do Not Intubate, No Antibiotics, and so on) can legally be entered by a physician whenever they are medically indicated or when they have been authorized by the patient or surrogate.

- **Confidentiality and Privacy:** The federal HIPAA law establishes sweeping regulations on the privacy and security of personal health information. But state laws about the treatment relationship also establish independent duties to protect patient confidences and private information.

- **Medical Futility:** A growing body of case law addresses the question whether a medical team can ever withhold life-sustaining medical treatment against the wishes of the patient or their surrogates. This question is among the most common to face HECs: The patient's family wants "everything" done, but the treatment team believes that further aggressive medical interventions would be pointless or even cruel. Frequently, the treatment team will accede to the family's wishes, even where they see no benefit to the treatment, out of fear of a lawsuit; and this can occur even after an ethics committee has agreed with the treatment team that the treatment is futile or medically inappropriate. In fact, state courts have increasingly favored treatment teams in such cases, granting permission to withdraw life-sustaining interventions in cases brought while the patient is still alive, and refusing to find medical liability in cases brought after the patient dies (Pope, 2008). Ethics committees should therefore make a special point of becoming familiar with any medical futility cases litigated in their state. Many hospitals and hospital systems also have their own in-house "futility" policies (often called "in appropriate care" policies); committee members should be familiar with these.

- **"Conscience" Laws:** Many states have passed laws or enacted regulations permitting doctors, pharmacists, and others to decline to provide certain kinds of health care (abortion, contraception, sterilization, assisted suicide) on grounds of moral or religious objection to the treatments in question.

- **"Standard of Care" and Medical Malpractice:** Any healthcare provider (hospital, physician, nurse, lab tech, occupational therapist, and so on) can be found liable to a patient for monetary damages if that provider breaches a duty toward the patient in a way that causes the patient harm. The most common duty involved in such liability lawsuits is the duty of care. (There are other duties – duties to avoid conflicts of interest, for example, and to maintain patient confidentiality – which can ground lawsuits, but these suits are not "malpractice" suits, and are not discussed here.)

The phrase "standard of care" refers, in the medical context, to the level of care at which a prudent medical professional with the same training and experience in the same (or a similar) community would practice under the same circumstances. Thus, if a pediatrician fails to diagnose an illness that a prudent pediatrician in their community would normally have diagnosed, they have failed to practice at the "standard of care," and have breached a duty to their patient. Note that the definition implies that specialized physicians are held to a higher standard within their specialty area than general practitioners practicing in that same area would be; that physicians who practice in a community where high-tech diagnostic equipment and consulting specialists are widely available might be held to a different standard than physicians in a remote and badly resourced region of the country; and that experienced physicians might be held to a higher standard than novices. Note, also, that the standard is not what the average physician would do, but what a prudent physician would do.

Physicians can depart from "standard of care" if, in their judgment, such departure is warranted by particular circumstances or by facts about the patient. For example, physicians are free to attempt innovative therapies with their patients' informed consent (see, e.g., American College of Obstetricians and Gynecologists, 2006), or to avoid standard interventions where the patients' particular characteristics make standard interventions inadvisable. In some cases, there may be multiple "standards of care" approaches to a given condition, with some physicians preferring one and some preferring another; or preferring one approach for one group of patients and the second for another. Finally, when a patient waives "standard of care" treatment – as, for example, when a competent adult patient or a qualified proxy decision maker refuses a life-sustaining intervention – the treatment team's duty is to respect the patient's wishes, rather than to stick to the standard of care.

Ethics committees should generally take care to assure that standard-of-care treatments are being offered. But they should also be aware that the treatment team may sometimes have a good justification for departing from standard of care, and that the patient or the patient's decision maker is free to decline standard-of-care interventions.

"Nonlegal" Ethics Standards

Nonlegal materials commonly shape the law. Courts routinely give deference to the established customs of private industry, to the arguments of experts, and to the rules of private associations. Part of the ethics committee's understanding of the law, therefore, ought to be an understanding of the important nonlegal standards from which the law will draw its content. No ethics committee should consider any case without looking to see whether any relevant professional bodies (the American Medical Association, the American Academy of Pediatrics, the American College of Physicians, and so on) have pronounced on similar cases in their ethics opinions or codes. Nor should the committee neglect any institutional standards that might apply: Catholic ethical standards in Catholic hospitals; Veterans Administration ethics opinions in federal Veterans Administration hospitals, and so on. The point is not that those pronouncements are necessarily binding on the commit-tee. Rather, consulting them makes sense both practically and legally. Practically, ethics codes, opinions, and standards are commonly the product of thoughtful persons of goodwill; they may well have something important to say about the matter at hand. Legally, such codes, opinions, and standards are quite likely to be cited by experts and consulted by judges in the unfortunate event that a committee decision is ever challenged in court. To ignore them is to ignore an important source of tomorrow's law.

Questions for Discussion

1. Conceptual: What laws are frequently implicated the HEC discusses cases and policies?
2. Pragmatic: To whom should the HEC turn and how might the HEC learn to interpret the meaning of laws and regulations in their ethical deliberations?
3. Strategic: Thinking about particular cases, when should committee discussion of legal standards occur–before or after discussion of the ethical issues?

References

American College of Obstetricians and Gynecologists. (2006). Innovative practice: Ethical guidelines. ACOG Committee Opinion No. 352. *Obstetrics and Gynecology*, 108(6): 1589–1595.

Pope TM (2008). Involuntary passive euthanasia in U.S. courts: Reassessing the judicial treatment of medical futility cases. *Marquette Elder's Advisor*, 9(): 229–268.

Pope TM (2011). Legal Briefing: Healthcare ethics committees. *Journal of Clinical Ethics*, 22(1): 74–93.

Pope TM (2017). Legal Briefing: New penalties for disregarding advance directives and DNR orders. *Journal of Clinical Ethics*, 28 (1): 74–81.

Prince AER, Davis, AM (2016). Navigating professional norms in an interprofessional environment: The "practice" of healthcare ethics committees. *Connecticut Public Interest Law Journal*, 15(1): 115–156.

US Department of Health and Human Services, Office of Civil Rights. (2017, October 12). HIPAA FAQs for professionals. www.hhs.gov/hipaa/for-professionals/faq/index.html.

Chapter 4

Understanding and Addressing Health Disparities through a Racial Paradigm

Jennifer L. McCurdy and Claretta Y. Dupree

Objectives

Upon reading and considering the content of this chapter, the reader should be able to

1. Associate health disparities with differential treatment in health care.
2. Describe the ethical challenges presented by social conditions and implicit bias in health care.
3. Formulate strategies to remedy implicit bias in ethical decision-making in health care.

Case 1

A 29-year-old Black female, Grace, is seen in the emergency room for vaginal bleeding in her 23rd week of pregnancy. Her fetus is in jeopardy and her obstetrician has called a neonatologist and the bioethics consultant to join a patient conference with Grace and her family to discuss options for care in case the fetus is delivered prematurely. Grace and her husband always wanted a child. Their current plan is for Grace to work while childcare is provided by her husband and his mother. Grace works for a nonprofit organization making $20,000 a year, and also works weekends at a grocery store in order to bring their income just above the federal poverty level. Grace's husband, Jim, is disabled from a gunshot wound sustained 3 years ago by a stray bullet that hit him while walking home one evening in their neighborhood. Grace has maintained a healthy diet and does not smoke or drink alcohol. Though Grace exhibits no symptoms, drug tests are ordered to rule out drug use as the cause of the pregnancy complications.

Case 2

A 48-year-old Inupiaq man, Frank, is admitted to the ICU in an Anchorage, Alaska hospital with respiratory failure. He is diagnosed with lung cancer and has a 30% chance of recovery with treatment. He is on a ventilator but is able to communicate and has the capacity to make his own decisions about his medical care. After consulting with his elders, Frank refuses treatment for the cancer. He lives in a rural Inupiaq community, and his income is below the poverty level. The village in which he lives is proximal to an oil drilling site and a toxic waste dump. His treatment would require him to stay in Anchorage, a thousand miles away from his family and community. Several members of the care team are distressed about his choice, especially at his age. They also wonder why he had not sought care sooner. They assume his lung cancer has been caused by smoking.

Introduction

Bioethics was founded on issues of justice over 50 years ago during the civil rights era. Its founding was in response not only to increasing technological advances, life-sustaining treatments in medicine, and physician paternalism, but also to the exploitation of vulnerable communities in research such as the commonly cited United States Public Health Service study on Black men in Tuskegee, Alabama and the New York School of Medicine hepatitis study on institutionalized children with disabilities at Willowbrook State School. Over the last few decades, the focus on justice in bioethics has faded in the shadow of emerging technologies. In clinical ethics, the primary focus has been on autonomous decision making and beneficent health care. Justice through the lens of health disparities has typically been addressed through public health, not bioethics, but this is changing. The American Society of Bioethics and Humanities' code of ethics states that HEC consultants should work with other healthcare professionals to reduce disparities, discrimination, and inequities when providing consultations (ASBH, 2014).

The purpose of this chapter is to provide a starting point for healthcare ethics committees (HECs) to understand the causes of, and to identify useful strategies to address, health disparities. Although this chapter focuses mainly on racial disparities, many of the concepts can be applied to disparities of any kind. It is important to keep in mind that each person or group experiencing health disparities will have unique historical contexts and local particularities that require their own focused attention.

Defining Disparity

Health disparities have historically been discussed in the narrow terms of health *care*, including access to hospitals, providers, and insurance. Society's responses toward health disparities are also often limited to arguments connecting individual behaviors to purported "essential qualities" of particular groups of people. The Centers for Disease Control and Prevention (CDC) defines health disparities as "preventable differences in the burden of disease, injury, violence, or in opportunities to achieve optimal health experienced by socially disadvantaged groups based on racialization, ethnicity, sex, sexual identity, disability, socioeconomic status, age, and geographic location" (CDC, 2017).

Racial healthcare disparities have been highlighted in the now widely circulated report by the Institute of Medicine's Committee on Understanding and Eliminating Racial and Ethnic Disparities in Healthcare. Published in 2003, this study reported racial and ethnic disparities at both the individual and systems levels in both patient outcomes and access to quality health care. Disparities were found across a wide range of disease areas and clinical services and in virtually all clinical settings, including preventative services, pain relief, cardiac care, cancer screening and treatment, diabetes management, end stage renal disease, treatment of HIV infection, pediatric care, maternal and child health, mental health, rehabilitative and nursing home services, and many surgical procedures (Smedley et al., 2003). These disparities remained even after factoring out socioeconomic and access-related causes, attributing some disparity to physician biases and stereotyping. This study on the discriminatory provision of health care highlighted one of many factors that cause widespread health disparities for racialized communities. Some of the most severe inequalities in health can be found in Native American and

Black communities. For instance, life expectancies of American Indians and Alaska Native (AIAN) people is approximately 5 years less than their white counterparts (US Department of Health and Human Services, Office of Minority Health, 2021). The rates of diabetes, adolescent female suicide, traumatic accidents, chronic liver disease, and death from hepatitis B and C for AIAN people are all roughly three times the rate of Caucasian counterparts in the USA (US Department of Health and Human Services, Office of Minority Health, 2021).

While disparities may be related to ethnicity, disability, sexuality, or gender, they are also intersectional, meaning structural discrimination and prejudicial attitudes may be experienced by the same person in relation to several categories. Those who fall into several marginalized groups, such as a Black person with a disability or who is transgender, will frequently have greater risk for experiencing poor health and differential treatment within the healthcare system.

The Root of Racial Disparities

Because all types of health disparities cannot be discussed here, this chapter will focus solely on racial disparities. Racial health disparities are caused not only by unequal access to quality health care, but also because of inequalities in social determinants of health such as socioeconomic status, education, employment, and racism, all of which exist due to the US history of maltreatment and marginalization of racialized groups. In addition to the continued existence of overt racism in the USA, an underlying worldview supporting the oppression of racialized groups continues to endure in more insidious forms such as structural and institutional mechanisms and unconscious biases. It is no coincidence that the people who disproportionately experience disparities today are those who have been racialized and colonized over the last 500 years. The lack of awareness of operating within a particular worldview has been called the "invisibility of whiteness," and is characterized by white people believing their reality is everyone's reality – that white and Western understandings of the world are the benchmarks of normalcy. Consider as examples of the "invisibility of whiteness" the concepts cultural competency, inclusion, resilience, pluralism, and multiculturalism (see Box 4.1 for further explanation). These well-intended concepts can be offensive and harmful to persons of color.

Box 4.1 Unexamined worldview in bioethics language

Cultural Competency: While meant to build sensitivity for those whose values and worldviews differ from the dominant set of values and worldviews, this approach assumes that those in the health professions are the norm, while "cultures" are those others who deviate from the norm. Culture is often considered only on the surface, lacks the critical analysis of power, and does not take seriously the sometimes-incompatible differences of worldview.

Inclusion: While including others can be a well-meaning gesture to bring people together, increase tolerance, and decrease social isolation, not all inclusion is welcome. For some AIAN people, for example, being included in mainstream society has historically meant (and continues to mean) assimilation: having one's own worldviews and values devalued or erased.

Box 4.1 (*cont.*)

Resilience: Resilience as a skill can help individuals build strength to cope with challenging situations like hardship and discrimination. But resilience cannot be a substitute for holding healthcare institutions accountable for the harms of discriminatory policies and practices.

Pluralism and Multiculturalism: We are a society of diverse people and communities with differing values, religions, ethnicities, and gender and sexual identities and preferences. Yet, discourses about pluralism and multiculturalism often represent difference superficially without changing the dominant rules or creating social and epistemic equality. People who constantly navigate between their own cultural context and the "white world" are already pluralistic, leaving one to question who benefits from these concepts. True pluralism is radical and challenges dominant values and worldviews.

The lack of worldview awareness can be found in the predisposition of those practicing healthcare ethics to seek similarities across groups. "Color blindness" is a claim, usually by a white person who says, "I don't see color. I treat everyone the same. We are all the same." Although well-meaning, this approach fails to acknowledge historical trauma, ignores the embodied experiences of differential treatment by people who have been stigmatized, and disregards knowledge derived from diverse perspectives.

Causes of Racial Disparities

In addition to the more obvious reasons for health and healthcare disparities such as access to quality care, disparities are also caused by the unique and enduring worldview that situates much of the USA. The thinking of the dominant culture contains an underlying racialized logic that manifests as both structural mechanisms and unconscious bias.

Structural Racism

Structural racism is "the totality of ways in which societies foster [racial] discrimination, via mutually reinforcing [inequitable] systems (housing, education, employment, earnings, benefits, credit, media, health care, criminal justice) that in turn reinforce discriminatory beliefs, values, and distribution of resources, reflected in history, culture, and interconnected institutions" (Bailey et al., 2017, 1454). In other words, structural racism is the continuation of the material colonial impacts on groups of people, particularly (but not limited to) Black, Latinx, and AIAN people in the USA. The stigmatization of marginalized groups affects members' ability to access needed resources. For instance, state and national policies are often written in ways that continue to maintain unequal access to the social determinants of health for such populations.

In the last few decades, the role of the social determinants of health has been framed largely by the field of public health, challenging both the limited notion of health equity as access to only health *care*, and repudiating the blaming of individuals and groups who are structurally oppressed. Social determinants of health are defined as "the conditions in which people are born, grow, live, work, and age" (World Health Organization, 2020) and include factors such as income, wealth, neighborhoods, housing, nutrition, education, environmental pollution, climate change, and social status. Evidence shows that socioeconomic status such as income, wealth, and education are most highly associated with health outcomes (Braveman and Gottlieb, 2014).

For example, attempts have been made for hundreds of years to eliminate Indigenous people from the land by destroying their food sources, cultures, and livelihoods. The resulting conditions continue to affect deeply Indigenous people's physical and mental health. In Alaska and elsewhere in the USA, many communities still rely on subsistence hunting and fishing. The availability of typical food sources is changing due to climate change, pollution, and the damming of waterways, making sustainable nutrition a challenge. We can see this in the case studies: The downstream effects of colonialism have had an effect on Frank's health at an early age. Frank and his family have had to rely on readily available high-calorie packaged foods that set them up for diseases such as diabetes and heart disease. Poverty also leads to the lack of access to transportation to get to medical facilities, decreasing the likelihood Frank's cancer could have been detected earlier. In addition, it is possible his lung cancer stems from the proximity of his community to oil fields and to toxic waste dumping grounds from military and industrial operations. The incidence of respiratory cancers where Frank lives is twice that of Alaska and the USA as a whole (Institute for Health Metrics and Evaluation, 2014). Yet, none of these socially determined factors are apparent when Frank seeks care.

Grace and Jim are also affected by socially determined inequalities. Wealth-building through an ability to save money and invest in the economic market was unattainable over the last few centuries for both enslaved Blacks diasphoric people and their descendants. The lack of wealth has implications for access to education, safe housing, higher-paying jobs, and healthier food. The couple's inability to move into a safe neighborhood put Jim in harm's way and has disabled him for life. Besides Jim's disability insurance they do not require public assistance; their level of income limits affordable housing choices, as does the need to outfit their house to be physically accessible for Jim. Grace and Jim endure constant financial stress, which has a direct effect on Grace's health and her pregnancy, despite her positive health-seeking behaviors.

Racism and Unconscious Bias

Racism is also a direct cause of health disparities, affecting the health of persons of color within social structures and within relationships between patients and healthcare providers. On a societal level, racism underlies access to health-promoting resources. Discrimination happens in individual sectors such as the housing market through the inability to secure loans and through residential segregation; through decreased access to, and discrimination within, school systems; and through job discrimination. Each one of these resources contributes to health. Second, racism at large directly affects one's psychological well-being. The psychological and emotional stress of dealing with racism in the world on a daily basis is chronic and compounding. These stressors include external factors such as violence, overt discrimination, and microaggressions. Racism also affects one's psychological well-being related to fear of rejection or retaliation, and the repression of one's thoughts and feelings in the face of racial profiling and stereotype threat. Psychological stressors can lead to maladaptive coping behaviors such as decreased self-worth, rumination, smoking, overeating, suicidality, and alcohol and drug use. Finally, the psychological effects of racism directly affect physical health through physiological responses including chronic cortisol output and diastolic blood pressure reactivity that contribute to diabetes, heart disease, premature births, increased maternal mortality, and a host of other chronic illnesses (Hatzenbuehler et al., 2013).

In the clinical setting, then, the experiences for Frank as well as for Grace and Jim, while not identical, are also affected by individual racism. The chronic stressors of maintaining hypervigilance about one's reception in a primarily white institution, the implicit biases (sometimes referred to as "unconscious racism") of healthcare providers, and the experience of microaggressions all continue to affect their health and health care even after they leave the facility. How patients are treated affects their trust. If Frank experiences disrespect or disregard for his culture and choices, and if Grace feels stereotyped by care providers, they are less likely to seek health care in the first place, further deepening the disparities already present.

Strategies for Ethics Committees

HECs cannot solve the problem of health disparity by themselves. But they have the opportunity to work collaboratively with others to continue to address the causes of disparities. A few general strategies are outlined below in Box 4.2.

Box 4.2 Strategies for HECs

Addressing structural racism:

- Radically diversify the ethics committee
- Create an ethics subcommittee to champion diversity and address disparity
- Review and revise ethics policies to counter structural discrimination potential
- Partner with hospital leadership in funding equity programming, research, quality metrics
- Partner with diverse communities
- Partner with public health practitioners to bridge clinical and public causes of disparities
- Create pipelines for increasing diversity in clinical and bioethics professions

Addressing unconscious bias:

- Raise awareness: take an implicit bias test
- Seek anti-bias training for HECs and hospital staff
- Create a culture of mutual accountability for recognizing implicit bias
- Start a hospital-wide effort to support staff in confronting discriminatory behaviors
- Practice recognizing and responding to microaggressions
- Read and apply the scholarship and advice of scholars of color
- Be morally courageous – speak up and speak out against discrimination
- Interrogate one's worldview and invest time learning alternative worldviews

---

Although structural racism is not easy to overcome, there are a few strategies for dealing with it. First, committees should have diverse membership, especially including those who are typically marginalized such as people with disabilities, LGBTQ persons, racialized and ethnically diverse people, and certain religious affiliations, from within and outside the institution who represent the patient population. Professional diversity may include not only the direct care providers, but also the hospital's chief equity officer, language interpreters, speech therapists, hospital police, and patient representatives.

Committees could consider creating a subcommittee to champion the committee's efforts at addressing diversity and disparity.

Second, committees can deliberately rework ethics policies so that they contain specific anti-racist and anti-discriminatory language. A systematic examination and restructuring with input from members of groups who experience discrimination would help to identify potential ways "colorblind" policies might be harmful.

Third and more broadly, the committee can partner with members of hospital administration to develop and fund equity programming, research, community outreach, and quality metrics to promote an anti-discriminatory ethical climate.

And fourth, structural changes outside the clinical arena include diversifying the healthcare student and professional pipelines, transforming healthcare curricula, and incorporating diverse worldviews and scholarship into the field of bioethics. HECs also have the opportunity to explore community partnerships in addressing the structural causes of disparity. Critical to the process of the inclusion of diverse viewpoints and in partnering with outside groups is the recognition that people of color have an insight that those in the dominant culture do not have. The navigation of two cultures, the dominant culture and their own, allows them to "see" the dominant culture. On the other hand, the dominant culture rarely experiences the discomfort associated with being the outsider, of not belonging, or of being oppressed. By listening and following the lead of those outside of the dominant worldview HEC members can become aware of their patterns of thinking and more deeply understand the experiences of people of color.

How might HECs address implicit bias? The covert nature of implicit bias comes from the messages received throughout a lifetime from school, media, family, and friends. Implicit biases may be triggered by the color of another's skin color, behaviors, or choices. Recognizing implicit bias requires self-reflection to separate ingrained and unconscious stereotypes from reality. Implicit bias tests that reveal one's unconscious bias can be found online. These tests gauge a test-taker's initial reactions to a rapid succession of pictures (for instance of Black and white faces) and their association with terms such as "good" or "bad." More broadly, HECs can seek anti-bias training and provide a safe space to question one another's biases and assumptions. For instance, in Frank's case an HEC member or care provider might assume, based on stereotypes, that Frank smokes, is lazy, or needs to become more modern and progressive (which are common stereotypes of Indigenous people). It might be assumed of Grace that she is an angry Black woman if she is not smiling, and that she and Jim chose poorly in getting pregnant, given their finances. These types of subconscious assumptions are commonplace and affect care providers' treatment decisions.

Implicit biases can also manifest as microaggressions. As defined by Sue et al., "racial microaggressions are everyday slights, insults, putdowns, invalidations, and offensive behaviors that people of color experience in daily interactions with generally well-intentioned white Americans who may be unaware that they have engaged in racially demeaning ways toward target groups" (Sue et al., 2019, 129). Targeted groups experience a constant flow of microaggressions, which take a cumulative toll on their psychological and physical well-being (Sue et al., 2019, 130). While some forms of microaggressions can be overtly and deliberately discriminatory, most are unintentional and implicit. Imagine if Grace overhears a physician commenting to another physician, "Her drug test was surprisingly negative" despite the fact that no one told her she was getting tested for narcotics. Or consider a nurse saying to Grace, "You are the whitest Black woman I know."

As with implicit bias, HEC members should acknowledge the existence of microaggressions and learn to recognize them. When a personal experience of microaggression is claimed, the claim should be acknowledged and accepted as valid. The HEC member's job is to try to understand the nature of what was said (or nonverbally expressed) and why it was harmful. Sue et al. (2019) proposed a helpful strategic framework for addressing microaggressions including making the "invisible" visible, disarming the microaggression, educating the offender, and seeking external support. For instance, consider the comment Grace overhears about being drug tested. Making the "invisible" visible (to the perpetrator) requires a bystander to educate the physician about the stereotype of Black women as drug users and of causing their own pregnancy complications. To disarm the microaggression, the physician would be encouraged to admit to using a microaggression and to have an honest discussion with Grace.

Conclusion

Social disparities have direct and challenging effects on the health care of individuals and groups. Racial disparities, in particular, are long-standing and can be traced from the beginning of the USA as a country. HECs are positioned to address individual and systemic issues of disparity on multiple levels, and to ultimately improve health equity. This starts with recognizing that equity can only be attained if those who comprise the healthcare system choose to acknowledge and take action against disparity.

Questions for Discussion

1. Conceptual: Should HECs act as neutral mediators on issues of racism and disparity, or should they take a normative stance?
2. Pragmatic: What policies and/or practices does your ethics committee and/or hospital presently have in place to address the causes of disparities?
3. Strategic: How can your HEC be more proactive about recognizing and responding to the multiple causes of disparities?

References

American Society for Bioethics and Humanities. (2014). Code of ethics and professional responsibilities for healthcare ethics consultants. In *Improving Competencies in Clinical Ethics Consultation: An Education Guide*, 4. https://asbh.org/uploads/ASBH_Code_of_Ethics.pdf

Bailey ZD, Krieger N, Agénor M, Graves J, Linos N, Bassett MT (2017). Structural racism and health inequities in the USA: Evidence and interventions. *The Lancet*, 389 (10077), 1453–1463.

Braveman P, Gottlieb L (2014). The social determinants of health: It's time to consider the causes of the causes. *Public Health Reports*, 129(1, Suppl. 2), 19–31.

Centers for Disease Control and Intervention. (2017). Health disparities. www.cdc.gov/aging/disparities/index.htm

Hatzenbuehler ML, Phelan JC, Link BG (2013). Stigma as a fundamental cause of population health inequalities. *American Journal of Public Health*, 103(5), 813–821.

Institute for Health Metrics and Evaluation. (2014). US County Profile: North Slope Borough,

Alaska. www.healthdata.org/sites/default/files/files/county_profiles/US/2015/County_Report_North_Slope_Borough_Alaska.pdf

Smedley BD, Stith AY, Nelson AR, eds. (2003). *Unequal Treatment: Confronting Racial and Ethnic Disparities in Health Care.* Institute of Medicine Committee on Understanding and Eliminating Racial and Ethnic Disparities in Health Care. Washington, DC: National Academies Press.

Sue DW, Alsaidi S, Awad MN, Glaeser E, Calle CZ, Mendez N (2019). Disarming racial microaggressions: Microintervention strategies for targets, White allies, and bystanders. *American Psychologist,* 74(1), 128–142.

US Department of Health and Human Services, Office of Minority Health. (2021). Profile: American Indian/Alaska Native. https://minorityhealth.hhs.gov/omh/browse.aspx?lvl=3&lvlid=62

World Health Organization. (2020). Social determinants of health. www.who.int/social_determinants/en/

Chapter

5

Cultural and Religious Issues in Health Care

Alissa Hurwitz Swota

Objectives

Upon reading and considering the content of this chapter, the reader should be able to:

1. Appreciate the profound influence culture has on how an individual approaches the healthcare encounter.
2. Describe how religious and cultural commitments may give rise to value tensions in health care.
3. Understand the role that healthcare ethics committee (HEC) members play in eliciting and addressing culturally relevant values of both patients and healthcare providers.

Case

Ms. A, 19, presents to the emergency department of a local hospital with high fever, cough, and a generally despondent demeanor. She is diagnosed with tuberculosis (TB), treated, and given a prescription for and information about the proper TB treatment regimen. Upon mandatory contact investigation from the county health department, Ms. A's father is identified as also having active tuberculosis.

Neither Mr. A nor his daughter are taking their TB medications routinely. Ultimately, they are both involuntarily committed to the appropriate institution (which was close to where they lived) for mandatory TB treatment. Ms. A, no longer ambulatory, was rolled into the institution on a gurney. Her father, though also ill, was ambulatory.

Adding to the complexities of this case was the fact that Mr. A and his daughter were both migrant workers who spoke very little English. Determining the precise dialect of Mixteca that they spoke and obtaining an appropriate interpreter was neither a quick nor an easy process. While in the hospital, on several occasions Mr. A attempted to remove the peripherally inserted central catheter line through which his daughter was receiving her TB medications. Healthcare team members were unsure why Mr. A was refusing medication that could so easily help his daughter, and uncertain as to how best to proceed in light of the current conflict.

Introduction

HEC members are often confronted by cases where communication breaks down. One particular type of case in which communication can break down is where patients speak a different language than care providers. In such cases something as simple as using the services of a trained medical interpreter can resolve many issues. More troubling for

HECs are patients whose cultural or religious commitments constitute a unique set of values and goals for the healthcare encounter. This is especially true in light of an increasingly culturally diverse patient population. More and more, health care is provided and negotiated across complex terrain. Often, operating in the background is the assumption that everyone comes to the table with a common understanding and shared expectations of the healthcare encounter (Sanchez et al., 1996). Such an assumption can easily lead to conflict and misunderstandings.

One laudable, but ultimately unsatisfactory, effort to deliver culturally effective care and avoid conflict and misunderstanding uses a kind of "cookbook" approach to understanding cultural values and differences. These kinds of approaches attempt to provide professionals with detailed tenets from as many different cultures or religions as possible, hoping to provide professionals with "competent" insight into a variety of cultural value-systems. While this approach may yield some good information and help to raise awareness of differences in values and goals, taking it as a sufficient step in providing culturally effective care is both unrealistic and misguided, as it is both impossible to achieve fully and may lead to stereotyping.[1] Ultimately, while there is benefit to learning about cultural values that can affect healthcare decisions, a more sensitive, nuanced, and personalized approach to gaining such awareness is needed.

Integrating Culture into the Ethics Encounter

Culture is a concept that has been defined in a multitude of ways.[2] Here, I will use the definition put forth by the US Department of Health and Human Services, Office of Minority Health (2001, 4), in which culture is understood as:

> the thoughts, communications, actions, customs, beliefs, values, and institutions of racial, ethnic, religious, or social groups. Culture defines how health care information is received, how rights and protections are exercised, what is considered to be a health problem, how symptoms and concerns about the problem are expressed, who should provide treatment for the problem, and what type of treatment should be given.

It is the lens through which an individual views the world, coloring everything from the most mundane to the exotic.

How, then, can members of an HEC understand culture in relation to their work on an ethics committee? First, HECs can facilitate inquiries into the ways culture may influence a patient's values and goals by engaging in meaningful discourse with the

---

[1] As Betancourt et al. (2003, 298–299) note,

> there may be certain helpful, culturally specific information that can be effectively taught while avoiding stereotypes. This includes particular folk illnesses among certain populations; ethnopharmacology; disease incidence, prevalence, and outcomes among distinct populations; the impact of the Tuskegee Syphilis Study and segregation as the cause of mistrust among African Americans; the effect of war and torture on certain refugee populations and how this shapes their interaction with the health care system; and the common cultural and spiritual practices that might interfere with prescribed therapies, to name a few.

[2] For the purposes of this chapter, I will employ a robust understanding of culture in which religion is a (type of) cultural tradition. For similar takes on the concept of culture, see www.calendow .org/uploadedFiles/principles_standards_cultural_competence.pdf and Lincoln (2003, esp. 51–61).

patient and family. Since culture and religion are tied to central features of patients' self-concepts, patients and families need to feel comfortable enough to reveal very personal information. Fearing criticism or negative judgments, some patients may not be forthcoming about particular cultural practices regarding health and illness that diverge from what providers traditionally see in the biomedical clinical context. Holding back information may interfere with the provision of optimal patient care, since a complete, accurate patient account of the situation is unable to be obtained. Inspiring trust and creating a strong foundation on which to base relationships with patients is crucial, but it is an inherently difficult endeavor – embarking on such an endeavor while navigating across cultures serves to increase the level of difficulty. Given this high degree of difficulty coupled with the deeply held values that are so often at stake, it is no surprise that breakdowns in communication occur and ethics consultations are called. To be sure, what is surprising is that ethics consultations are not called more frequently.

Add to this the current healthcare environment in which long-term relationships with healthcare providers are the exception as opposed to the rule, the encounter between patient and provider is all too brief, the focus too often shifted to one of "managing clients" instead of "caring for individual patients," and the importance of good, clear communication is even more striking.[3] However, there is a delicate balance that must be struck between accommodating any and all practices because they are part of a patient's culture and adopting an ethnocentric view in which only the biomedical model of Western medicine is accepted. Turner (2002, 298–299) does well in summarizing the difficulties faced in striking this balance in the clinical setting:

> The dual dangers in addressing the moral obligations of health care providers in multicultural, pluralistic settings are those of falling into a facile acceptance of all cultural and religious norms, even when some practices cause great harm and violate basic human rights, and insisting upon a narrow understanding of acceptable moral reasoning, when there is good reason to think that a plurality of human religious and cultural practices should be accommodated.

Greene et al. describe myriad factors providers may need to consider to provide culturally effective care: "assessing patients' understanding of their illness, identifying mistrust, negotiating treatment plans, assessing English proficiency, identifying relevant cultural and religious beliefs, understanding decision-making roles, working with interpreters, and counseling patients about their use of complementary or alternative medicine" (Green et al., 2017, 17). The case of Mr. A and his daughter highlights the importance of providing culturally effective care, the centrality of good communication, and the difficulties involved in achieving both.

Recognizing the influence of culture on oneself and the way one engages with the world is equally as important as understanding the influence of culture on others. As such, it is as important for HEC members to gain an understanding of their own culture. Such self-awareness serves to alert HEC members to the biases and preconceptions they bring to the consideration of the ethical issue. This awareness will not only help to minimize the influence of such biases and preconceptions, it will also allow the ethics consultant to reflect more critically on the judgments they make. As an ethics committee member grappling with complex value conflicts, such self-awareness is imperative in

---

[3] For a nice review of studies demonstrating "a correlation between effective physician-patient communication and improved patient health outcomes" see Stewart (1995, 1423).

setting the stage for a transparent ethics consultation. Ultimately, recognizing the considerable influence of culture in one's own life facilitates the acknowledgment of the same in others.

Providing Culturally Effective Care: Tools for Practice

Language differences layered with disparate notions of the cause of illness were just some of the factors that served to make the case of Mr. A and his daughter incredibly complex. To be sure, it would have been "easier" for healthcare providers to go ahead with the standard tuberculosis treatment regimen, relying solely on their authority to impose such treatments on a patient in Ms. A's condition. In an effort to avoid such a restrictive option and try to build trust in the relationship, healthcare providers put forth great efforts to understand and appreciate Mr. A's position, respect his role as his daughter's surrogate, and negotiate a mutually agreed upon plan of care that demonstrated such an appreciation. Engaging Mr. A in dialogue gave providers a chance not only to gain insight into Mr. A's understanding of the situation, but also afforded an opportunity for healthcare providers to answer questions from Mr. A and convey their understanding of the situation.

In this case, different conceptions concerning what was causing Mr. A's daughter to be ill proved to be a source of great tension, arising from differences in the explanatory models of illness held by Mr. A and the healthcare team. Briefly, an individual's "explanatory model of illness reflect[s] the cultural understanding of what illness is, how it occurs, why it exists and what measures can be taken to prevent or control it" (Bowman, 2005).

Ethics consultations often serve a clarifying function, helping to elucidate the issues at play in a situation, highlighting the values that are in conflict, or, possibly, identifying which perspectives are not being given sufficient voice. Indeed, an HEC member may have been the one to discover Mr. A's explanatory model from the case described above. Cultural and religious values often bring these clarifying functions into stark relief precisely because providers, patients, and families may approach decisions from very different perspectives. For example, patients whose religious commitments prevent them from accepting blood products for fear of losing ultimate salvation may seem unreasonable from the perspective of healthcare providers whose goals are to restore form and functioning through physiological mechanisms.

Once the team began to ask questions that helped to elicit Mr. A's explanatory model in a way that demonstrated respect for Mr. A's input, a resolution to the conflict became possible. From the outset, Mr. A refused to believe that tuberculosis was the cause of his daughter's illness, or that his daughter even had tuberculosis in the first place. Instead, Mr. A maintained that someone back in their village in Mexico had put a hex on his daughter, and that was the cause of his daughter's poor condition. Remedying her condition would therefore require sending money back to someone in his village who could counter the hex. Further, far from helping his daughter, Mr. A maintained that the medicines for tuberculosis were making her worse.

The HEC member's task under such conditions is to help healthcare providers recognize that further education for patients/families about the medical facts and necessities will not resolve this conflict. Rather, the conflict exists precisely because of a difference in values and goals that are generated by cultural and religious commitments. In addition, the HEC member also has the responsibility to help patients/ families articulate these values and their grounding, as well as to help them understand why the providers see the picture differently.

Asking the right questions, in a culturally sensitive manner, with humility and authenticity, at the right time, is a crucial skill that must be honed. To this end, having a reserve of questions from which to draw is invaluable during the process of an ethics consultation. Several such resources exist to help ethics committee members gain an understanding of a patient and their perceptions of the healthcare encounter (see, for example, LEARN [Berlin and Fowkes, 1983], HOPE [Anandarajah and Hight, 2001], and FICA [Borneman et al., 2010]). One such useful tool, which can be used alone or in combination with other tools, is Arthur Kleinman's (1980, 106 fn4) set of questions for obtaining explanatory models. To be sure, all of Kleinman's questions need not be asked in every encounter and can be amended in order to best serve the purpose at hand.[4]

- What do you call your problem? What name does it have?
- What do you think has caused your problem? (etiology)
- Why do you think it started when it did? (time of onset)
- What does your sickness do to you? How does it work? (pathophysiology)
- How severe is it? Will it have a short or long course? (course)
- What do you fear most about your sickness?
- What are the chief problems your sickness has caused for you? (personally, in your family, and at work)
- What kind of treatment do you think you should receive?
- What are the most important results you hope to receive from the treatment?

As important as knowing which questions to ask, ethics consultants must make it clear to patients and families that they genuinely want to know the answers and that the information gleaned is an essential component in developing a treatment plan. Such interest can be demonstrated by an ethics committee member who takes time to engage patients and families in dialogue, is an active listener, and answers questions clearly and consistently. When ethical conflict is the result of misunderstanding the sources of values that give rise to conflicts of care, HEC members can be well-served by considering some of the aforementioned tools as a way to identify the foundation of the difference in position. To be sure, resolution in Mr. A's case was made possible, in part, because one of the healthcare providers knew Kleinman's questions, their value, and how to ask them. Specifically, by eliciting Mr. A's understanding of the cause of his daughter's illness and his thoughts regarding appropriate treatments, crucial insight was gained and a more robust narrative of the situation was developed.

With this and other information gleaned from continued dialogue, the healthcare team was able to negotiate a plan of care with which everyone was satisfied. Continuing to administer the TB medications to his daughter during negotiations provided the time necessary for the medications to work and Ms. A's condition to improve. This in turn helped Mr. A realize that the medications themselves were not causing his daughter's problems. At the same time the tuberculosis medications were continued for Mr. A's

---

[4] Other useful "tools" include the LEARN Model (from Berlin and Fowkes, 1983; Carrillo et al., 1999); see also BELIEF (Dobbie et al., 2003).

daughter, arrangements were made for Mr. A to have money wired back to someone in his village in Mexico who would reverse the hex that Mr. A believed to be causing his daughter to be ill. As expected by the healthcare team, administering the proper medications without further interference allowed Mr. A's daughter to make a full recovery. Even at discharge, Mr. A refused to believe that his daughter had had tuberculosis or that the medications she was given caused her to recover. Nonetheless, whether Mr. A believed this change in condition was due to medication or a "counter-hex" did not seem to matter. In this case, the information provided by Mr. A served to help direct the actions of the healthcare providers (e.g., wiring Mr. A's money to Mexico), and at the same time, helped healthcare providers negotiate a change in Mr. A's behaviors (e.g., he agreed to refrain from interfering with the administering of medications to his daughter). By not making assumptions, engaging decision makers in a dialogue, and weighing the values of all stakeholders, providers were able to avoid extreme restrictions on the patient, deescalate the conflict, and deliver effective patient and family-centered care.

Responding to a Cultural Misunderstanding

Vigilance in spotting cultural misunderstandings is necessary. However, such vigilance would not be nearly as valuable without the knowledge of how to proceed after a misunderstanding is identified. The following recommendations have been developed to help those in a healthcare setting restore an effective working relationship with patients and families after a conflict has developed (Flaming and Towey, 2003, 37–38):

- Be direct and apologize for the behavior that may have distanced the patient or family member
- Explain how the behavior is appropriate in the physician's culture as a way to provide a rationale for the behavior
- Acknowledge that the patient and family members know more about their own cultural background than the physician. Ask about ways to generate appropriate and acceptable solutions
- Complex situations with unclear solutions may necessitate bringing in an additional person or persons to mediate or act as a "culture broker"

While these recommendations refer to physicians specifically, they are useful for HEC members as well. Ethics consults are often called when the conflict is already quite intense. These tips can help deescalate tensions in such situations. In addition, HEC members can refer to these recommendations when providing advice and guidance to members of the healthcare team involved in a conflict born out of cultural differences. Overall, these recommendations provide guidance as to how to proceed when, in spite of good intentions and a solid knowledge base, a cultural misunderstanding is identified.

Implications for Policy and Education

While this chapter has primarily focused on the consultative role of the HEC in regard to religious and cultural values, there are important implications for both policy and education that merit consideration. There are some religious and cultural practices that are either ubiquitous generally, or that are common enough in a particular region that they ought to be considered in policy development and revision. For example, any policy about blood transfusion should make explicit the institution's approach to refusals of blood products by Jehovah's Witnesses on behalf of themselves or on behalf of their minor child; this latter piece is particularly important because there may be different policies and/or procedures for these two different populations. As another example, members of some populations (e.g., a subset of the Orthodox Jewish population) may object to policies of brain death, preferring to rely on a cardiopulmonary definition of death. Any brain death policy should state clearly how providers should approach situations where an individual's religious commitments prevent a shared understanding of the meaning of physical signs and symptoms.

In addition, there may be instances where a policy exists but there are good reasons for permitting exceptions. Consider the patient whose care has been deemed medically futile, but who insists on aggressive therapies for an additional few days so that they will not expire during the current phase of the moon – an event that is spiritually anathema to them (Rubin, 1998). Once an HEC member elicits the values that support the request, there may be ways to accommodate patient requests that at first seem untenable. Sometimes this results in a compromise, as seen with Mr. A above, and sometimes the patient's request can be honored as-is once providers understand the request was not born out of a misunderstanding of the medical situation.

Finally, all of these instances of culturally or religiously based values are excellent opportunities for education. Certainly, providers who are likely to encounter decision-making influenced by such values need to know some information about those cultures (e.g., the practice of coining when practiced by a significant cultural presence in town, or refusals to accept brain death criteria among a certain population). But more than this, it is important for the HEC to educate the institution at large about such practices. Education can serve as an action of preventive ethics not simply by avoiding instances of misunderstanding, but rather by reminding providers to elicit the value-systems and explanatory models of patients and families on a routine basis. Taking a proactive approach toward cultural awareness will enable providers to provide culturally effective care and to avoid the conflicts that are likely to arise from a (sometimes erroneous) presumption about shared models of health and disease.

Conclusion

Eliciting the values and preferences of patients and families is a necessary step in respecting the autonomy of patients and families. While this is a crucial function of the ethics committee, the task is not easy amid the plurality of cultures present in the healthcare setting. In order to resolve conflicts raised by differences in values, HEC members must engage in a process that fosters respect and understanding for patients, families, and healthcare providers alike. While I have offered some tools to assist the HEC member in this role, the use of such tools will only be successful if it is coupled with genuine dialogue, authentic inquiry, and institutional support. The latter can best be achieved through policy development and organizational education; both of these practices will prepare members of the institution to address a variety of culturally inspired conflicts that may arise in healthcare delivery.

Questions for Discussion

1. Conceptual: What are the most common cultural or religious misunderstandings/conflicts that you see in your institution? How might you address them proactively?

2. Pragmatic: How might an HEC member deescalate conflict in the face of a cultural misunderstanding?
3. Strategic: At the beginning of Ms. A's case, what are some tactics that could have been employed to avoid conflict?

References

Anandarajah G, Hight E (2001). Spirituality and medical practice: Using the HOPE questions as a practical tool for spiritual assessment. *American Family Physician*, 63 (1): 81–89.

Berlin EA, Fowkes WC Jr (1983). A teaching framework for cross-cultural health care: Application in family practice. *Western Journal of Medicine*, 139(6): 934–938.

Betancourt JR, Green AR, Carrillo JE, Ananeh-Firempong O, II (2003). Defining cultural competence: A practical framework for addressing racial/ethnic disparities in health and health care. *Public Health Reports*, 118 (4): 293–302.

Borneman T, Ferrell B, Pulchaski CM (2010). Evaluation of the FICA Tool for Spiritual Assessment. *Journal of Pain and Symptom Management*, 40(2): 163–173.

Bowman K (2005). Bioethics and cultural pluralism. *Humane Health Care*, 13(2). www.humanehealthcare.com/Article.asp?art_id=776

Carrillo JE, Green AR, Betancourt JR (1999). Cross-cultural primary care: A patient-based approach. *Annals of Internal Medicine*, 130(10): 829–834.

Dobbie AE, Medrano M, Tysinger J, Olney C (2003). The BELIEF Instrument: A preclinical teaching tool to elicit patients' health beliefs. *Family Medicine*, 35(5): 316–319.

Flaming M, Towey K (2003). *Delivering Culturally Effective Health Care to Adolescents*. Chicago: American Medical Association. www.ama-assn.org/resources/doc/ad-hlth/culturallyeffective.pdf

Green AR, Chun MBJ, Cervantes MC, et al. (2017). Measuring medical students' preparedness and skills to provide cross-cultural care. *Health Equity*, 1(1): 15–22.

Kleinman A (1980). *Patients and Healers in the Context of Culture*. Berkeley: University of California Press.

Lincoln B (2003). *Holy Terrors: Thinking about Religion after September 11*. Chicago: University of Chicago Press.

Rubin S (1998). *When Doctors Say No*. Bloomington: Indiana University Press.

Sanchez TR, Plawecki JA, Plawecki HM (1996). The delivery of culturally sensitive health care to Native Americans. *Journal of Holistic Nursing*, 14(4): 295–307.

Stewart MA (1995). Effective physician-patient communication and health outcomes: A review. *Canadian Medical Association Journal*, 152(9): 1423–1433.

Turner L (2002). Bioethics and end-of-life care in multi-ethnic settings: Cultural diversity in Canada and the United States of America. *Mortality*, 7(3): 285–301.

US Department of Health and Human Services, Office of Minority Health. (2001). *National standards for culturally and linguistically appropriate services in health care: Final report*. http://minorityhealth.hhs.gov/assets/pdf/checked/finalreport.pdf

Chapter

6

Moral Distress

Lucia Wocial

Objectives

Upon reading and considering the content of this chapter, the reader should be able to:

1. Differentiate moral distress from other kinds of distress that healthcare providers face routinely.
2. Identify strategies to prevent, mitigate, or address issues of moral distress in healthcare providers.
3. Identify elements of hospital policy and standard operating procedures that support navigation of moral distress in healthcare providers.

Case 1

Liz is 78 years old and has had fragile health for many years. She is now dying from terminal cancer. Her daughter Mia has been her full-time caregiver. As Liz's health deteriorates, Mia increasingly becomes agitated and disruptive. She brings in information from the Internet about new cures and treatments that can save her mother and insists the team try what she has found. She demands that her mother be resuscitated if she goes into cardiac arrest. When Liz suffers a cardiac arrest, attempts to resuscitate her are unsuccessful. During the resuscitation, Liz's ribs are broken and she is bleeding from multiple sites. Mia insists the team continue for more than 30 minutes, despite no return of spontaneous circulation. Whenever Dr. Baker attempts to "call the code," Mia begs them to continue, threatening to sue if they stop.

Case 2

Dr. Adams, concerned about moral distress, contacts the healthcare ethics committee (HEC) regarding one of his patients. Mr. Sinclair is a 75-year-old man who experienced a hemorrhagic stroke resulting in right-sided paralysis, difficulty speaking and understanding language, and partial loss of vision in both eyes. He is unable to swallow and overall appears frail. His wife insists that he be resuscitated if he arrests and demands that Dr. Adams place a feeding tube so he can be transferred to a rehab facility and continue to fight for his recovery. When the HEC responds, Dr. Adams expresses exasperation, stating, "This is the 10th patient in this condition for whom I have placed a feeding tube. This has got to stop. We should stop allowing spouses to make these decisions!"

Case 3

Gary suffers from multiple chronic illnesses. He has run out of insurance and his complex medical needs make him virtually undischargeable from the acute inpatient hospital setting. His current medical interventions are prolonging his life; however, they will not restore his health. He has full capacity and is content to remain in the hospital. He behaves belligerently toward the staff, periodically throwing things at them and is consistently verbally abusive. He is intermittently uncooperative with treatments yet clearly states he wants to live as long as possible.

Introduction

When healthcare providers (HCPs) feel a violation of their core values or a violation of their integrity, this can lead to the experience of moral distress. First discussed and studied among critical care nurses, the growing body of research now confirms that moral distress is an issue that affects all HCPs and ultimately the quality of patient care (Austin et al., 2017). The three cases above illustrate some of the ethically challenging situations that may lead to HCP distress and a request for assistance from healthcare ethics committees (HECs). Not all distress is moral distress. Likewise, a claim of moral distress is not evidence that the individual experiencing moral distress has moral privilege or that there is an ethical violation. HECs need skills in differentiating moral distress from other types of distress so that they can identify how to intervene to support the HCP who is in distress. The most essential skill is helping HCPs explore their distress. Left unexplored, HCPs may fail to appreciate the ethical nuances of a situation and prematurely judge their or others' actions. They may conclude that moral distress is only their problem and not understand that oftentimes, moral distress reflects systems issues within an organization. This chapter will explore moral distress and the potential role HECs can play in addressing this prevalent problem in health care.

Moral Distress

It is the moral judgment about the rightness or wrongness inherent in a situation that can lead to an emotional response commonly referred to as moral distress. Despite being discussed for decades and in multiple research studies, a precise definition of moral distress remains elusive (Dudzinski, 2016). For the purposes of the discussion in this chapter, moral distress is the psychological response experienced by an individual who believes they have a responsibility to act, believes they know the ethical thing to do, and perceives barriers that prevent them from acting ethically. Thus, moral distress has three essential components: emotional, cognitive (the judgment of the morality of the situation), and behavioral (how an individual acts on the judgment). The experience is grounded in a perception that the individual has a responsibility to act (or avoid acting) in a particular way in a given situation.

HCPs experience moral distress when they believe they are responsible for acting ethically and something compels them either to act against their conscience or to fail to act on their conscience where their choice has ethical consequences. There are many situations that contribute to HCPs' experience of moral distress. For example, moral distress is common when HCPs and patients/families have differing opinions about what is the best course of action when caring for a patient. The most frequently identified situation is when HCPs feel compelled to provide treatment that seems ineffective and potentially causes more harm than benefit for patients facing terminal illness (Musto and Rodney, 2018). Personal values, the limits of medicine, lack of resources, and perceptions of suffering are examples of the many things that can contribute to HCP moral distress in end-of-life situations.

Case 1 illustrates the complexity HCPs may encounter in these situations. Mia's insistence that the resuscitation continue long past where Dr. Baker believes it is appropriate challenges Dr. Baker's sense of moral integrity. Mia's threat to sue if the attempts at resuscitation stop poses a significant barrier to Dr. Baker acting on her judgment about the resuscitation. The nurses caring for Liz may feel a strong obligation to provide appropriate end-of-life care for her and the prolonged efforts to attempt resuscitation thwart those efforts. In addition, when Liz's ribs break and she begins bleeding, all the HCPs may believe they are causing unnecessary harm, a clear violation of their obligation to a patient. They may feel powerless to stop the resuscitation.

Before Liz's resuscitation, there were signs that the situation was at risk for ethical conflict (Pavlish et al., 2011). Ideally, HCPs caring for Liz would have seen the signs and contacted the HEC for assistance in navigating anticipated conflict. Without preparation for an inevitable confrontation when the patient died, the team will feel constrained. Believing they should stop, yet uncertain how to demonstrate compassion toward Mia and still provide dignified care to Liz as she is dying, the team continues resuscitation efforts long after recognizing they offer no benefit to Liz. HECs may not be able to intervene to support HCPs during the resuscitation, yet they can play a powerful role in unpacking the ethical complexity of the situation by providing debriefing for HCPs following such a difficult event.

The emotion associated with the experience of moral distress is what first captured the attention of many, particularly nurses. Consequently, moral distress is often lumped together with other negative psychological states, specifically burnout and compassion fatigue (CF). Constant exposure to excessive stress leads to burnout, causing an individual to feel overwhelmed, frustrated, exhausted, and unable to meet demands. CF is a secondary traumatic stress (STS) response that occurs when individuals are exposed indirectly to traumatic events; witness to the trauma others must endure (Austin et al., 2017).

The manifestations of burnout and CF are similar to those for HCPs who report high levels of moral distress. Two things differentiate moral distress from other types of distress: The harm to the HCP comes secondary to their sense of responsibility, and there is a judgment about conflicting professional obligations and responsibilities. Ultimately, it is the compromise to integrity that differentiates moral distress from other types of distress (Thomas and McCullough, 2017; Berger et al., 2019). To distinguish the experience of moral distress from these other negative psychological states it is necessary to explore both the emotional distress of the individual experiencing it and the moral dimensions of the experience (Musto et al., 2015; Dudzinski, 2016; Austin et al., 2017). Table 6.1 illustrates how burnout, CF, and moral distress compare.

Case 2 above provides an illustration of distress that is not necessarily moral distress. In this case, Dr. Adams is clearly distressed. The revelation about the number of similar cases suggests there may be more burnout here than moral distress. Stating that spouses should not be allowed to make decisions is an opinion that is inconsistent with shared decision-making and respecting surrogates' role in decision-making. It is likely sad to

Table 6.1 A comparison of burnout, compassion fatigue, and moral distress

Variable	Burnout	Compassion Fatigue	Moral Distress
Etiology	Reactional: response to work or environmental stressors (i.e., staffing, workload, managerial decision-making, inadequate supplies or resources)	Relational: consequences of caring for those who are suffering (i.e., inability to change course of painful scenario or trajectory)	Judgment about the ethical rightness or wrongness of a situation, violation of integrity
Chronology	Gradual, over time	Sudden, acute onset	May be acute in response to a situation or be the accumulation of multiple experiences (moral residue leading to a crescendo)
Outcomes	Decreased empathic responses	Imbalance of empathy and objectivity	Variable
Common manifestations	Emotional exhaustion, mental exhaustion, physical exhaustion, decreased interactions with others, depersonalization, decline in ability and desire to care, contributes to job turnover		

care for so many patients who face significant challenges regarding recovery from stroke and may lead an HCP to become frustrated or discouraged. The distress is real; however, it is not necessarily moral distress. Members of an HEC are in a position to help Dr. Adams acknowledge the distress in the situation and appreciate that it may be sad and difficult, yet the spouse's decisions are ethically permissible. It would be important to explore with Dr. Adams what makes this case different from the previous ones. Only with exploration about the moral judgments regarding the spouse's chosen treatment can the HEC assist Dr. Adams to appreciate what is causing the distress and, if indicated, attend to the integrity violation.

Some authors suggest that moral distress is essentially a relational construct, intrinsic to healthcare settings rather than a property of a distressed individual alone (Musto and Rodney, 2018; Sanderson et al., 2019). The emphasis is more on the features of an organization rather than characteristics of individuals. For example, poor communication and lack of collaboration frequently contribute to moral distress, indicating a strong relationship between the environment where HCPs practice and the experience of moral distress (Hamric and Epstein, 2017). As part of the structure of institutions, HECs are in a position to create opportunities for moral reflection and dialogue as a means to build and foster meaningful relationships among members of the healthcare team.

Moral Agency

Moral agency is an individual's ability to act on a judgment using a commonly held notion of right and wrong and be accountable for those actions (Traudt et al., 2016).

While individual patient situations often trigger moral distress, the constraints to actions typically reside in the intricate relational interplay between HCPs and the complex environments within which they practice (Musto and Rodney, 2018). Beyond the institutional, it may be the broader sociopolitical contexts that exert more barriers to acting as a moral agent, thus leading to moral distress. Case 3 above illustrates just such an example.

The patient in this example exhibits unpleasant behaviors that no doubt challenge an HCP's ability to meet a basic ethical standard, treating patients with dignity and compassion. The broader challenges with the healthcare system contribute to an inability to move the patient to a location outside of an acute care setting where structures and processes are not designed to care for patients long-term. It is beyond the scope of HECs to resolve the larger systemic challenges that led to this situation. It is well within the sphere of influence of an HEC to address how an organization supports HCPs caring for this patient.

HECs are in a position to work with the organization's leaders to create structures and policies that help HCPs navigate the challenges of ethical care for such patients. For example, they can participate in a standard response team or training for how to set clear boundaries and respond when patients become aggressive toward staff (e.g., restriction of privilege for the patient, additional chaplain, social work and behavioral health experts for the team caring for the patient, and engaging institutional leaders in regular discussions about and when necessary with such patients to demonstrate meaningful support for the front-line staff). HECs are in a position to ensure that the leadership response to HCP moral distress in this situation is more than telling the HCPs they have to be tough and continue to provide care to the patient no matter what.

Consequences of Moral Distress

The increased prevalence of moral distress among HCPs likely is contributing to an overall increase in burnout (National Academies of Science, Engineering, and Medicine, 2019). With a renewed interest in promoting the well-being of HCPs, there has been a surge of interest in endorsing resilience and enhancing individual coping skills as strategies to combat moral distress. These and other self-care strategies can improve an individual's sense of well-being but will do little to reduce the occurrence of moral distress. Placing all the emphasis on resolving the emotional aspects of moral distress without addressing the ethical nature of the situation treats the symptom not the problem (Musto et al., 2015). This approach unfairly puts the onus squarely on individuals to remedy the situation and ignores the moral responsibility of organizations to support HCPs in providing patient care in ethically complex contexts.

Beyond the well-documented immediate consequences of moral distress (Austin et al., 2017; Hamric, 2017), Hamric and Epstein (2017) theorize about the consequences of unaddressed moral distress. HCP moral distress may diminish when the immediate situation resolves. However, unaddressed HCP moral distress will likely contribute to residual moral distress, referred to as moral residue. Over time, repeated exposure to situations that trigger moral distress may lead to a crescendo, evoking a more intense emotional response to ethically challenging situations. Even though the residual crescendo may be more problematic, the best opportunity for intervention is likely when HCPs experience a moral distress crescendo (Epstein and Hamric, 2009). HECs have a responsibility to track instances of moral distress and identify patterns that may indicate institutional factors that contribute to HCP moral distress.

The evidence is overwhelming that failing to address HCPs' moral distress has negative consequences for them and consequently for the quality of care patients receive (Musto and Rodney, 2018). Given the complexity of moral distress, it is essential that HCPs learn to move beyond simply claiming they are experiencing moral distress. Listening to and validating the feelings of moral distress does not address what triggered the emotional response in the first place: The judgment that a moral harm is occurring. It is therefore essential that HECs learn to discern moral distress from other negative emotional experiences and offer interventions that assist HCPs to reflect on their moral judgments.

A Tool for Navigating Moral Distress

Mapping moral distress may be an effective strategy both to alleviate the feelings of moral distress and to explore the moral dimensions of the situation that caused it. Creating a map helps to avoid a blaming approach and lays the foundation for creative and responsible actions in the face of an ethically challenging situation (Dudzinski, 2016). HECs can use a map to reduce the emphasis on the emotional aspects of moral distress and discourage HCPs from oversimplifying a situation. To assist HCPs in mapping their moral distress, HEC members need skill beyond the ability to name the ethical elements of a situation (e.g., capacity, surrogate decision-making, benefit burden analysis). HEC members must be prepared to acknowledge intense emotion and direct discussion to focus on the ethical issue.

Mapping moral distress fosters a degree of self-reflection and encourages HCPs to exercise moral imagination. It challenges them to first acknowledge the emotion and then step back from it and explore the nature of the distress, including an examination of the moral judgments associated with the negative feelings. This process may help to alleviate the negative feelings experienced and to identify potential interventions to address the contextual features of the situation that led to the moral distress. Table 6.2 shows elements of a moral distress map and includes some common examples.

A Strategy for Building Moral Communities

HECs can lead the way in establishing environments that support HCPs to voice concerns freely, where they are appreciated for having ethics sensitivity rather than criticized for having moral weakness. Research studies show that HCPs often identify talking to others as a helpful strategy for making sense of and working through the experience of moral distress (Musto et al., 2015). This provides support for understanding moral distress as a relational concept. Talking in the form of discussions around personal and professional values creates opportunity for enhancing communication skills, building relationships, and creating shared understanding (Traudt et al., 2016). Such discussions can facilitate agreement on shared beliefs and team building to better support HCPs as moral agents. Environments that foster these types of discussions help HCPs develop a sense of empowerment that is essential for exercising moral agency (Hamric and Epstein, 2017).

Open discussions to address moral distress with key stakeholders are essential to creating shared notions of right and wrong that form the basis of HCPs' moral

Table 6.2 Elements of Dudzinski (2016)'s moral distress map with examples

Map Elements	Examples
Emotions	Frustration, anger, guilt, self-blame
Situation	Feeling compelled to provide treatment thought to be ineffective (potentially inappropriate)
Personal values	Quality of life
Professional responsibilities	Avoid unnecessary harm
Internal constraints	Feeling powerless, socialized to follow orders
External constraints	Diminished patient care due to poor team communication
Conflicting professional obligations/responsibilities	Socialized to follow orders vs. advocate for diminished patient suffering
Possible courses of actions	Seek an ethics consultation, collaborate with others to identify strategies

judgments (Traudt et al., 2015). Because of the emotional nature of moral distress, it is beneficial to have a neutral facilitator, one who can promote an environment that allows for questioning and tolerates the expression of uncertainty as participants explore the ethical complexity of situations. Members of HECs may serve a valuable role in such discussions.

Beyond Individual HCP Moral Distress

One thing is certain, strategies to alleviate moral distress must be multifaceted, addressing the relationship between HCPs as individual moral agents and the organizational structures within which they practice (Musto et al., 2015). Moral distress may occur in ethically challenging situations where the "solution" depends on a broader health system solution, much like Case 3 at the beginning of this chapter. There are multiple factors in play contributing to provider moral distress, and likely burnout and compassion fatigue. The situation in Case 3 has multiple indicators that could predictably lead to moral distress.

HECs can be instrumental in shifting organizational culture when in addition to providing (reactive) resources to resolve ethical conflict they develop (proactive) resources to help HCPs identify early indicators of situations that are at risk for ethical conflict (Pavlish et al., 2011). HECs are in a position to help HCPs peel back the layers of complexity, revealing not an ethical conflict but rather moral distress that is resolved with improved communication and exploration of different ethically permissible perspectives.

HECs have a responsibility to foster environments where HCPs and organizational leaders recognize the presence of moral distress as an indication that people of good conscience face ethical challenges within a flawed healthcare system. It is incumbent upon members of HECs to

- create and advertise policies that allow open access to resources for HCPs
- ensure that the people who serve as ethics resources are trained in ethical reasoning and are skilled at facilitating emotionally charged discussions about ethically complex situations

- support the 24/7 availability of meaningful resources
- build relationships with organizational leaders such that they are seen as trusted advisors

In this way, HECs can act more as architects of moral space not just arbitrators in the face of moral conflict (Hamric & Wocial, 2016). HECs can be instrumental in helping to focus attention on broader structural power dynamics within organizations that contribute to the experience of moral distress and move away from focusing on abilities of individuals.

Conclusion

Failing to address HCP moral distress will have serious consequences for patients, their families, and staff. It is unreasonable to expect HCPs to navigate repeated exposure to ethically challenging situations without providing some meaningful support to help them navigate the accompanying moral distress. HCPs must acknowledge moral distress first as an indication of moral sensitivity and a reason to explore the ethical complexities of a given situation, not as evidence alone of a moral harm.

If HECs are to fulfill their intended purposes, namely to provide a mechanism that allows staff members, patients, and families to address ethical issues, then they must develop systems and processes to address HCP moral distress. They have an obligation to move beyond a reactive model, acting only when a conflict has occurred. When HECs foster open discussion where participants respect each other even when they disagree, the HEC will promote a proactive approach to navigating ethically challenging situations. Addressing moral distress depends on creating work environments that foster open communication and collaboration all the time, and especially in ethically challenging situations.

Questions for Discussion

1. Conceptual: What are the essential elements of moral distress? How can HEC members help individual healthcare providers navigate the experience of moral distress?
2. Pragmatic: What resources exist within your institution that support clinicians who are experiencing moral distress? What processes are in place to address organizational factors that contribute to healthcare provider moral distress?
3. Strategic: What training and education do HEC members need to be able to help clinicians navigate the experience of moral distress? What resources does your institution need to address clinician moral distress?

References

Austin CL, Saylor R, Finley PJ (2017). Moral distress in physicians and nurses: Impact on professional quality of life and turnover. *Psychological Trauma: Theory, Research, Practice, and Policy*, 9(4): 399–406.

Berger JT, Hamric AB, Epstein E (2019). Self-inflicted moral distress: Opportunity for a fuller exercise of professionalism. *Journal of Clinical Ethics*, 30(4): 314–317.

Dudzinski DM (2016). Navigating moral distress using the moral distress map. *Journal of Medical Ethics*, 42(5): 321–324.

Epstein EG, Hamric AB (2009). Moral distress, moral residue, and the crescendo effect. *Journal of Clinical Ethics*, 20(4): 330–342.

Hamric AB, Epstein EG (2017). A health system-wide moral distress consultation service: Development and evaluation. *HEC Forum*, 29(2): 127–143.

Hamric AB, Wocial LD (2016). Institutional ethics resources: Creating moral spaces. *Hastings Center Report*, 46(Suppl. 1): S22–S27.

Musto LC, Rodney PA, Vanderheide R (2015). Toward interventions to address moral distress: Navigating structure and agency. *Nursing Ethics*, 22(1): 91–102.

Musto M, Rodney P (2018). What we know about moral distress. In Ulrich CM, Grady C, eds., *Moral Distress in the Health Professions*. Cham, Switzerland: Springer, 21–58.

National Academies of Sciences, Engineering, and Medicine. (2019). *Taking Action against Clinician Burnout: A Systems Approach to Professional Well-Being.*

Washington, DC: The National Academies Press.

Pavlish C, Brown-Saltzman K, Hersh M, Shirk M, Nudelman O (2011). Early indicators and risk factors for ethical issues in clinical practice. *Journal of Nursing Scholarship*, 43(1): 13–21.

Sanderson C, Sheahan L, Kochovska S, et al. (2019). Re-defining moral distress: A systematic review and critical re-appraisal of the argument-based bioethics literature. *Clinical Ethics*, 14(4): 195–210.

Thomas TA, McCullough LB (2017). Focus more on causes and less on symptoms of moral distress. *Journal of Clinical Ethics*, 28 (1): 30–32.

Traudt T, Liaschenko J, Peden-McAlpine C (2016). Moral agency, moral imagination, and moral community: Antidotes to moral distress. *Journal of Clinical Ethics*, 27(3): 201–213.

Ethics Consultation Mission, Vision, Goals, and Process

Georgina D. Campelia and Denise M. Dudzinski

Objectives

Upon reading and considering the content of this chapter, the reader should be able to:

1. Describe the goals, scope, and limits of clinical ethics consultation.
2. Discuss the similarities and differences between ethics consultation and other services whose roles may overlap with ethics consultation.
3. Outline the steps necessary for any ethics consultation to be considered adequate, fair, and complete.
4. Compare the strengths and weaknesses of the three types of consulting models (individual, team, and committee).
5. Identify the skills and knowledge that different professions can bring to an ethics consult.

Case

Mr. B, 60 years old, has end-stage renal disease (ESRD) and is on hemodialysis (HD) three times per week. Mr. B was admitted to the hospital in renal failure due to decline from having missed three of the past seven dialysis appointments. Mr. B faces several difficulties adhering to HD. He takes a bus that unreliably runs every hour to the outpatient center, and a late arrival often means missing his appointment. He typically goes to appointments alone and quickly becomes agitated about having to sit still for so long. He often chooses to stop his session within the first 1–2 hours.

While inpatient, Mr. B does not face the same difficulties keeping dialysis appointments. He feels that he has greater support and coaching from his clinicians in the hospital, and he more frequently tolerates longer runs, though he only intermittently completes the entire run. He still sometimes declines HD because he's "too tired" or feels he "doesn't want to do it today." At the same time, he'll affirm that he does not want to die and understands that he will die without HD.

Mr. B's clinicians and hospital administrators have met multiple times over the past few admissions to determine optimal therapy for Mr. B. They have tried to find support from his family and local community to accompany him to appointments. They offered to arrange transportation so that Mr. B would not need to take the bus. With each new admission, Mr. B affirms his desire to continue with treatment and is adherent upon discharge for a time, but quickly returns to a pattern of declining or incompletely adhering to the recommended treatment. Healthcare providers are becoming frustrated by the tension between what seem to be Mr. B's autonomous preferences and their inability to provide the standard of care that is likely to achieve Mr. B's health goals.

Introduction: Complex Values in Clinical Care

The challenges of Mr. B's clinical care are integrally tied to tensions in his own values and between his values and those of his clinicians. It is important to understand if Mr. B really wants to receive dialysis, but circumstances make it challenging to do so, such as trouble with transportation or lack of work accommodations. Alternatively, Mr. B's intermittent participation may be a sign of ambivalence toward the value of the treatment. Exploring Mr. B's values may help to determine what constitutes best care *for him*, even when clinically optimal treatment is not possible.

Clinical ethics consultation (CEC)[1] resides in this value-laden terrain. The American Society for Bioethics and Humanities (ASBH) describes CEC as "a set of services provided by an individual or group in response to questions from patients, families, surrogates, health-care professionals, or other involved parties who seek to resolve uncertainty or conflict regarding value-laden concerns that emerge in health care" (ASBH, 2011, 2). Mr. B's desire to live is challenged by the difficulty of getting to dialysis appointments and his discomfort of staying on dialysis runs. Clinicians want to help Mr. B meet his goal to live, which requires dialysis, but they may find themselves struggling to meet his needs. They might try to adjust the timing of dialysis and find better transportation and other ways to support Mr. B's adherence with treatment; still Mr. B's difficulty remaining on dialysis runs may persist. Mr. B and his clinicians might have to decide between two ethically and clinically suboptimal pathways. Compelling dialysis over Mr. B's *autonomous* refusals would be disrespectful, though it would honor his preference to live longer. Should his cognitive capacity decline, proceeding over his *nonautonomous* refusals may not be disrespectful in the short term, but it would become so with ongoing and frequent repetition of compelling dialysis. On the other hand, Mr. B's consistent refusals may demonstrate a preference for comfort over longevity. If so, honoring this preference would mean not proceeding with dialysis and transitioning to comfort measures only, since not dialyzing will lead to Mr. B's death. CEC offers a means of understanding complex values like Mr. B's, negotiating different moral responsibilities, and facilitating a path forward by employing moral reasoning.

What Is the Role of Clinical Ethics Consultation?

Although there is a long history of theoretical and practical deliberation at the intersection of ethics and medicine, its formalization through institutional committees and ethics consultation services is relatively recent. It happened in the wake of the broader Civil Rights movement in the United States in the mid-twentieth century, which challenged systems of oppression and demanded greater attention of the respect owed to all persons. CEC helps to ensure this respect in clinical settings by attending to the values of all stakeholders and facilitating resolutions when those values conflict.

Goals and Scope

CEC distinctly addresses ethical conflicts and uncertainties. This means identifying relevant moral values and tensions between them (e.g., a tension between the value of

---

[1] HEC is often used as an abbreviation for 'healthcare ethics consultation' (cf. https://heccertification.org/); however, in this book, we will use the abbreviation CEC so as not to be confused with HEC standing for 'healthcare ethics committee'.

comfort and the value of longevity for Mr. B), exploring different ways of applying those values in the context of the consult, and facilitating a resolution that is respectful of all involved parties (ASBH, 2011, 3). As the American Medical Association defines the role,

> The goal of ethics consultation is to support informed, deliberative decision making on the part of patients, families, physicians, and the health care team. By helping to clarify ethical issues and values, facilitating discussion, and providing expertise and educational resources, ethics consultants promote respect for the values, needs, and interests of all participants, especially when there is disagreement or uncertainty about treatment decisions.
>
> (American Medical Association, 2019)

This goal is typically actualized through three overlapping functions of ethics committees and consultation services: consultation, education, and policy analysis (Fletcher and Siegler, 1996, 122–126). This chapter focuses on the role of ethics consultation services in particular. In the case of Mr. B, an *ethics consultation* might be called to help discern Mr. B's values and those of his clinicians. When there are tensions among these values, ethics consultants help clinicians work with Mr. B to find the best path forward.

Ethics consultations are different from other consultation services, insofar as their role is not to dictate clinical decisions or recommend a clinical pathway. For instance, it is beyond the scope of ethics consultation to respond to medical questions, such as "what are Mr. B's medical risks and benefits with ongoing intermittent adherence to dialysis?" Rather, ethics consultation is meant to respond to ethical questions, such as "what are clinicians' ethical responsibilities to Mr. B?" "How should the benefits of continuing HD be weighed against the harms of withholding this treatment?" "Is it ethically permissible to withhold HD for Mr. B, why or why not?" While these questions and their resolutions depend on clinical and contextual facts, they are fundamentally about moral values and responsibilities. As such, they often have a different normative force than clinical recommendations. So, when a nephrology consult might recommend dialysis, the *force* of that recommendation acts more like an expectation or requirement (trading off of unspoken "standards of care"). However, when a clinical ethics consult recommends that a family meeting occur with the goal of establishing a surrogate decision maker, such a recommendation may not lead to such a meeting. While the lack of such a meeting is regrettable, it typically does not put a clinician in any sort of institutional or legal peril. This depends on hospital policies, which sometimes require involvement from ethics in specified contexts.

When requests extend beyond ethical considerations, then they are beyond the scope of an ethics consultation and should be referred to the appropriate service. This can take two forms: (1) when there is an underlying ethics concern that is coincident with other concerns (e.g., legal concerns), ethics consultants can work collaboratively with other services; (2) when there is no underlying ethics concern, then ethics should refer to the appropriate service. Collaborating while also maintaining professional boundaries helps build trust (ASBH, 2011, 4).

Three Ethics Consultation Models

Ethics consultation is typically a central role of CEC services. ASBH endorses a *facilitation approach* to CEC, as opposed to an authoritarian or pure consensus approach (ASBH, 2011, 3, 6–10). Though there are variations within this approach (ASBH, 2011, 8), it generally means that consultants guide consensus while ensuring coherence with core ethical principles. CEC services typically adopt one or more of the following models:

1. Individual ethics consultant
2. Whole committee
3. Team (subcommittee)

There is little empirical research comparing these models, but there are identifiable advantages and disadvantages to each. For instance, individual consultation is more nimble, responding promptly and gathering perspectives firsthand. This model is also attractive because it is consistent with how other clinical consultations are sought. At the same time, this model entails a great deal of responsibility and expertise.

Alternatively, a subcommittee or whole committee approach might offer greater diversity in perspective because ethics expertise is "pooled" (ASBH, 2011, 20), which can be especially valuable when the ethical conflict is unique and difficult to resolve. Depending on the institution, there will be variance in how teams negotiate responding to consults. For instance, it may be that there is a primary consultant who will be responsible for contacting the requester or who will do "curbside" consults alone, but then involve the rest of the team for more complex cases. Additionally, while some institutions will rely on a small core team alone, at other institutions the core team may recruit and collaborate with others as needed to strengthen the team's expertise. This approach can have advantages over the individual ethics consultant model because it fosters collaboration across different perspectives. It may also be more expedient than a whole committee model if there are fewer consultants to coordinate.

A whole committee model can be the most effective model for fostering thorough reasoning and structuring ethical justification on diverse perspectives and expertise, though actualizing these values ultimately depends on the makeup of the committee. In both whole committee and team models, there is a risk that it will be more difficult to reach a resolution, especially if there is no clear leader in the discussion or if the committee is large. There are also practical challenges and delays in scheduling meetings for multiple busy professionals from diverse disciplines.

Ultimately, for any given ethics consultation service it is likely that the use of these models will vary with need. For more challenging consults, an individual ethics consultant benefits from seeking input from a subcommittee or full committee. Likewise, when a patient and family will be intimidated by a large group, one to two consultants can represent the larger service or committee. Importantly, the model itself cannot guarantee a fair process. Fairness depends on procedural justice practices, the competence of the consultants, and the inclusion of all key stakeholders.

Foundational Knowledge, Skills and Virtues in Ethics Consultation

CEC services, like other clinical consultation services, depend on a consultant's ability to draw on expertise in the field. Although a variety of academic and professional degrees qualify one to be an ethics consultant, CEC has been increasingly professionalized (Tarzian et al., 2015). Ethics consultants must be able to identify, understand, and facilitate resolution of ethical dilemmas, so the role requires some grounding knowledge in ethical theory and moral reasoning as it relates to health care. This involves understanding different moral frameworks or theoretical approaches and their application in different clinical contexts. For instance, one need not understand the nuances of different theories of consequentialism, but one should have enough of a grasp of the consequentialist approach to recognize and reason through different applications of it. In Mr. B's case it will be important to understand not only the different possible clinical risks and

Table 7.1 Examples of knowledge, skills, and virtues in CEC (ASBH, 2011)

Skills	Knowledge	Virtues
• Identify stakeholder values • Identify value-based conflict or uncertainty • Access ethics literature, policies, guidelines, and standards • Communicate and collaborate effectively • Facilitate meetings • Elicit moral views • Facilitate communication between involved parties	• Moral reasoning and ethical theory as it relates to CEC • Bioethical issues and concepts that typically emerge in CEC • Clinical context as it relates to CEC • Healthcare institution services, resources, and policies as they relate to CEC • Perspectives, values, and resources of local communities	• Creativity • Curiosity • Empathy/sympathy • Generosity • Honesty/transparency • Humility • Openness • Patience • Self-reflection • Trustworthiness • Respectfulness

benefits of discontinuing dialysis, but the ability to facilitate consideration of personal, social, and spiritual risks and benefits for Mr. B, his family, and his clinicians. Knowledge of and experience with ethical issues that typically arise in CEC is also critical, such as standard value-based tensions in withholding and withdrawing life-sustaining treatment or difficult clinician–patient encounters. Ethics consultants should also be able to apply relevant ethics concepts in order to articulate the ethical dilemma and analysis (e.g., "rights," "autonomy," "beneficence," "substitute judgment," etc.).

Of course, the consultant should understand institutional and communal norms enacted in policy and practice. In order to help Mr. B, the consultant needs to understand the clinical details as well as institutional policies (e.g., a policy to guide patient care when patients face challenges adhering to medically recommended treatment), relationships between inpatient and outpatient services (e.g., options if the outpatient dialysis clinic refuses to dialyze Mr. B for being late to his appointment), relevant laws (e.g., Mr. B's legal right to decline life-sustaining treatment), and potential support services (e.g., resources to help Mr. B arrive at his appointments on time).

The *Core Competencies in Healthcare Ethics Consultation* addresses domains of knowledge that are important to CEC (ASBH, 2011, 26–31) as well as many of the critical skills; see Table 7.1 (ASBH, 2011, 22–25). Skills in this arena are partly related to foundational knowledge in clinical ethics and moral theory, such as the ability to identify relevant values and articulate ethical conflicts. These skills relate to identifying and analyzing ethical uncertainty and conflict. Other skills relate to facilitating conflict resolution, including collaborating well, active listening, demonstrating respect, empathizing, perspective-taking, facility with communicating across differences, cultural competency, educating, eliciting different views, and recognizing bias.

An ethics consultant might find themselves intuitively aligned with a particular clinician's moral perspective and may have to work to ensure that competing perspectives are given adequate respect and attention. Additionally, it can be challenging to boil down quickly the central ethics question in a complex case. The tasks of identifying values, understanding conflict, and facilitating a resolution become even more challenging in settings where relationships are frayed, medical decisions are typically fast-paced, and emotions are reasonably intense. Unsurprisingly, honing these skills takes practice and ongoing education in both ethical analysis and facilitating complex value-laden discourses.

Overlap and Limits

Some of the skills employed by CEC services may intersect with other services in the healthcare setting. Palliative and spiritual care, for instance, both routinely clarify patient values and goals. Likewise, empathy, curiosity, humility, self-reflection, honesty, and trustworthiness are important in all aspects of patient care. CEC services, in particular, must be able to invite differing perspectives by modeling respectful curiosity, empathizing with all stakeholders, and naming unarticulated values. Consultants also engender trust by being conscious of the limits of their role/authority (e.g., leaving final treatment decisions to the treating team and patient/surrogate).

Risk management will typically weigh in when ethical tensions are intertwined with legal obligations and consequences. While ethics consults must demonstrate familiarity with relevant laws, ethics recommendations can sometimes conflict with legal advice. Likewise, CEC services do not dictate medical decisions. Instead, they facilitate deliberation and consensus building and make recommendations when there is conflict or uncertainty. It is then up to clinicians, patients, and their support persons/legal surrogates to have ongoing discussions and determine together the best path forward. Ethics consultants can have an ongoing role in this process, but they do not have the authority to make treatment decisions.

Additionally, clinicians routinely make day-to-day ethical decisions and may need support from CEC from time to time. Chief executive officers and management teams may need guidance on organizational ethics issues (see Chapter 27). CEC can foster an ethical climate by encouraging transparency and respectful discussion when differences of opinion arise. Defining the role of CEC services and adeptly referring to other services when ethics lacks the requisite expertise is crucial to this endeavor. Healthcare ethics committees and consultation services should also provide education around common ethical conflicts and uncertainties. Finally, as demand for CEC increases, garnering financial resources and leadership support protects the quality and integrity of the service.

What Is an Adequate and Fair Process for Healthcare Ethics Consultation?

CEC requires multidisciplinary deliberation. So, when ethics consultation is done by a team or committee the process benefits from having members that represent diverse professional backgrounds (academics, administrators, chaplains, nurses, physicians, social workers, etc.), social identities (gender, race, spirituality, etc.), and experiential perspectives (values, cultures, communities, upbringing, etc.). A diverse group in all of these regards encourages creativity, critical analysis, and empathy. Even on an individual model of ethics consultation, a committee with diverse backgrounds and expertise can facilitate quality improvement and quality assurance for individual ethics consultants. This occurs when individual consultants report out and seek feedback at committee meetings, as well as when individual chart notes or recurring ethics issues are reviewed by the committee.

While training of core knowledge and skills is increasing (ASBH, 2015), there continues to be variation in the extent to which different CEC services use formal analytic tools, such as the four principles (Beauchamp and Childress, 2019) or Jonsen et al.'s casuistic method (Jonsen et al., 2015). There are professional debates about strategy. For example, should ethics consultants act as mediators or facilitators? In response to wide variations in ethics consultation practice, in 2017 ASBH formed the Healthcare Ethics Consultant (HCEC) Certification Commission to establish a process for certifying members of CEC services. The Healthcare Ethics Consultant-Certified (HEC-C) certification is available to those with a certain number of hours in ethics consultation activities and after passing a multiple-choice test (HCEC Certification Commission, n.d.).

While there is some variation across CEC services, the ethics consultation process typically involves (1) gathering information, (2) facilitating ethical deliberation and analysis, and (3) making a recommendation. While the practice of ethics consultation is far from uniform, there is some agreement about the best ways of accomplishing these three steps.

Gathering Information

CEC services should be available to all healthcare professionals as well as patients and families. Depending on the type of hospital and available personnel, it may be preferable for ethics consultation to be available 24 hours a day. Requests for ethics consults can be done via phone, pager, or email. The initial conversation with the requestor will help to determine the next steps.

As a matter of fairness, ethics consultants should speak with key stakeholders in the case. One can ask clinicians specific questions, such as "what is the ethical conflict or uncertainty here?", and open-ended discussion prompts, such as "tell me about what's going on for Mr. B from your perspective." It is also critical to speak with Mr. B and any support persons about their perspectives, goals, preferences, and values. This dialogue is necessary because it can change the ethics question, ethics analysis, and ethics recommendation in significant ways. For instance, it is possible that Mr. B's "difficulty adhering to dialysis" is primarily related to challenges in getting to his appointments. It is also possible that his discomfort with remaining on dialysis runs is related to discrimination he faces from staff at the outpatient clinic, such as that based on socioeconomic status, citizenship, race, gender, or ability. One would have to talk with Mr. B personally to know more about his version of the narrative, which may be very different from the narrative as described by clinicians and the medical chart. Speaking directly with Mr. B, his physicians, nurses, and social worker allows for a richer and more accurate understanding of Mr. B's experience as well as the challenges he faces. Failure to speak with patients will undermine patients' and their families' trust. Trust building is crucial to finding a resolution but can be immensely challenging if tensions have already escalated.

Gathering information for an ethics consultation requires, among other skills, an ability to read a medical chart and extract relevant information. It is important for ethics consultants to be able to understand and interpret notes from all disciplines (social work, nursing, palliative care, primary team, consulting services, etc.) and to scan the past history of the patient for salient events or discussions (sometimes spanning years). When the consultant does not have clinical training or is unfamiliar with the electronic medical record, both self-driven learning and mentorship are necessary to develop these skills. Clinician consultants teach humanities-trained consultants and vice versa. Well-functioning ethics consultation services are multidisciplinary and encourage calling a colleague – and those colleagues are responsive and collegial.

Finally, many consults will depend on gathering information from hospital policy, professional guidelines, and city, state, or federal law. A consultant might begin by finding relevant legal cases or related paradigm cases that can help establish a baseline of medical, legal, and ethical analysis. This can help establish which policies, laws, or guidelines will be relevant to the ethical analysis. For instance, in Mr. B's case it may be important to know if outpatient dialysis units have policies regarding patients who miss appointments or end runs early. Likewise, it would be important to know Mr. B's rights regarding declining a life-sustaining medical intervention. While the weight of his statements will hinge on his decisional capacity, even without full decisional capacity he retains rights that others, including ethics consultants, must protect.

Ethical Deliberation and Analysis

Once ethics consultants have gathered information from the chart, policy/law, and relevant stakeholders (Mr. B, Mr. B's chosen support persons, physicians, nurses, social workers, etc.), they must articulate the ethical question, clarify relevant values and obligations, and ethically justify one or more pathways by employing multiple ethical frameworks. Talking with others throughout this process is critical for robust ethical deliberation, especially when it engages multiple perspectives, articulates points of disagreement, and detects bias.

In Mr. B's case, ethics consultation should help to elucidate the meaning of benefi-cence from multiple perspectives. While intermittent adherence may not optimize longevity, perhaps it would contribute to both longevity and palliation of symptoms while also affording Mr. B the benefit of having control over his care. On the other hand, physically manifested agitation during dialysis could suggest a new or chronic clinical issue, pose risks to Mr. B, and, in extreme circumstances, to the staff. Likewise, under-standing what it means to respect Mr. B is not just about respecting autonomous decisions, but also about recognizing his vulnerability as a patient, being honest with him about the challenges facing the team, carefully considering Mr. B's preferences and concerns, and expressing the genuine desire to do what is best for him. Sometimes, being respectful means setting clear expectations or boundaries for patients. Ultimately, a robust individual and collective analysis of Mr. B's case will clarify how the treating team might understand competing obligations, nurture therapeutic relationships, and find an ethically justified, though perhaps clinically suboptimal, resolution.

Making Ethics Recommendations

Ideally, collective deliberation, either in a multidisciplinary meeting or through one-on-one conversations with multiple people, will lead to a resolution that all parties have helped formulate and endorse. Sometimes ethics consultation recommendation(s) will acknowledge consensus, for example, "consensus among Mr. B and his clinicians at a family meeting on xx/xx/xx, was that..." The recommendation should be succinct and articulate an action plan with reasons that ethically justify it. For instance, "We recommend that Mr. B's outpatient dialysis be transitioned from clinic X to clinic Y because Mr. B is more likely to be adherent at clinic Y; it respects his autonomous preference for that clinic and supports our commitment to beneficence."

In some cases, recommendation(s) may be made in the context of ongoing uncertainty or lack of full consensus. Under these circumstances, ethics recommendations may not offer resolution, but rather clarity on the ethical conflict or uncertainty. Openly acknowledging challenges or ongoing disagreement may offer moral perspective, understanding, and relief of moral distress, even as conflict persists.

Legal recommendations may be at odds with ethics recommendations or individual stakeholders may continue to disagree with one another. Ethics consultants describe the potential paths forward, laying out the challenges and reasonable disagreements, while ultimately supporting recommendations that withstand the scrutiny of multiple ethics frameworks. For instance, in Mr. B's case there might be different perspectives on what it means to be respectful of Mr. B's autonomy, what it means for dialysis to benefit or harm Mr. B, and what rights patients and clinicians have in the context of dialysis. The recommendations in the case should reflect robust consideration of different stakeholder perspectives, deliberation among stakeholders, and, ultimately, sound reasoning using multiple ethical principles or frameworks.

Document in the Medical Chart

The deliberation, analysis, and resulting recommendations should be documented in the medical chart. Ethics notes and/or consultation records may include more narrative and take on more of an essay format than typical chart notes. While it is good to be concise, various stakeholders will look for the ethicist to define and elucidate obligations, values, and reasons supporting a particular clinical pathway. The note could be important to clinicians as well as hospital administrators and may be of interest if legal adjudication ensues. On the whole, the goal is for the reasoning expressed in a chart note to be sound enough to withstand criticism, especially when the note supports a path that may be objectionable to some.

Review Process and Outcome

In order to maintain strong relationships with other healthcare disciplines, ethics consultants should follow up with key members of the healthcare team, as well as the patient and support persons where feasible. At a minimum, this practice ensures that ethics recommendations have been communicated back to decision makers, allows for debriefing and/or potential correction of misunderstandings, and addresses lingering moral distress.

Additionally, it is important for ethics consultations to be reviewed by the CEC service and/or ethics committee for the purposes of the professional development of individual consultants and for the quality improvement of the service (ASBH, 2011, 34–50). It is advisable to have a separate database for keeping track of all ethics consultations for purposes of review and quality improvement. These can be enhanced consult notes that articulate the ethical issue, the process that was used to resolve it, ethics recommendations, and clear reasoning in a way that is accessible to a wide audience. While notes in the chart are accessible to relevant medical personnel, a database enables a more thorough review by other members of the team or committee; it can help to track occurrences of similar types of consultations and promote cooperation among different consultants when there are multiple consultations for the same issue or same patient.

Potential Obstacles to a Fair Healthcare Ethics Consultation Process

Two of the primary obstacles to a fair consultation process are "groupthink" and bias. Groupthink is the phenomenon that occurs when the drive for conformity overpowers the drive for creativity and independent thinking (Lo, 1987). Ethical deliberation among stakeholders might tend toward confirming group decisions even when individuals have reservations or disagree. The conjunction of groupthink and implicit (unconscious) or explicit (conscious) bias can cause those with marginalized voices to be silenced by the dominant beliefs in the group. There might be inadvertent pressure to reach consensus (e.g., because of medical urgency), some may try to avoid controversial issues, and others might underestimate risks and objections, or fail to consider alternatives or to search for additional information.

Fortunately, there are a number of tools and methods for ensuring a fair ethics consultation process in the face of these obstacles. CEC leadership can foster a safe environment and spirit of deliberation by reminding members that what is said in meetings is protected by the Health Information Portability and Accountability Act (HIPAA) and other confidentiality standards and by routinely encouraging dissenting opinions. CEC leaders must also keep dialogue open and promote the participation of all members (Hester, 2008, 290). This can be challenging, especially when one must balance the need for marginalized voices to occupy space typically taken up by more powerful voices in the group. Along these lines, it is crucial for leaders and members to be cognizant of silence. When a group as a whole or particular member is silent, then work must be done to examine power dynamics, determine if voices are being oppressed, and understand the "etiology of the oppression" (Hester, 2008, 291).

Individual consultants can foster this same environment in interdisciplinary and family meetings by involving diverse perspectives in meetings, asking for doubts and objections, encouraging silent voices to speak up, and ensuring that the case against the majority is stated and considered. These strategies can promote disagreement as a crucial part of the process and thus work against both groupthink and bias (Wilkinson and Truog, 2015).

Finally, including patients and their support persons/legal surrogates is a fundamental part of ensuring fairness in the process. For instance, doing one's best to understand Mr. B's reasoning for sometimes declining treatment is necessary to responding fairly. Open-ended questions, such as "tell me what going to dialysis is like for you?" and empathic questions, such as "We can certainly understand that you want to get better but also don't want to sit for 4 hours multiple times per week, unfortunately we can't meet both preferences at the same time. Can you help us come up with some compromises?" can engender trust, engage Mr. B in a shared decision-making process, and support equitable perspective-taking.

Conclusion

While national and international standards for CEC are still in development, there is broad agreement regarding the key components of adequate and fair ethics consultation processes. And with increasing awareness of and research on obstacles related to bias and groupthink, there is a multitude of practical ways to ensure that CEC directly addresses these issues. These endeavors are central to CEC services because they regularly engage in consultation and policy formation that affects marginalized groups and may be asked to lead education efforts related to injustices in medicine. As CEC services become more prevalent and standardized throughout the USA and internationally, it is a pivotal moment to partner with diverse healthcare professionals and members of the healthcare community to formalize inclusive structures of ethical deliberation going forward.

Questions for Discussion

1. Conceptual: In what ways should ethical frameworks guide ethics consultations (use Mr. B's case as an example)?
2. Pragmatic: If your CEC service was presented with the case of Mr. B, what steps would it take to complete the ethics consultation and what ethical recommendations might you make?
3. Strategic: What steps can your CEC service take to guard against obstacles related to groupthink and implicit or explicit bias?

References

American Medical Association. (2019). Code of Medical Ethics Opinion 10.7.1. www.ama-assn .org/delivering-care/ethics/ethics-consultations#targetText=Code%20of% 20Medical%20Ethics%20Opinion,and%20the %20health%20care%20team.&targetText=(a) %20Seek%20to%20balance%20the,the% 20patient's%20needs%20and%20values

American Society for Bioethics and Humanities (ASBH). (2011). *Core Competencies for Healthcare Ethics Consultation*, 2nd ed. Glenview, IL: American Society for Bioethics and Humanities.

American Society for Bioethics and Humanities (ASBH). (2015). *Improving Competencies in Clinical Ethics Consultation: An Education Guide*, 2nd ed. Chicago: American Society for Bioethics and Humanities.

Beauchamp TL, Childress JF (2019). *Principles of Biomedical Ethics*. New York: Oxford University Press.

Fletcher C, Siegler M (1996). What are the goals of ethics consultation? A consensus statement. *Journal of Clinical Ethics*; 7(2): 122–126.

HCEC Certification Commission. (n.d.). Healthcare Ethics Consultant-Certified Program. https://asbh.org/certification/ hcec-certification

Hester DM. (2008). *Ethics by Committee.* Lanham, MD: Rowman & Littlefield Publishers, Inc.

Jonsen A, Siegler M, Winslade WJ (2015). *Clinical Ethics: A Practical Approach to Ethical Decisions in Clinical Medicine*, 8th ed. New York: McGraw-Hill.

Lo B (1987). Behind closed doors. *The New England Journal of Medicine*, 317(1): 46–50.

Tarzian AJ, Wocial L, The ASBH Clinical Ethics Consultation Affairs Committee. (2015). A code of ethics for health care ethics consultants: Journey to the present and implications for the field. *The American Journal of Bioethics*, 15(5): 38–51.

Wilkinson D, Truog R (2015). In favour of medical dissensus: Why we should agree to disagree about end-of-life decisions. *Bioethics*, 30(2): 109–118.

A Method of Consultation

8

D. Micah Hester

Objectives

Upon reading and considering the content of this chapter, the reader should be able to:

1. Recognize characteristics of moral deliberation during a consultation.
2. Use a tool (like GRACE considerations) to identify facts, obligations, consequences, and character considerations affecting and affected by ethically challenging cases.
3. Develop well-considered moral arguments in light of the conditions of the case during a consultation.

Case

Mr. Q, 26, was brought to a local medical facility with severe head pain. He was referred to the academic medical center (AMC) 45 miles away after a CT scan at the local facility indicated a large brain mass. At the AMC, the patient arrived at the emergency department and was immediately admitted for surgery on a brain tumor.

During his stay, his brain hemorrhaged, rendering him completely unresponsive and requiring a ventilator, tracheotomy, and feeding tube. Mr. Q remained in the ICU for 3 weeks and was able to be moved to a step-down unit on week 4. He remained unable to respond meaningfully to questions, and part of his skull was removed until his head stopped swelling.

Now in the step-down unit in a stable condition, the neurosurgeon indicates that Mr. Q can be moved out of the hospital, though it will be many months before another surgery will be performed to replace the missing part of his skull. Case management has discussed future discharge options with family who expressed concern that the patient was being moved out prematurely. The case manager discussed nursing home options and noted that his state-based insurance was going to stop paying for his care in the hospital within a couple of weeks.

The patient lives with his grandmother, and his father lives nearby. There are conflicting reports from both family and healthcare providers about whether Mr. Q suffered from some mild form of developmental delay prior to this hospitalization.

Ethics was initially contacted by risk management, which had learned that the family contacted the newspaper to complain about the patient being discharged because they could not pay. The risk manager's concern was that the hospital's resources were being unduly taxed by caring for a patient who could be served in a rehab or long-term care facility.

The clinical ethics consultant talked with bedside nursing, a resident, and the attending physician to understand the medical situation better. He also discussed the patient's situation with the family every day for a week. These discussions led to three healthcare team conferences.

Through this process it was learned that the family felt obligated to protect the patient from undue harm that they believed would more easily occur if not in the hospital. They were not interested in moving him to a nursing home, believing that nursing homes would not be able to provide adequate care. They were confused by why their loved one was being sent somewhere else when his head was still not fully recovered, and they were not clear on how long it would be until that recovery might occur.

While the healthcare providers recognized the family's distress, they also did not believe that keeping the patient in the hospital was, in fact, protecting him from undue harm. Hospital-acquired infections and other problems can arise in acute care facilities. They also believed that as an acute care facility, they should not be obligated to take on chronic care patients whenever the family was uncomfortable with long-term care options.

The risk manager was concerned that the hospital's reputation had taken a hit that it did not deserve, that it was obligated to find an appropriate long-term care facility, and once one was found that could take the patient, funding would run out.

Introduction

As noted in Chapter 7, most clinical ethics consultations stimulate moral reflection on different aspects of the case at hand. Moral reflection is an important and complex process. It aims at better understanding morally challenging situations and providing insight and direction for morally acceptable responses to those challenges.

Bioethicists have developed methods, tools, and approaches to help healthcare professionals systematically identify, assess, and address ethical issues as they arise in health care. For instance, a frequently cited approach is the "Four Box" method of Jonsen et al. (2015) (or its variation by Orr and Shelton [Shelton and Bjarnadottir, 2008]) where one systematically assesses the medical indications, patient preferences, quality of life, and context in a given case. The US Department of Veterans Affairs developed and implemented the CASES approach, which is another variation on a systematic framework to assess ethical values (National Center for Ethics in Health Care, 2015). Finally, in the previous edition of this textbook, Jeffrey Spike offered up GiNO'S DiCE as another method (Spike, 2012).

Each of these has its benefits and detriments, and in Chapter 7 Campelia and Dudzinski described the important features, models, and processes that every consultation should consider. In this chapter, then, I will break down the process of moral reflection itself – moral evaluation, moral considerations, moral instrumentation, and moral argumentation – in order to provide a comprehensive accounting for what goes into the moral analysis of a case.

Moral Evaluation

Clinical ethics consultations are forms of moral evaluation in which consultants identify ethical problems and explore solutions. Some of these consultations result in ethically grounded recommendations, and others simply provide the opportunity to think through the ethical issues and values at play. But either way, a multifaceted moral evaluation occurs.

Clinical ethics consultations may begin as a hallway conversation, a phone call, an email, or an order in the electronic system. A nurse or resident physician, an attending physician or social worker, or even a patient or family member is troubled by some aspect of a situation in the organization. People wonder whether what is going on is "right" or "good," and this leads them to reach out. The clinical ethics consultant, then, is confronted by a request for help and that request typically is predicated on there being a problem to avoid or solve. In fact, a frequent question the ethicist will ask early on is, "What do you think the ethical problem is or what ethically is at issue here?"

Problems are puzzles to be solved, irritations to be eliminated, or concerns to be met. They are the stimulants for reflective thought, and they set the agenda for that reflection. Every identified problem only admits to a finite set of solutions, and thus, a well-developed problem is half-solved. Thus, carefully understanding and investigating the problem itself is an important first step in consultation.

Once an issue (or set of issues) has been identified, consultants begin to explore the range of possible, reasonable ways to address it. Any ethically challenging situation is precisely a challenge because goods compete or obligations conflict. In such situations, obviously acceptable solutions are not readily identified because multiple, competing solutions have their supporters and detractors. For a physician to tell the wife that she is at risk of a sexually transmitted disease from a patient who is her philandering husband would meet the good of protecting her. At the same time, it would violate the obligation of confidentiality. Both meeting her good and fulfilling the obligation to him have good reasons that would support going in one direction or the other. Is it clear on its face which should win? If not, then we must investigate both further before making a final morally based decision. If so, what do you tell the party whose good you denied or obligation you violated were the reasons for doing so?

This last question, then, leads to another aspect of moral evaluation – justification. To say something is wrong or bad versus right or good simply stimulates the next question: What makes it wrong or bad versus right or good? "It just is" is the weakest answer possible, for the claim is one of moral ontology and intuition – that is, the claim is that some things just *are* good or *are* bad. But again, in the face of competing possible solutions to the moral problem, such a response rings hollow. What is required are reasons and justification. In the development of reasonable solutions, careful exploration of the issues ensues. Strengths and weaknesses are considered. Values and principles are brought to bear. And this all provides the support for any of the reasonable solutions being investigated, and justifications are required precisely because competing values and solutions are at play.

Moral Considerations

In explaining moral evaluation above, I provided no description of what should be explored and what kinds of data and concepts make for moral justification. What, then, is the content of a moral evaluation? In order to look at content comprehensively, I suggest the use of GRACE considerations – an acronym intended to remind consultants of the major ethics content of most any moral evaluation.

G – Get the Whole Story

As mentioned earlier, ethics consultants will often ask what the requestor believes is the moral problem, but why take their word for it? Furthermore, problems lead to solutions, but what solutions are reasonably available in any given situation? To answer these questions, the ethics consultant must find out what is going on. Individual lives and communal or cultural experiences can be seen as different life stories or narratives. Clinical situations are no different. What is the medical condition of the patient? What is the prognosis, and on what evidence is it based? Who are the stakeholders, decision makers, and affected parties? What are their personal stories? How do the values and beliefs of those people affect the actions and choices in the case? What are the policies and laws that are implicated by the situation?

For example, in the consultation about Mr. Q, the medical facts are that his neurological condition requires long-term nursing care. Furthermore, his grandmother is ill-equipped to provide that care at home. Neither his grandmother nor father want him to go to a nursing home in part because they believe that high-end hospital care is safer than the care he would get at a nursing home. All this, and much more, is part of the story that shapes the decisions to be made.

Clinical ethics addresses real-life issues that happen in real time. To understand the ethical issues at play, the concerns to be addressed, and the problems to be solved, the ethics consultant must investigate the ongoing narratives in the situation because it is from those narratives that the moral issues arise, and those narratives will be affected by the process and product of clinical ethics evaluation.

To put it differently, a common claim made by ethics consultants is this: Good ethics begin with good facts.

R – Recognize Obligations

One set of facts (debatable as they may be) is the collection of obligations that each of us carries with us. As mentioned in Chapter 2, each of us takes on roles and commitments that obligate us. If we have a spouse, we are obligated through marriage to meet certain expectations of that spouse. If we practice a religion, religious maxims and tenets exist that we should fulfill. And if we are professionals, the professions we serve require that we act and practice in particular ways to remain within the bounds of the profession.

All of these, and many more, are obligations that come out in ethics consultations. You can see in Mr. Q's case that his grandmother, as his caregiver, is deeply concerned about making decisions that might put her grandchild in harm's way. She feels obligated to fight to provide him the best care available. Physicians, nurses, and other healthcare providers all experience the constraint of obligations – whether that be keeping patient conversations confidential or demanding blood transfusions for pediatric patients whose parents refuse but allowing such refusals by adult patients.

The ethics consultant, then, must attempt to map out the many obligations at play in the situation. To fulfill or violate an obligation takes an understanding of its value in relation to other obligations and ethical considerations. Although they may not be determinative by themselves, these obligations have moral weight in any ethical evaluation.

A – Accept Responsibilities and Avoid Overreaching

One of the challenging things about obligations is that sometimes they compete. A physician, for example, may need to be home when school gets out to pick up their children and feed them dinner. That same physician may also get a page at 4:00 p.m. that requests their expertise on a patient matter right away. Determining which obligation to fulfill will be based on a number of factors: Is the physician the only one available to take the call? Can the children remain at school in an after-care program? Is there another parent? Are they available? However it gets worked out, there are responsibilities to be fulfilled, and the physician *must* fulfill them. If the physician decides to pick up the children, they must find another physician to cover the call. If the physician decides to stay at work, the children or spouse need to be alerted to the change in familial planning. Accepting these responsibilities, not just merely acknowledging them, is of vital importance.

Furthermore, in determining obligations to be fulfilled, professionals often are confronted by their own personal values – that is, values they have come to hold because of their lives outside their profession, whether from families, religions, or education. As professionals, however, the ethical situations that call forth consultations must be navigated carefully so that the professional does not "overreach." In health care, there is a concept known as "scope of practice," in which professionals are expected to do only what is in their training to do. Moral agents in the role of physicians are not spiritual guides. Persons in the role of nurses are not psychotherapists. Individuals when acting in the role of social workers are not police officers. This, too, holds for ethical considerations. While physicians may be persons with strong religious beliefs, when they are acting in the role of a physician they cannot let the belief in the healing power of a deity interfere with providing evidence-based medical care. Nurses who may have a spouse in their personal lives cannot let their concern for a wife's unknown risk of a sexually transmitted disease undermine their obligation to confidentiality of their patient. Social workers who are also civically engaged outside the hospital cannot have hospital security hold an adult patient against their will simply because the patient has a mental illness.

In a clinical ethics consultation, not only is it necessary to map out the obligations at play but to look at what responsibilities will need to be fulfilled. Who owes what to whom? How will that reckoning take place? And what happens when some responsibilities go unfulfilled?

C – Consider Consequences

Whichever obligations are fulfilled or responsibilities accepted, all choices promote actions that lead to consequences. Even the best of intentions to fulfill necessary obligations can go astray – as the saying goes, the road to hell is paved with such intentions. Consequences matter. In fact, whatever our motivations, they lead us to an attempt to achieve some end, and those ends should be evaluated, not simply accepted.

Admittedly, in ethical deliberation, although some consequences have more evidence and some much less, all consequences under consideration are speculative. Thus, consequential considerations are challenging. Will Mr. Q get an infection in the hospital? Will the nursing home meet its obligations to care for him properly? We must act on probability and pragmatics – that is, what we think will happen and what we believe is most worth our efforts in trying to achieve it given our lack of certainty that it will, in fact, come to pass. The former turns on evidence, the latter on character.

E – Evaluate Character

A final consideration, then, concerns who we are and who we want to be – personally, professionally, and institutionally. As with Mr. Q's situation, risk managers, while primarily managing risk, are often concerned about "how will it look?" This can smack of being unduly self-serving, but all our actions say something about us – as people, as professionals, and as institutions. The obligations we fulfill or violate say something about us and about our roles. The consequences that follow our actions affect our future pursuits – validating or undermining our values, beliefs, decisions, and processes. To make choices is to express our values through the choices we make. And the results of actions are ours to own.

Each clinical ethics consultation has the potential to say something about the many parties at play. But even further, the decisions and outcomes say something about the institution in which they occur. The consultant needs to keep this in mind to fashion an outcome that can be owned by the institution (or, more precisely, must be owned by the institution). For this reason, some ethics consultations lead to policy review and development.

Moral Instrumentation

Moral considerations are but one aspect of evaluation. With obligations seemingly coming from every direction and consequences of all stripes following from actions, how do we take all these considerations and begin to reason through them? Moral considerations function in a moral evaluation like wood, drywall, cement, and paint do in building a house. They are the raw material. The material becomes a structure (or becomes structured) using instruments or tools. In homebuilding, those tools are hammers, power drills, mixers, and brushes. The tools of moral evaluation are values, principles, maxims, rules, and more.

Elsewhere in this text you will read about basic biomedical principles, such as respect for autonomy, beneficence, and justice. We might also enumerate principles of utility and fidelity, among others. But even more broadly, we might use principles to guide action, such as only act so as to promote good and minimize harm to all those affected by the proposed action or cultivate habits that moderate among extreme outcomes. We also follow maxims such as treat others as you would want to be treated or act in a way that you would be willing for anyone else to act under similar circumstances. Furthermore, we abide by moral rules like do not harm innocent others, tell the truth, and be kind.

Each of these concepts are moral instruments (i.e., ethical norms) that can be applied in situations given the moral considerations under scrutiny. Which ones to bring to bear, however, remains challenging. Ethics consultants, like their theoretical counterparts, come in all ethical stripes. Every ethicist should do as comprehensive a job as possible rooting through and out the moral considerations in a case, but which tools to use to put those considerations into an evaluation is highly individualized. Some ethicists are primarily worried about meeting certain moral demands or duties; others are moved mostly by consequences; still others find that focusing on moral virtues best moves thought forward. Whichever approach is taken, ultimately, decisions must be made and justification given.

Moral Argumentation

Moral evaluation as a process of identifying moral problems and attempting solutions results in taking a moral position. To do so requires comprehensive work on moral considerations honed by moral instrumentation both crafted by and resulting in moral argumentation. An argument is not simply a dispute between people. In fact, some arguments are so well done that they result in no dispute at all. What is meant, then, by argument is a logical structure that puts data and evidence (sometimes called *premises*) together to support a claim (or *conclusion*).

Data and evidence can be physical facts or moral beliefs, cultural norms or statistical outcomes, emotional responses, or scientific discoveries. In an argument, they are connected up with principles of support – whether of the kinds of moral instruments just mentioned or logical tools such as creating valid deductive arguments or identifying argument fallacies. Without the fit, data are bare and meaningless. Principles give data meaning. For example, an argument could be made as follows:

> *Kareem Abdul-Jabbar scored more points than any other NBA player (38,387). (this is a premise)*
> *He won six NBA and three NCAA championships. (this is another premise)*
> *Therefore, he is the greatest basketball player ever. (this is the conclusion)*

This is an argument because it contains both data and evidence for support and a conclusion from that data. Now, you might disagree. Some, in fact, argue that Michael Jordan (1963–) is the greatest basketball player ever. But how can that be? The data given about Kareem Abdul-Jabbar (1947–) are true; they are facts that cannot be contested. So, how can we contest the conclusion? Simple, really. We can contest the *meaning* of the given data. Why should we accept that both (or either) 38,000-plus points and winning championships mean that you are the greatest basketball player? Well, hidden in the argument are a number of unstated premises that are doing a lot of the logical work. These premises are what are making the data meaningful for the purpose of the argument. They might go something like this:

> *Winning games, championship games, is the whole point of playing competitive sports. (this is an unstated premise)*
>
> *Basketball games are only won if points are scored. (this is an unstated premise)*
>
> *A player scoring more points puts you in the position to win. (this is an unstated premise)*

Other options for unstated premises would still give useful meaning to the data in relation to the conclusion, but the point is that whatever the unstated premises are, they are doing the work of what has been called a *warrant* – that is, what makes bare data meaningful in an argument.

Summing It Up

The case at the beginning of the chapter is an example of how some of these elements come together (both explicitly and implicitly) irrespective of the method (GRACE, CASES, etc.) used. To understand, then, where cases sometimes end up, below is how the deliberations in a consultation might conclude:

> *Recommendation:* Mr. Q's situation highlights ethical tensions among doing what is best for the patient, what his decision makers are requesting, and the appropriate stewardship of medical resource. The hospital is obligated to provide the best care possible, but tertiary, acute care hospitals are not the best environment for long-term care patients. The family's concern about nursing homes is motivated, in part, by having very little knowledge of what kinds of nursing homes are available in

their area. It is recommended that the family be given the opportunity to visit nursing homes in their area in order to identify a suitable long-term care facility. Further, the family would like better head protection of the patient before leaving the hospital, and it is recommended an occupational therapy helmet be ordered and fitted. Finally, the family appreciates the work of the neurosurgeon, and so it is recommended that the neurosurgeon take the time to explain carefully, slowly, and comprehensively the current situation, short-term processes, and long-term prognosis.

Resolution: After three care conferences with the family and different members of the healthcare team, the family indicates that they understand that Mr. Q's care is going to take months, maybe even years, and that the hospital is not the best place for that kind of care to occur. They are assured that he will be given more surgery for his head and skull, but only after his brain had recovered enough.

The patient was eventually moved to a nursing home within 10 miles of his family, and the latter surgery was successful. While Mr. Q never recovered to his pre-injury baseline, he did recover enough to work around the house and enjoy his time with family and friends. The family never did talk on the record with the media, and they continued to use the hospital and healthcare team for future care for Mr. Q.

* * *

There are a great many parts to an ethics consultation, and in the throes of the consultation, careful deliberative processes must occur to assure comprehensive ethical reflections. Data and evidence are gathered through the efforts to get the whole story (talking with professionals, families, friends, and the patients – where possible) while recognizing the obligations at play, accepting responsibilities that flow from those obligations, considering possible consequences that would follow from proposed actions, and evaluating the character of those people and institutions affected by the decisions to be made. But that is not enough. Ethics consultations must connect all these elements up into an argument wherein moral instruments bring ethical meaning to the data, and in bringing meaning insights arise, conclusions are drawn, and recommendations are made.

Questions for Discussion

1. Conceptual: When identifying the facts and various ethical norms related to a case, what makes something a "fact" and which values become "norms" ... and why?
2. Pragmatic: Given that GRACE considerations do not privilege duties over consequences or character over outcomes, how should the healthcare ethics committee *reason through* and *weigh* considerations? How should a healthcare ethics committee determine what facts and values matter more?
3. Strategic: In order to maintain consistency of process, what would a checklist or rubric for working through the ethical considerations of a case look like? Would a checklist or rubric stifle or promote comprehensive ethical analysis?

References

Jonsen AR, Siegler M, Winslade WJ (2015). *Clinical Ethics: A Practical Approach to Ethical Decisions in Clinical Medicine*, 8th ed. New York: McGraw Hill.

National Center for Ethics in Health Care. (2015). *Ethics Consultation: Responding to Ethics Questions in Health Care*, 2nd ed. Washington, DC: US Department of Veterans Affairs.

Shelton W, Bjarnadottir D (2008). Ethics consultation and the committee. In Hester DM, ed., *Ethics by Committee: A Textbook on Consultation, Organization, and Education for Hospital Ethics Committees*. Lanham, MD: Rowman & Littlefield, 49–77.

Spike J (2012). Ethics consultation process. In Hester DM and Schonfeld TL, eds., *Guidance for Healthcare Ethics Committees*. Cambridge University Press, 41–47.

Informed Consent

Jessica Berg

Objectives

Upon reading and considering the content of this chapter, the reader should be able to:

1. Define and analyze the elements of informed consent and its variations.
2. Distinguish between ethical and legal considerations for informed consent.
3. Explain shared decision-making and how the process should incorporate respect for patient autonomy, professional authority, and informed consent.

Case

Mr. A is 45 years old. During surgery to remove a failing kidney, the operating surgeon detected a tumor on the distal portion of Mr. A's pancreas. His wife gave consent to resecting the pancreas and removing the spleen and kidney. Pathology confirms the malignancy of the tissue after the operation. Mr. A is referred to an oncologist for follow-up care. The oncologist discusses with both Mr. and Ms. A the advisability of using a combination of experimental drugs and radiation, which has shown promise in treating the cancer at issue. They are told that most pancreatic cancer patients die of the disease, that Mr. A is at great risk of recurrence (at which point his cancer would be deemed incurable), that the therapy in question is unproven in cases such as Mr. A's, that adverse side effects are possible (e.g., the treatments are prolonged, difficult, and painful), and that no treatment is an option. At no time are the As told the overall statistical life expectancy for patients with pancreatic cancer. However, statistical life expectancy is not clear in this case since most pancreatic cancers are not discovered until well after they metastasize, whereas here the tumor is comparatively localized and discovered in the course of another surgery. Moreover, the operating surgeon was able to completely excise the tumor and leave a margin around the surgical site that appeared clinically free of cancer.

(Case adapted from *Arato v. Avedon*, 1993)

Introduction

Informed consent has become a standard part of medical practice over the past half-century (Berg et al., 2001). In the twentieth century, at a high point of other movements toward expansion of civil and individual rights, a series of court cases delineated the doctrine of "informed consent" for the first time. Prior to this time, consent, if it existed at all, was based on a concept of a simple consent – disclosure of information was not considered necessary; the patient just had to agree to treatment. In some situations, merely the fact that a patient sought treatment in the first place, along with the fact that they did not leave when treatment was begun, was deemed adequate consent.

The idea that explicit authorization to proceed was required might seem obvious today, but it was anything but that when New York Court of Appeals Justice Cardozo in the 1914 case of *Scholendorff* v. *New York Hospital* stated that "every human being of adult years and sound mind has a right to determine what should be done with his body." Little was said about disclosure requirements until a series of cases almost 40 years later that emphasized the need to disclose risks (*Salgo* v. *Leland Stanford Junior University Board of Trustees*, 1957; *Mitchell* v. *Robinson*, 1960) and the "nature and probable consequences of the ... recommended ... treatment" (*Natanson* v. *Kline*, 1960).

The ethical doctrine of informed consent developed out of the legal one, with the courts sometimes referring to ethical standards as if they were well established when, in fact, information disclosure and patient consent played little role in medical care before the emergence of the legal doctrine. The idea of autonomy, which underpins the ethical doctrine, is a distinctly Western (if not North American) value and may not fit well with other cultures and practices. Even within Western culture, the principle of autonomy may be weighed against other principles such as justice, which can limit the distribution of scarce medical resources across society regardless of individual preferences; or by the principle of beneficence, which may weigh in favor of treatment even over the individual's objections. But regardless of the absence of informed consent in historical codes of medical ethics, it has become a bedrock of current practice. There are at least four reasons for emphasizing the importance of facilitating individual decision-making in medicine:

1. Individuals are most likely to know their own interests and thus make better choices for their health and well-being
2. The information requirement may increase the likelihood that the intervention will be successful since the individual better understands what to expect, including being prepared to recognize problems that may arise
3. Even if individuals err in their choices, we are better off as a society if we encourage individual decision-making, and thus develop autonomous citizens
4. Individuals have a basic right to control what happens to their bodies

Informed Consent Requirements

In practice, informed consent has two important elements – a provider disclosure requirement and a patient choice requirement. Note that the latter is a *choice* requirement, not merely a consent requirement. Patients should make informed decisions about care – both consents and refusals. Moreover, these choices should be voluntary. Voluntariness does not mean that there are no factors that are likely to weigh on the patient's choice. The mere fact that the patient needs care can be a determining factor, and life-or-death situations make the patient feel as though choices are limited. For example, Mr. A faces a very poor prognosis if his cancer is untreated, and the only treatment option is experimental and of limited potential benefit. But these factors do not make his choice about whether to proceed with treatment involuntary. A lack of care options can limit choices, as can a lack of financial or other resources. These pressures do not invalidate a choice on the ground of involuntariness. Rather, the voluntariness aspect of informed consent to treatment focuses on external pressures, most of which come from other people. So, consent would not be deemed voluntary if an individual were threatened by a healthcare provider or family member. Outside of the requirement that individuals must have capacity to consent (an issue addressed in Chapter 11), voluntariness has not been a large focus in the treatment context. It is much more commonly discussed when talking about consent to research participation.

Significantly more attention has been paid to the disclosure aspect than the voluntary choice aspect. When the landmark case of *Canterbury* v. *Spence* was decided in 1972 the court identified the elements of disclosure that still apply today:

- Condition or diagnosis
- Nature and character of proposed treatment
- Anticipated benefits of treatment and expected results
- Known possible risks and complications
- Potential alternatives, including nontreatment

Healthcare providers are usually focused on the scope and nature of their obligations to provide information. Under a shared decision-making model, while the bulk of disclosure obligations fall to the provider, ideally informed consent should entail a dialogue between the provider and the patient. The provider shares information about the medical options, while the patient identifies priorities and goals for treatment. The patient must also be given time to ask questions, seek additional information, and/or involve other people in the decision-making.

In the case described above, Mr. A was told he has pancreatic cancer (condition), and an experimental combination of chemotherapy and radiation was proposed (treatment). If successful, the treatment would allow him to live longer, but it may not work. Even if it does work, the cancer could come back and then would be incurable (benefits), the treatment would be long, difficult, and painful (risks), and no treatment was an option (alternative). Should statistical life expectancy have been disclosed?

The key issue is determining whether disclosure of a particular piece of information is needed to make a fully informed choice regarding care options. Ethically, the provider should consider the patient's subjective values in determining what to disclose, although in practice this may prove impossible to implement. Legally, this is defined in terms of whether the information is "material" – which is the information a reasonable patient would want to know before deciding. In other words, would most (typical) patients want to know the information? Applying this to our case, would most patients want to know statistical life expectancy? But the question may not be that simple. Perhaps the better question is whether most patients with atypical pancreatic cancer that is found earlier than normal would want to know statistical life expectancy. Alternatively, we might just say we disclose if most patients would want to know, but also disclose that the statistics we have are not clearly applicable to the case in question.

Even though we might talk in terms of a "reasonable" or "typical" patient in setting standards, there are both objective and subjective elements of disclosure. Some information should be disclosed to all patients – for example, the nature of the treatment in question – and some information may be particularly relevant to certain patients – for example, a very rare mild hand tremor to an artist. There are some elements of information that would always be considered relevant (see bullet points above). But even within the categories of information that should be shared with all patients, there are elements of discretion. Take, for example, the question about disclosure of alternatives – how extensive is this requirement and how much does a provider (or institution) need to explore what different options exist so as to inform the patient? Do you need to disclose an alternative that is not covered by the particular patient's insurance? Or an alternative that is not readily available? Or a homeopathic alternative if you are an allopathic provider? Or an alternative that is only available as part of a research protocol? The answer is – it depends. In part it depends on subjective factors – is this a patient for whom the information in question would be deemed material? This is an almost impossible inquiry after the fact. Once a patient experiences a bad outcome they may claim that of course they would have wanted information on other options, even those that are extremely difficult to obtain. This is part of the paradox of informed consent.

So how do we determine what to disclose beyond the basic elements bullet-pointed above? The answer is that this is part of the process of shared decision-making. When in doubt, ask a patient whether they want more information about a particular topic. For example, a patient may be told that experimental treatments exist, but only in the context of participation in a research protocol. Instead of providing immediate details, the patient might be told how to get more information on access to research protocols. For simple procedures, it may be sufficient simply to identify the most common procedure and let the patient know that they are free to refuse care and/or explore additional/alternative treatment options. Thus, a patient who presents with an initial bacterial sinus infection may be offered amoxicillin. The provider is not required to explore multiple alternatives, although they may choose to do so. In other cases, such as for cancer treatment, a more in-depth discussion of various alternatives may be warranted. Mr. A, for example, could have been asked how much detail he wants about the likelihood of success since the recommended treatment was experimental. He might have even been asked whether he wanted details like statistical life expectancy, even though those statistics may not have been as relevant to him individually.

Disclosure of cost of care is another area that can be confusing. While most people would say their out-of-pocket costs are relevant to their decision-making, providers are not required to understand and discuss the intricate details of all insurance plans. These obligations fall to the healthcare institution generally, and patients may be encouraged to seek more information from their insurer about specific factors. Ethics committees will want to ensure that institutions have mechanisms in place to provide general financial counseling for patients (including a breakdown of costs that will be charged), and that patients can easily access the service.

Shared Decision-Making

The fact that the ethical doctrine of informed consent drew almost directly from the legal doctrine led to some difficulties as healthcare providers (both individuals and institutions) sometimes conflated the legal requirements with ethical ones. So, while the legal doctrine seemed to delineate disclosure and consent requirements as if the two aspects were separate parts and all obligations were on the provider (to disclose information and "get" patient consent), ethically, informed consent requires a dialogue between the provider and the patient. Patients need to be given time to ask questions, absorb information, and consult with others of their choosing. Additionally, because the doctrine was created in a legal setting, documentation often takes on unusual significance. Consent forms proliferate throughout organizations. While these forms may constitute prima facie evidence (evidence that on its face shows something) that the legal requirements are met, they do not establish that the ethical requirements are met. In fact, getting a signature on a consent form does not mean that the patient gave either legally or ethically valid consent to treatment. Similarly, the lack of a form might be strong evidence that no consent was obtained but is not definitive (at least not ethically and often not legally).

The ethical doctrine of informed consent has shifted since its inception to focus more recently on the concept of *shared* decision-making rather than on individual consent (Beach and Sugarman, 2019). Most people do not make decisions in a vacuum, particularly not important life decisions. Many people may be involved – family, friends, and multiple treatment providers, and the information flow is not unilateral. A concept of shared, rather than individual, decision-making better reflects this reality. It also serves to reinforce the obligations and roles of the individuals involved. Providers are required to share, in understandable terms, their medical and health expertise. Providers should also try to elicit from the patients their values, goals, and concerns. Patients may want to choose to involve other parties in the decision-making process (such as family, friends, religious leaders, additional health professionals). Together the parties should determine the best option(s) for the specific person under the specific circumstances. Providers should not make choices for patients and need to accept that some patients will make choices that are not, strictly, in their best medical interests. Patients cannot demand any treatment – only those that are medically appropriate (and, currently, for which they have a mechanism to cover the costs). While shared decision-making may seem like an ideal, it is an ideal worth striving for, even if in practice some parts may fall short.

Ethics committees will play an important role in effecting shared decision-making and in prioritizing the ethical doctrine over the legal one. Education will be an important part of this. It can be very helpful to facilitate discussions about disclosure using specific case examples, such as the one described at the beginning of this chapter. Asking questions about the roles of the providers, patient, and family can help draw out the contours of a shared decision-making approach to informed consent. In addition, ethics committees may want to develop guidance documents to help providers understand informed consent requirements and variations, discussed in the sections below.

Shared decision-making tools should be designed to encourage patients to explore and request information about areas of importance, both those that are important to most patients and those that might be important to the specific patient. Guidance documents can identify questions that providers can pose to patients, or that patients can consider on their own (or with family members). For some standard procedures, ethics committees may want to develop guidance documents delineating the specific information to be disclosed, including information related to the procedure itself, the facility in which the procedure will be undertaken, and the provider(s) who will be involved in the care.

There are some excellent resources designed to facilitate shared decision-making, many of which have been developed by academic medical organizations. Ethics committees will want to compile resources for easy access by providers.[1] In larger institutions,

---

[1] For examples see: Agency for Healthcare Research and Quality, *The Share Approach: Putting Shared Decisionmaking into Practice – A User's Guide for Clinical Teams*, April 2014, www.ahrq .gov/sites/default/files/wysiwyg/professionals/education/curriculum-tools/shareddecisionmaking/

ethics committees may even want to create their own tools. These can include decision aids (video, electronic, and print) for specific procedures; educational modules for patients, families, and providers; guidelines for legal and ethical requirements; and shared decision-making toolkits.

Variations on the Basic Doctrine

Even as it described the initial parameters of informed consent, the *Canterbury* court identified some variation on the doctrine and later cases expanded the list. These include incompetence, emergency, therapeutic privilege, waiver, and public health (Berg et al., 2001). Competence is a legal status and is considered a core requirement for the exercise of autonomy and thus medical decision-making, so incompetence is an unusual "exception" (Berg et al., 1996). Lack of competence does not obviate all informed consent obligations; rather, the obligations usually shift to a substitute decision maker, who must then be provided with all relevant disclosures and be afforded the necessary support to make a decision regarding care. (Competence, capacity, and substitute decision makers are discussed in more detail in other chapters herein.)

The other areas function more traditionally, allowing a modification of the regular requirements when the conditions are met. For example, in emergency situations we do not require the same level of disclosure, if any disclosure at all. In part this is a recognition that most people would rather be treated in an emergency without disclosure and consent than provided an opportunity to engage in shared decision-making. In some cases, the individual in the emergent situation lacks capacity to make a decision, so the two areas can overlap. While emergency is probably the most recognized and established exception, it is worth stressing that providers cannot engineer an emergency to avoid informed consent obligations. So, if there are anticipated treatment choices, a provider cannot wait until the patient deteriorates and then claim it is an emergency and informed consent cannot be obtained. Similarly, if something unexpected is discovered in the course of another procedure, the provider may need to consult with a substitute decision maker. This is what happened with Mr. A – the pancreatic cancer was discovered during another surgery and his decision maker (his wife) was informed and then asked to consent to the additional excision. Moreover, the authorization for care in the emergency situation is only to the extent needed to address the emergency in question. Finally, emergencies are not coterminous with care received in emergency departments. Not all care in an emergency department is an actual emergency and even in cases where care is needed quickly, there may be time for disclosure (or limited disclosure) and choice.

Therapeutic privilege is a more controversial exception; it is designed to allow a provider to choose not to disclose otherwise required information out of a concern that the disclosure will be so upsetting that it would prevent the patient from being able to make a decision. Based on an anachronistic conception of patient decision-making (and linked back to the times when physicians routinely withheld material information such as cancer diagnoses for fear of upsetting patients), the exception still exists but should be rarely used in practice. The physicians involved in Mr. A's case might claim that if they

tools/tool-8/share-tool8.pdf; Dartmouth-Hitchcock, Center for Shared Decision Making, www.dartmouth-hitchcock.org/shared-decision-making/resources; Mayo Clinic, Shared Decision Making National Resource Center, https://carethatfits.org/.

disclosed the extremely low life expectancy of pancreatic cancer patients they would have taken away all hope and thereby harmed Mr. A. Ethics committees should be aware that providers may misuse the therapeutic exception to withhold information they would rather not disclose; patients have a much better ability to handle difficult disclosure than providers may think. The only time this exception should apply is when information is truly so harmful that disclosure would, in fact, paralyze the patient's decision-making process. It is hard to imagine a situation in which that would occur. Carefully putting the information in context could have helped Mr. A incorporate the information into his decision-making process.[2] The mere fact that providers are aware that a therapeutic privilege exception exists may make some wary of disclosing information. Difficult or upsetting information can be offered in a variety of settings, in a variety of ways, and over varying periods of time. It is almost never the case that the mere disclosure of a piece of information would completely prevent decision-making. There are better and worse ways to provide information, including "bad news." Providers should be well versed in the options (Paladino et al., 2019) and ethics committees should offer guidance, arrange for training, and provide resources about how to disclose difficult information.

Waiver is perhaps the most interesting of the exceptions, as it is based on the idea that respecting autonomy includes not only the right to make decisions, but the right to choose not to make decisions (Berg, 2003). In theory, waiver can apply to both the disclosure and choice aspects of informed consent. A patient can choose not to get certain information ("I don't want to hear about the alternatives" or "I don't want to hear about a risk of death"), or choose not to make a choice, or both. The first is the hardest to reconcile with the underlying doctrine. Waiver of material information means that the resulting decision is not fully informed. The result is an "uninformed" consent, which is hard to reconcile with the underlying concept of autonomy upon which the doctrine is based. Waiver of the choice aspect of informed consent, or waiver of both elements, essentially means that the patient is saying "I consent to whatever X recommends." As long as X's decision meets the requirements of informed consent this functions similarly to substitute decision-making in the context of incompetence, but has the added benefit of having the patient's imprimatur. If X is an individual who we would likely identify as a substitute decision maker (e.g., spouse), this raises few questions. If X is a healthcare provider, it may be more complicated, although still permissible. The patient who basically says "whatever you say, doctor" is clearly not meeting the autonomous decision-making goals of informed consent, nor reflecting the ideal goal of shared decision-making (see discussion above). At the same time, it is hard to understand how we would force patients to hear information or make decisions in the name of promoting autonomy. So, waiver continues to be a recognized exception and perhaps worth some time from ethics committees in terms of educating providers in their institution.

Finally, there are some circumstances where societal interest in public health goals overrides the interests in promoting autonomous decision-making (Berg, 2012). In these

---

[2] This assumes that the statistical life expectancy information should have been disclosed and that the therapeutic privilege would have applied to create an exception – it is not at all clear that the exception would even have been needed if the information was not deemed material at the outset.

settings, individual informed consent may be completely unnecessary (e.g., addition of fluoride to public water sources), or modified to focus less on whether the consent is fully autonomous (e.g., access to sexually transmitted infection [STI] treatment by minors). Different states have different laws relating to these public health exceptions and institutions should make sure that providers are well aware of the contexts in which this exception operates.

Not only are there state laws that may describe exceptions to informed consent, but there are also state laws that require specific disclosures for certain procedures, specific consent forms or documentation, or which may limit some kinds of substitute decision-making. While the general framework is described above, it is worth investigating the law of the state in question. Ethics committees should make sure to gather this information and ensure it is easily accessible to providers, particularly those practicing in areas in which the laws are relevant (e.g., STI minor consent laws for pediatricians and OB/GYNs).

Ethics Committee Role

Ethics committees and their members should educate themselves about informed consent standards in their state and consider taking the following steps for their institution:

1. Create short summary documents listing and describing the laws relating to informed consent in the state in question including requirements for:
   a. Consent for specific procedures (if statutes on this exist)
   b. Consent documentation
   c. Consent variations, including standards for things like incapacity and guidelines for substitute decision makers

2. Identify resources and/or create toolkits to facilitate shared decision-making. There are a number of decision-making tools now available for different treatments, and ethics committees will want to compile resources to facilitate shared decision-making. In larger institutions they may even want to create their own tools. These can include decision aids (video, electronic, and print) for specific procedures; educational modules for patients, families, and providers; guidelines for legal and ethical requirements; and toolkits.

3. Conduct training sessions for healthcare providers regarding how to use the tools created, how to deal with difficult cases, and when to call for an ethics consultation

Questions for Discussion

1. Conceptual: How do we reconcile the legal requirements for informed consent (and the goal of promoting autonomy) with the ideal of shared decision-making?
2. Pragmatic: Is there a way to structure consent requirements, including consent forms and consent aids, to facilitate interaction and engagement between providers and patients?
3. Strategic: What kinds of guidance documents or tools could your ethics committee develop to facilitate informed consent and shared decision-making? What aspects of informed consent do you think are the most challenging for providers in your institution? Can you address those?

References

Beach MC, Sugarman J (2019). Realizing shared decision-making in practice. *JAMA*, 322(9): 811–812.

Berg JW (2003). Understanding waiver. *Houston Law Review*, 40(2): 281–344.

Berg JW (2012). All for one and one for all: Informed consent and public health. *Houston Law Review*, 50(1): 1–40.

Berg JW, Appelbaum PS, Grisso T (1996). Constructing competence: Formulating standards of legal competence to make medical decisions. *Rutgers Law Review*, 48 (2): 345–396.

Berg JW, Appelbaum PS, Lidz C, Parker L (2001). *Informed Consent: Legal Theory and Clinical Practice*, 2nd ed. New York: Oxford University Press.

Paladino J, Lakin JR, Sanders JJ (2019). Communication strategies for sharing prognostic information with patients. *JAMA*, 322(14): 1345–1346.

Confidentiality and Privacy
Traditional Concerns and Digital Challenges

Kenneth W. Goodman

Objectives

Upon reading and considering the content of this chapter, the reader should be able to:

1. Define confidentiality and privacy in health care, and identify applicable laws, regulations, and institutional policies.
2. Explain why privacy and confidentiality are important in the clinical setting, and the harms that may result from data or information breaches.
3. Describe behaviors that respect and promote privacy and confidentiality and that address sensitively the tension between the duty to warn at-risk third parties and the desire to honor patient confidentiality.
4. Identify challenges in maintaining confidentiality given the use of communication technologies (e.g., texting, email) and electronic medical records in patient care.

Case 1

Mr. Varela is a 67-year-old man recently discharged from your hospital after treatment for complications from his diabetes. Ambulatory care is provided by the hospital's clinicians. One day Mr. Varela uses his personal, commercial account to email a physician. He does not have a telephone. In the email, he describes recent symptoms, including dangerous blood glucose levels and diet. The physician contacts the ethics committee seeking advice about whether and how to reply, given that Mr. Varela's email account is not encrypted, as required by law.

Case 2

The Marketing Department wants to begin advertising the hospital's new patient portal, and staffers there seek guidance about how to manage requests by parents to access their children's records. One of the marketers says, "I can tell you that I'd insist that I have access to my kid's record no matter what. We're not that patient-centered." The ethics committee is asked to develop a "points to consider" document.

Introduction

Medicine has had a long-standing tradition requiring that clinicians keep the private concerns of patients in confidence. However, the traditional duties to safeguard health information and respect for privacy rights face new, interesting, and difficult challenges.

The scope of health information technology and its ability to store and analyze vast amounts of information have, as is often the case in bioethics, outstripped efforts to keep up both ethically and legally.

Since the times of Hippocrates (at least), protecting "holy secrets" has been a deeply held and celebrated value. As such, the value of keeping information "in confidence" has been central to the practice of Western medicine. Without successful protection of health information, patients may be less than forthcoming with, and even lie about, their lives and health status. That can, in turn, impede diagnosis and treatment, which then entails worse clinical outcomes. As such, the central social and ethical principle is sound: Privacy, in part the right to control who has access to information about you, is essential for social relationships, for enjoying anonymity, and, indeed, for most important connections between and among people. But further, this principle has legal implications – namely, "a right not protected by law might not be much of a right" (Goodman, 2016, 39).

Generally, then, we might say that "privacy" is a broad concept that entails an entitlement (or "right") to control that access, including disclosure of data and information, and, largely, to be free of unwanted intrusion. Relatedly, "confidentiality" is an expectation (read: "obligation") concerning personal or "owned" information, protecting it from access unless the "owner" agrees to access. And yet, given the value that even secure information has for improving the health of populations or specific individuals, neither the obligation of confidentiality nor the right to privacy should be regarded as absolute.

Privacy in the Clinical Setting

Given the importance of protecting patient privacy, then, the inappropriate release or disclosure of personal health information is an ongoing and vexing concern. Patients deserve a safe space in which to express and expose intimate aspects of their lives for the benefit of their health. As such, disclosures – intentional or not – can constitute a moral transgression, or a *wrong*. It does not matter whether the information is about a trivial malady or a stigma-inducing one. In contrast, if an illicit disclosure causes someone to lose a benefit, incur a cost, be subjected to public stigma, or fail to seek future medical attention, then that person has suffered a *harm*.

In the clinical setting, a patient can be wronged, harmed, or both by incautious and unguarded conversations, by failures to follow basic electronic health record (EHR) hygiene (do not share your password, log off, do not make copies), and by efforts to trick users or attack systems. The risk of both wrongs and harms is mitigated or reduced when good education and reminders for providers are in place and when data breaches are prevented. Breaches of any kind or size can erode trust and undermine universal values that shape the clinician–patient relationship.

On the other side of this coin, a key privacy component, recognized in well-known legislation, is the right to access one's own information. Adults and most minors should have complete and nimble access to all their health information, including lab results, images, progress notes, etc. Internal or institutional impediments to such access are likely products of the structure of patient "portals" provided by vendors of EHRs.

Limits on Privacy: The "Duty to Warn"

Most privacy protections are straightforward and, generally, uncontroversial: The value of privacy is ancient and sound, and the steps taken to honor it are subject to the usual institutional processes and oversight. Yet laws and institutional policies are sometimes either inapplicable or impotent in the face of novel cases or new technologies. The correct action or stance can be unclear when values are in conflict.

The classic exemplars of such a problem are the Tarasoff case from California in the mid-1970s and the early days of HIV-AIDS. The Tarasoff case concerned a mental health professional confronted with the challenge of whether or not to inform an innocent third party who had been threatened by a client. The California Supreme Court ruled that there are some cases in which the obligation to retain patient information in confidence should be breached, particularly when there was a clear threat of imminent harm to an identifiable other person. While this was a ruling by a state court, it has had national repercussions, with many states implementing Tarasoff-based statutes creating a legal "duty to warn" in a narrow set of circumstances.

Further, in the late 1980s–early 1990s, providers and states wondered what the duty was regarding disclosures of HIV-AIDS to persons outside the therapeutic relationship. Should confidential diagnostic or treatment information be disclosed to someone who is at risk of contracting the disease? On whom or what, if anywhere, does an obligation to report patient HIV-AIDS status fall – on the patient themself, on the practitioner, or on the state through health agencies or even police? States have taken different approaches to this issue – sometimes specifically calling out HIV-AIDS under separate laws and policies, and sometimes folding it into laws regarding infectious disease reporting, writ large.

In the decades since the emergence of HIV-AIDS, genetic information has come to elicit tensions between privacy and a duty to warn, though there are key differences between infectious diseases and genetic conditions. Importantly, someone "at risk" in genetic cases has already been "exposed" to whatever genetic malady is in question. The questions of whether and when to disclose a genetic risk to a child, sibling, or parent is best answered by modeling privacy-enhancing behaviors and achieving clarity about putative duties to warn. For example, it might be one can warn those at risk after obtaining consent from those whose confidentiality is at stake. The point is, there may be carefully crafted solutions that can eliminate the moral tensions while preserving many, if not all, of the moral values at stake.

Healthcare ethics committees (HECs) in their education, policy review, and consultation roles can adopt several strategies to help mitigate these concerns. First, learn about and acknowledge both privacy rights and duties to protect the public. Next, improve communication about risks before they are incurred. For instance, genetic analysis will almost always produce results of use or interest to relatives, and wise use of genetic counselors can prepare patients for these possibilities and their consequences. Third and relatedly, remember the foundations of valid consent. Adequate information is a powerful tool in motivating people to think clearly about their duties and rights.

Legal Considerations and the Role of HIPAA

Legally, the history of privacy laws in the USA has had the states owning jurisdiction over such matters – that is, until the 1996 federal statute, the Health Insurance Portability and Accountability Act (HIPAA). This statute was written in order to make it easier to pass information among different parties to provide better coverage for employees with preexisting conditions.[1] However, this meant that patient information, whether on paper or, increasingly, computers, needed some protection and security. While the various state privacy laws have remained in effect and take precedence when they are stricter, the HIPAA Privacy Rule came into effect in 2003, with specific guidance and restrictions for how information is to be passed among parties.[2] Under HIPAA, healthcare institutions must have policies to govern and procedures to guide use and disclosure of what the law calls "protected health information" (PHI): individually identifiable health information, including information about a person's mental or physical health or condition or treatment or payment for such care (US Department of Health and Human Services, 2017). PHI covers both health information and other "common identifiers" such as name, address, birth date, etc.

Key provisions of the Privacy Rule include:

- Patients should have easy and secure access to their own health information, and have the right to request an accounting of who has accessed their health records. HECs should work to foster improved ease of access to EHR information.
- The sharing and exchange of health information should be guided by the "minimum necessary standard." This means that one should not share more information than needed for a particular purpose.
- Institutions must establish policies to govern interactions between people or organizations that provide or pay for health care ("covered entities").

Importantly, HIPAA requires the appointment of institutional privacy officers to take responsibility for all HIPAA compliance, and the HEC should know who has that responsibility in the institution.

Compliance versus Ethics

We began with the observation that privacy has ancient origins and, moreover, is fundamentally internal to the health professions. To be sure, privacy and confidentiality came to be legal requirements in most jurisdictions, but it was not until HIPAA came into force that there were nationwide rules and increasingly severe penalties for violations (US Department of Health and Human Services, 2015).

The enforcement of HIPAA's Privacy Rule paralleled and contributed to the emergence of a kind of "compliance culture" in healthcare organizations. Hospitals now all have compliance offices. Such institutional offices arose because of billing fraud, research misconduct, and sexual harassment. What followed was a blossoming of new HIPAA

---

[1] The use of such tools for internal ethics committee communication is similarly constrained. Absent a dedicated and secure internal system, it is likely inappropriate for ethics committee members to send or receive texts containing protected health information.

[2] An important ethical issue unrelated to privacy is shaped by the extent to which any new technology should be regarded as suitable for use with humans. The evolution of telemedicine was accelerated by initial uses in rural areas and prisons – with no evidence base to suggest it was as good as face-to-face interactions. Indeed, more attention has been devoted to solving billing questions – consider a physician in one state and a patient in another – than to addressing, say, research in vulnerable populations, evidence of efficacy, and training.

policies, which were drafted by consultants and lawyers, not ethics committees; mandatory "training" sessions, which were conducted by privacy office officials, not ethics committees; and hotlines for HIPAA questions and consultations, which were staffed by lawyers, not ethics committees. These constitute a suite of missed opportunities for HECs.

Compliance, though, remains a matter of interpretation. For instance, many EHR vendors structure their systems so that all psychotherapy notes are coded as "super-confidential" with access permitted only to other psychotherapists. There is no basis in the law requiring such a stricture. Indeed, any rule that would prevent a pediatrician from seeing a psychologist's note could be harmful to the patient.

Now consider Case 1 above. A physician in your institution would like to communicate with their patient on a time-sensitive matter using a texting application. May they? The compliance answer is "no" – commercial texting apps are provided by companies lacking HIPAA-approved "covered entity" business associate status; it does not matter that any particular company promises encryption. However, HECs, focused on ethics rather than compliance, may have alternative responses. They could propose to obtain patient permission/consent to use an unencrypted medium; or advocate for adoption of secure messaging tools, as some institutions have already done. To be sure, it is not being suggested that HECs alone would come up with these alternatives; and either option would require the concurrence and approval of other internal entities, including the compliance or privacy office. The point is that a competent and engaged ethics service is perfectly placed to advise colleagues and institutions and, in the process, to signal that values can guide decision-making.

Patient presumptions of confidentiality are varied. An ethics committee asked to consult in a case involving a clinician's monitoring of social media posts must consider whether, despite the public utterance, the patient would regard their physician accessing it to be illicit. Veracity and transparency are the values to bring to bear.

Addressing the Use of Technology

Digital technologies (from wearable monitoring devices to ease-of-access EHR portal to e-health apps to telehealth) are unlike other technologies in health care, for not only do they transmit and store a great deal of personal data but also their use is often advanced and advocated by patients themselves. Whether the use of these technologies improves care or outcomes is an ongoing empirical question. What is clear is that each presents novel privacy and confidentiality challenges.

HECs can help meet these challenges. First, assuming a fundamental level of institutional security, an HEC should ensure that it has familiarity with digital and mobile health tools. Some of this will depend on context: How is patient data from a wearable fitness device or blood glucose monitor transmitted, and where is it stored? What secure encryption is used when data are transmitted? Are data shared with the EHR?

Among the virtues of health information systems, for example, is that they make it easy for clinicians and other appropriate personnel to find and add to a patient's record. But that virtue has an evil twin: Absent robust security measures and parallel policies, it also makes it easy for sightseers and hackers to view and copy records.

Similar concerns need to be addressed with the rise of telehealth (or "telemedicine" or "remote presence health care"). Though these clinical modalities can vary from a telephone to the use of high-fidelity cameras, voice connections, and the Internet, privacy challenges arise. For example, clinicians need to disclose to patients if anyone else is on the line or in the room. And further they should note whether or not the software being used to transmit the visit is encrypted or not. Moreover, privacy-protecting processes and policies are needed to govern storage and sharing of information collected from patients at some remove from any clinician or institution.

Other issues arise when, say, a patient or clinician uses an e-health app or device. Whatever the benefits of such apps, HECs should be aware of whether there is any evidence to suggest it is useful and secure. Are there privacy risks, harms, or unintended consequences to consider? It is reasonable for an institution to maintain control over the use of electronic (even commercially produced) media? Even those most passionate in advocating patient-centered care and systems must concede that anything that imperils security systems or introduces novel risks to confidentiality needs to be scrutinized carefully.

The use of all these technologies entails that HECs have an opportunity to develop policies to identify and govern appropriate uses and users. At a minimum, HECs should encourage their members to be familiar with the ways in which patients, guardians, and clinicians use these tools. Ethical issues that arise and which can be addressed by nimble policies include:

- **Privacy and Confidentiality:** Are the tools secure? Are they provided by a (trusted) covered entity? HECs can develop policies that make clear the need for risk disclosure and consent.
- **Appropriate Uses:** The growth of e-health and telehealth has in many cases outstripped the evidence for their efficacy, let alone their superiority or noninferiority compared to face-to-face interactions. As these technologies evolve, HECs should note that ethical issues can arise given quality issues, and corresponding policies might address these concerns.
- **Minors' Rights:** Provisions should be made to manage minors' rights to privacy in cases in which parent or guardian rights might conflict. However, policies to address these issues will be tricky (see below).

Consider the practice of Googling patients for clinically relevant information in their or others' online posts. The practice is apparently not addressed by any law or regulation. But questions arise regarding the veracity of online information, as well as how to incorporate appropriately (presumably verified) online information into clinical care – an effort that can turn a clinician into a trust-eroding spy.

The common practice of texting also raises concerns: The ability to communicate rapidly and easily with patients has a number of virtues. Some pediatricians, for example, have made good use of text and SMS tools to urge or dissuade a visit to an emergency department. But not all experiences are positive, and there are questions regarding whether and how to document these exchanges and how to prevent abuses such as trivial texting at inappropriate times.

Both issues are fertile ground for HEC education efforts and policy development. For instance, a policy governing searches for patients in social media should at a minimum require a justification balanced against risks; a review process might be considered. A policy for texting should address documentation of consent to use a medium not provided by a covered entity as well as recording key content in texts.

Example of Ethical Challenges with Technology: Personal Health Records or "Portals"

EHR software makes patient records accessible online, thus making it possible for both system-users and tech-savvy data hackers to see personal information of patients. On the latter side of this issue, HECs have little say, and institutions must use well-encrypted software and excellent firewalls. But on the former side, HECs should be aware of all the ways in which those with login ability can see patient information, and when it would be wrong for some persons, be they professionals or family, to view such data.

An important development for easing access for patients to their own health information are "personal health records" (PHRs), accessible through online portals that enable patients to track their health information, communicate with clinicians, and tend to their health just as they tend to professional, financial, and other affairs. While the adoption of portals in the United States is driven in part by the government's "meaningful use" requirements and incentives (Neuner et al., 2015; Zhao et al., 2018), many portals remain cumbersome and incomplete.

Evidence suggests that portals can improve care, but that such improvements are impeded by a number of factors. They also raise important policy challenges for HECs. There is much we do not know about PHR use and preferences: how such use measures up to face-to-face communication or whether, indeed, it might be superior for precisely the kinds of health issues minors encounter. We also do not yet know if there is a nontrivial difference between portal use by patients with chronic maladies and those with less frequent medical needs.

The challenges to the fundamental right to privacy posed by PHRs is brought into stark relief when we look at the use of portals for minor/teenage patients, since both patient and parents have legitimate interest in the information and concerns for protecting confidentiality.

Take the following points into consideration:

- Portal use is increasing, with nearly one-fifth of pediatric patients having their own accounts; secure messaging is the most frequently used tool, followed by test result access; and more than four-fifths of logins are by parents or guardians (Steitz et al., 2017).
- Likely because of greater familiarity and comfort with information technology, as well as a more carefree stance toward privacy, "younger patients are more willing to enter all the required data to complete a robust PHR and share this data" (Cushman et al., 2010).
- In at least some populations, adolescents have misconceptions about the clinician–patient relationship, are not aware of their ability to obtain care, and do not fully understand EHRs or portals (Miklin et al., 2019).

Getting portal design and access right for minors is exquisitely difficult. There are two major reasons for this. First, there is no agreement on or standard for determining conditions (legal or moral) for when parents or guardians can be excluded from access to their child's personal health records. The American Academy of Pediatrics recommends that "Adolescents should have the right to exclude parents from their PHRs when law dictates that they may be treated without parental consent. When these features are used, health care professionals need to know that these exclusions are in place" (American

Academy of Pediatrics, 2009, 407). However, few states have so-called mature minor doctrines in either statutory or case law, and while many states do allow minors to consent to, say, reproductive health interventions (contraception, STD treatments), many states explicitly allow for confidentiality to be breached by providers if they believe it is in the minor's best interest. This problem is supported by the fact that adolescent autonomy and maturity evolve in idiosyncratic ways and, in parallel, many parents will be displeased by – and even protest – a minor's decision to block their access; or they might disagree with a diagnosis or treatment plan (Bourgeois et al., 2018).

There are, therefore, legitimate grounds for debate about (1) when (or whether) minors should first be asked to grant parental access and (2) the frequency with which they thereafter should be asked. A 12-year-old might agree to such access but change their mind in a year or two. (At least one electronic medical record vendor stipulates that its portal access can be restricted only beginning at the age of 13.) As above, this is an opportunity for HECs to incorporate practical guidance into institutional policies.

Second, the American Academy of Pediatrics observes, "most systems are not capable of allowing dual (or plural) consent to allow or restrict access to different portions of a patient's electronic health information," and it attributes this to a lack of standards, including standards "for electronic medical technology regarding privacy issues and care for the adolescent patient where rights of minors are protected by state laws or precedent court cases ... [or] for electronic medical technology when states remain silent on the issue of care around sensitive area issues for the adolescent, and care is routinely provided to teenagers as mature minors" (American Academy of Pediatrics, 2012), 988. So, while disclosure to parents through insurance and billing information still persists as a potential breach of confidentiality, EHRs compound this problem as they are often inadequately designed in order to protect fully patient privacy. This is especially true in the case of teenage patients. System software must be able to partition or segment specific aspects of the record in an environment in which there is no agreement on what discussions, diagnoses, tests, or maladies legitimately fall within the scope for denying parental access, and in fact, some rules vary by state.

Conversely, parents may legitimately seek to ensure that such information that has made its way into a child's chart not be accessible to the child – to protect the *parent's* confidentiality. And yet, there is no consensus on how to manage information ranging from disclosures about paternity to previous abortions and parental behavior as risk factors. There is, moreover, no clear guidance on how to address genetic information such that disclosure to a child might violate a parent's privacy rights.

Privacy, Confidentiality, and the Twenty-First-Century Healthcare Ethics Committee

The following are steps an HEC can take to be a full partner in protecting confidentiality, especially in the Digital Age:

- Learn about health information technology and become familiar with its growing ethics literature
- Reconnect with or reach out to the institution's privacy officer, a compliance official, and chief medical information officer (often in charge of computer systems and their

security), and consider inviting them to meetings, or even offer full membership about ethical issues related to privacy and confidentiality

- Become familiar with institutional privacy policies and special cases they address (e.g., prisoners and students), and become reacquainted with HIPAA
- Create an ethics curriculum that is available to all clinicians, trainees, and students; offer it regularly to accommodate newcomers; and perhaps include periodic refresher sessions. This might also be an opportunity to collaborate with institutional privacy officers and patients themselves.

This work may expand the HEC's activities, especially if the committee is included in efforts to update or draft new institutional privacy policies and undertakes to provide educational or in-service sessions on contemporary confidentiality issues.

Conclusion

The number and variety of privacy and confidentiality issues raised by health information technology will continue to increase, not least given growing recognition of the utility of "patient-generated health information." Patients who embrace their health apps and portal contributions might produce data and information at least as valuable as lab reports, especially for chronic conditions. Information from patients might support clinicians' efforts to monitor patients between visits (Ancker et al., 2019).

Managing this vast tide of information is challenge enough. But ensuring that patients can later review it and that the institution will protect it appropriately signal new and exciting opportunities for HECs to continue to contribute to wellness and to honor and safeguard patient rights.

Questions for Discussion

1. Conceptual: It can be difficult to protect privacy and safeguard information. Is that a good enough reason to declare, as many now do, that "privacy is dead"? Should we give up on privacy?
2. Pragmatic: Ethics committees are well advised not to take on issues outside their competence. What steps are needed to bring your committee up to speed with biomedical informatics?
3. Strategic: How might the HEC maintain good relations with the general counsel, risk management, and privacy offices at your institution in order to be able to discuss both case-based and system concerns regarding privacy?

References

American Academy of Pediatrics (2009). Policy statement – using personal health records to improve the quality of health care for children. *Pediatrics*, 124(1): 403–409.

American Academy of Pediatrics (2012). Policy statement – standards for health information technology to ensure adolescent privacy. *Pediatrics*, 130(5): 987–990.

Ancker JS, Mauer E, Kalish RB, Vest JR, Gossey JT (2019). Early adopters of patient-generated health data upload in an electronic patient portal. *Applied Clinical Informatics*, 10(2): 254–260.

Bourgeois FC, DesRoches CM, Bell SK (2018). Ethical challenges raised by OpenNotes for pediatric and adolescent patients. *Pediatrics*, 141(6): e20172745.

Cushman R, Froomkin AM, Cava A, Abril P, Goodman KW (2010). Ethical, legal and social issues for personal health records and applications. *Journal of Biomedical Informatics*, 43(5 Suppl.): S51–S55.

Goodman KW (2016). *Ethics, Medicine and Information Technology: Intelligent Machines and the Transformation of Health Care.* Cambridge University Press.

Miklin DJ, Vangara SS, Delamater AM, Goodman KW (2019). Understanding of and barriers to electronic health record patient portal access in a culturally diverse pediatric population. *JMIR Medical Informatics*, 7(2): e11570.

Neuner J, Fedders M, Caravella M, Bradford L, Schapira M (2015). Meaningful use and the patient portal: Patient enrollment, use, and satisfaction with patient portals at a later-adopting center. *American Journal of Medical Quality*, 20(2): 105–113.

Steitz B, Cronin RM, Davis SE, Yan E, Jackson GP (2017). Long-term patterns of patient portal use for pediatric patients at an academic medical center. *Applied Clinical Informatics*, 8(3): 779–793.

US Department of Health and Human Services. (2015). The HIPAA Privacy Rule. www.hhs.gov/hipaa/for-professionals/privacy/index.html

US Department of Health and Human Services. (2017). Summary of the HIPAA Privacy Rule. www.hhs.gov/hipaa/for-professionals/privacy/laws-regulations/index.html

Zhao JY, Song B, Anand E, et al.. Barriers, facilitators, and solutions to optimal patient portal and personal health record use: A systematic review of the literature. *AMIA Annual Symposium Proceedings*: 1913–1922.

Chapter

11

Decision-Making Capacity

Arthur R. Derse

Objectives

This chapter will help the healthcare ethics committee (HEC) member:

1. Summarize the elements of decision-making capacity.
2. Describe why determination of decision-making capacity is essential for respecting autonomous patient choices.
3. Describe a standard method and mnemonic for determination of decision-making capacity.
4. Describe the procedure to address any unresolved questions about the patient's ability to make medical decisions.

Case

A 93-year-old woman with early dementia is brought in with cachexia (extreme weight loss). She is widowed. Her sole daughter assists her and is attentive to her. According to her daughter, the patient does not have a guardian. She has been bedbound for the past 2 months, has continued to lose weight, and refuses offered oral feeding, saying she will eat when she is hungry. The patient doesn't know the date or year but knows the season, and that she is in a hospital. She recognizes and responds to her daughter and to the physician but doesn't know the medications she is taking or her medical problems. "My daughter knows all that, and you should know it, too, since it's somewhere in my chart in this place and you're the doctor," she says.

The physician discusses with the patient and daughter whether a feeding tube might be an option to help her regain weight. The physician tells the patient she may die if she continues to lose weight. The patient adamantly refuses. "I've said all my life, no tubes for me. I'd rather die than be stuck on tubes." The daughter agrees, saying "she's said that to me many times before." There is no evidence of depression.

Does the patient have the capacity to understand the medical decision? Should the physician accept the patient's expressed statement refusing a feeding tube? The physician consults the HEC for advice.

Introduction: Definition and Significance of Decision-Making Capacity

Decision-making capacity is the ability to make autonomous and reasoned decisions about medical care. The presence of this ability to make decisions about medical care is crucial to recognizing autonomy. Recognizing autonomy supports the ethical right of individuals to make decisions about their medical care. Although informed consent is essential to the exercise of autonomous decision- making, informed consent rests not only upon the information needed to make a decision, but also upon the capacity of the individual to make a medical decision. Thus, individuals must possess decision-making capacity in order to exercise their right to make autonomous decisions about their medical care.

Individuals who are unable to make autonomous decisions due to conditions such as dementia, delirium, or coma, cannot exercise their legal right to make these decisions. Their medical decisions must be made by others, based on either what the patient would have wanted under the circumstances, or what is best for the patient. Those who are unable to make decisions because they have never possessed decision-making capacity due to developmental disability, or because they are too young to have developed it, will need a determination of what medical course of action should be taken in the absence of their ability to make decisions.

Elements of Decision-Making Capacity

Decision-making capacity consists of three essential elements. The first element is the patient's ability to understand the information provided about medical treatment and the consequences of their choices. The second element is the patient's ability to evaluate the information, comparing the benefits of the proposed treatment and alternatives against the risks (including the benefits and risks of choosing to forgo treatment) with an appreciation of the consequences for the individual. The third element of decision-making capacity is the patient's ability to communicate a treatment decision that remains consistent over time. Lack of any of these three elements constitutes an overall lack of decision-making capacity (Derse and Schiedermayer, 2015, 21–24).

When determining decision-making capacity, it is important to note that not all patients have the same ability to understand and analyze the information presented by the clinician. Impairments include medical conditions such as advanced dementia, delirium, or developmental disability. Care must also be taken to provide medical information to patients that is compatible with their educational background, reading level, and ability to hear. Impairments that may be accommodated should be addressed before concluding that a patient cannot understand the information and consequences.

The second element, the ability to evaluate information, comparing the benefits of the proposed treatment and alternatives against their risks (including the benefits and risks of choosing to forgo treatment) is complex. It requires the patient to evaluate outcomes using probabilistic thinking (determining the likelihood of risks, e.g., the ability to weigh the significant benefit of surgery against the overwhelming risk of not treating appendicitis). The patient must also measure the likelihood of these outcomes against the patient's set of values. The third element of decision-making capacity is the ability of the patient to communicate a decision to the clinician. Impairments that can be overcome or accommodated should be addressed before concluding that the patient cannot communicate. An extreme example would be a patient with "locked-in" syndrome. The patient has decision-making capacity, but is able to communicate only by moving the eyelids and eyes (as depicted in the book and film, *The Diving Bell and the Butterfly*). Even in this extreme state, accommodations can be made so that the patient can communicate.

Generally, patients should communicate the same medical treatment decision over time. Patients with decision-making capacity may change their minds, perhaps even frequently, as new information is presented. However, patients' random responses over time should serve as a warning that the patient may not have decision-making capacity.

A simple analogy to remember the elements of decision-making capacity is a computer that receives information about a problem, compares it against a set of internal values, makes a determination, appreciates the consequences of that determination, and communicates that determination. Of course, human beings are not computers, and their values are not expressed in such a mathematical or strictly logical way. Their family, community, faith, and culture will also influence their values.

Differentiation of Decision-Making Capacity from Competence

Although they may be frequently used interchangeably, the concept of decision-making capacity is different than the term "competence." "Competence" describes the ability to do something effectively. The law presumes that adults are competent to make decisions unless they have been legally determined to be incompetent. A legal determination of incompetence is dependent upon evidence and testimony that the individual is no longer able (or never was able) to make decisions about their personal individual choices, their finances, or both. Once a court rules a person to be incompetent, a guardian or conservator will be appointed to make decisions in the person's best interests.

The differentiation between lack of decision-making capacity in the medical context and incompetence as determined by a court can be illustrated by two examples. In the first instance, a patient who has never been declared legally incompetent may temporarily lose decision-making capacity, for example, a patient who experiences disorientation from a metabolic disease. On the other hand, a patient who has been declared legally incompetent to make financial decisions may still have the capacity to make and express decisions about important medical matters, still retaining the necessary elements of decision-making capacity, and the ability to express preferences to the clinician based on an understanding of the consequences. For example, a patient who has a developmental disability or mental illness, who has a guardian, may still be able to make some medical decisions.

Many clinicians and attorneys use the terms interchangeably, so the HEC member should consider whether the patient has the essential elements of decision-making capacity and should ask the clinician or attorney if the patient has been determined by a court to be incompetent.

Decision-Making Capacity Characteristics

Decision-making capacity is dependent upon patients' abilities, the requirements of the task at hand, and the consequences of the decision. When those consequences are substantial, the need for certainty about the presence of decision-making capacity is even greater. Decision-making capacity is not necessarily established by simply expressing a preference by stating "yes" or "no," because that does not indicate that the patient understands the consequences of the decision. Also, there is no particular "objectively correct" standard delineating what the patient must decide. Patients may make choices that may not be what the majority of people would choose. That does not necessarily mean that the patient lacks capacity. On the other hand, concurrence with the clinician's recommendation is not a sign that the patient has decision-making capacity (President's Commission, 1992, 55–68).

Questions regarding patients' capacity to make medical decisions often arise when a patient chooses a course other than the one the clinician suggests, especially when it is a refusal of recommended treatment (Roth et al., 1977). However, clinicians tend not to question decision-making capacity when the patient agrees with the suggested treatment plan. It is important to note that patients with decision-making capacity are allowed to refuse all treatment, including life-sustaining medical treatment (Cruzan, 1990). Therefore, if a patient makes a choice to refuse a recommended treatment and that refusal might result in the patient's death, the ethical practitioner – and the HEC member – understandably wishes to be sure that the patient's decision is autonomous.

Patients with decision-making capacity may also refuse treatment due to religious beliefs. The ability of patients to choose to forgo life-sustaining medical treatment on the basis of religious beliefs has been affirmed in many legal cases. As an example, adult Jehovah's Witness patients have won the right to refuse life-sustaining blood transfusions.

Determination of Decision-Making Capacity

Who should determine whether a patient possesses decision-making capacity? All clinicians should be able to perform routine capacity assessments. Clinicians perform informal assessments of decision-making capacity during their conversations with patients, noting ability to understand information, reason, and communicate. However, when decision-making is called into question, a formal assessment should be performed. In many cases, the patient's primary clinician may be the best assessor of decision-making capacity, since the evaluation is made in the context of a long-standing relationship with knowledge of the patient's values and goals. For more complex cases, psychiatric or neuropsychological expertise may be necessary. Additionally, when clinicians differ in their evaluations as to whether a patient possesses decision-making capacity, a mental health professional's assessment may be necessary.

At times, HEC members and consultants are asked to give their opinion about a patient's decision-making capacity. HEC members who are clinicians, including those with mental health expertise, may have the skill to assess the patient's decision-making capacity, and may have additional expertise for helpful insight into issues of decision-making capacity that may arise during HEC case deliberations. As well, ethics committee members who are not clinicians may have an opinion based on the apparent presence or absence of the elements of decision-making capacity.

When decision-making capacity is central to the ethical issues at hand, decision-making capacity determination may be best done by a clinician or mental health professional who is not a member of the HEC, so that HEC members may objectively weigh the clinician's evaluation of decision-making capacity in their deliberations.

There is no "gold standard" test for determining decision-making capacity. A common historical test with some correlation to capacity has been the Mini-Mental Status Exam (MMSE), which tests orientation, memory, attention, and reasoning ability (Folstein et al., 1975). MMSE score (range 0–30) has been correlated with clinical judgment of incapacity, with lower scores (generally less than 19) correlated with decreased cognitive function. The MMSE may be helpful in establishing certain cognitive benchmarks, though it may not address critical issues of decision-making capacity, such as the kind of complex reasoning that must occur in an individual considering choices and personal values. One must register and pay a fee for each form in order to use the MMSE, now in its second edition. Another common test for cognition for use with patients without charge is the Montreal Cognitive Assessment (MoCA) tool that also has a 30-point scale (Nasreddine et al., 2005). The Aid to Capacity Evaluation form (ACE) (Joint Centre for Bioethics, n.d.) is designed to test decision-making capacity specifically, with scoring based on the ability to understand the medical problem, the proposed treatment, alternatives, and the consequences of refusal, including withholding or withdrawal. The MacArthur Competence Assessment Tool for Treatment incorporates information for the individual patient's specific medical decision through a structured interview. For patients with dementia, there are special rating scales such as the Dementia Rating Scale and the Alzheimer Disease Rating Scale. Though these instruments have increased the reliability of the evaluation process, there is no clear widely accepted professional standard (Appelbaum, 2007). The Commission on Law and Aging of the American Bar Association has useful resources for clinicians and attorneys about assessment of decision-making capacity (American Bar Association Commission on Law and Aging, 2021).

The most vexing challenges of decision-making capacity may be helped by a formal neuropsychological evaluation, with evaluation of reasoning and problem-solving ability, processing speed, and memory (both short term and long term), visual-spatial organization and visual-motor coordination, and so-called executive function, including the ability to plan, synthesize, and organize. Since decision-making capacity is task-specific, the neuropsychological evaluation can provide supporting evidence and opinion as to the presence or absence of the ability of the patient to make a specific kind of medical decision.

Irrational Choices

Individuals frequently make choices that may not seem logical. For instance, an individual may prefer to drive a long distance rather than go by air travel because of a fear of flying, even though driving the same distance is statistically far more dangerous. Even though patients make illogical choices like this in many domains of life, when making medical decisions with significant life-threatening risks and life-saving benefits, there is an expectation that patients choose carefully, and rationally, in accord with their values. However, their reasoning should be consistent with their own values, and not necessarily with what the majority of society would deem rational. Patients may have their own level of willingness to undergo certain risks. Nonetheless, patients who refuse treatment on the basis of seemingly irrational considerations can present challenges to treatment teams and HEC members, who wish to assure that the refusal is consistent with the individual patient's values. The type of reasoning about these choices can be organized by various categories.

Making a so-called irrational choice can be due to a number of factors, including a bias toward the present and near future (e.g., forgoing injections for a life-threatening problem because of the immediate pain of the injection), unrealistic attitudes toward risk (e.g., forgoing a life-saving operation for appendicitis because of the wish to avoid the extremely minor risks of a reaction to the anesthesia), fear of pain or the medical experience (e.g., forgoing all medical treatment because of fear of hospitals – "that's where people die!"), and "framing effects" where the losses loom larger than gains (e.g., forgoing a life-saving operation for appendicitis because of the wish to avoid the extremely small risk of death from surgery) (Brock and Wartman, 1990).

Clinicians must evaluate decision-making capacity carefully, since the results of an irrational choice may be serious injury, disability, or death. HEC members must weigh carefully the assessment of decision-making capacity, such as in the case example at the beginning of this chapter.

Decision-Making for Those without Decision-Making Capacity

If a patient is determined by a clinician to be incapacitated for the purpose of making medical decisions, who may make decisions for the patient? The standard for decision-making for an incapacitated patient who has never indicated what they would want in the particular circumstances, and who does not have a legislated or court-appointed decision maker to assist in decision-making, is that actions be taken according to the patient's best interests.

If the patient has already been declared incompetent by a court and has an appointed guardian, the guardian may be authorized under state law to make medical decisions for the patient, based on the patient's best interests, or on the wishes expressed by the patient before declaration of incompetence. If the patient does not have a guardian, the patient may have a power of attorney for health care that appoints an agent and may have also included instructions for the agent in the directive. The power of attorney for health care is activated when the patient has lost decision-making capacity. Alternatively, the patient may have a "living will," or "direction to physicians," that expresses the patient's wishes concerning withholding or withdrawing of life-sustaining medical treatment, as well as other wishes, that is activated when the patient has a terminal condition and has lost decision-making capacity (see Chapters 13 and 14 for more information). If none of these exist, there may be a state-authorized hierarchy of individuals who may act as decision maker under the circumstances. If none of the above exist, and a temporary guardian is unable to be appointed in a timely way, physicians and caregivers should identify the person most involved and knowledgeable about the patient's feelings and preferences. Absent the above, a decision should be based on what is determined to be in the patient's best interests.

Common Misunderstandings of Decision-Making Capacity

Decision-making capacity is not an all-or-none phenomenon. Patients who lack decision-making capacity for one healthcare decision do not necessarily lack the ability to make all of them. For example, patients who lack decision-making capacity for complex healthcare decisions may not lack the ability to make other more straightforward healthcare decisions, where the benefits of treatment are great and the burdens and risks are low. This calibration has been described as a "sliding scale" (Buchanan and Brock, 1989).

Cognitive impairment does not automatically entail a lack of decision-making capacity. Decision-making capacity and cognitive ability are related, but not equivalent. Decision-making capacity is the ability to make a particular healthcare decision, while cognitive ability encompasses a broad range of facilities including attention, comprehension, memory, and problem-solving. Tests of cognitive ability alone should not be used as a substitute for decision-making capacity assessment.

A lack of decision-making capacity may not be a permanent condition. Decision-making capacity may wax and wane, or will be temporarily impaired, such as in patients who are experiencing delirium or other temporary disorders of consciousness. For such patients, repeated determination of decision-making capacity should be done at appropriate intervals when the patient's medical condition changes. Importantly, when a patient with an advance directive regains decision-making capacity, the patient is able to make medical decisions, and the patient's advance directive is deactivated.

Appropriate provision of information is crucial for a patient to be able to make medical decisions. Patients should be given relevant information about their treatment on a consistent basis. A patient who can make medical decisions may not be able to do so if there is not enough information, if the information is inconsistent, or given at an inappropriate intellectual level for the patient, or if there are language barriers.

Patients with psychiatric or neurological conditions do not necessarily lack decision-making capacity. Even patients who have dementia or schizophrenia may retain some decision-making capacity. When patients have been involuntarily committed for mental illness because of danger to self or others, these patients typically have lost the ability to make some medical decisions. However, even if patients have been involuntarily committed, they may still retain the legal right to refuse psychotropic medications, unless there is continued imminent danger to themselves or others or a court has ordered otherwise. Nonetheless, despite their ability to refuse psychotropic medications, these patients generally do not have the same ability to refuse continued life-sustaining medical treatment that was implemented to reverse a life-threatening condition the patients intentionally caused when they were under the influence of the mental illness that resulted in their commitment. Nonetheless, patients should be allowed to make those decisions that they can. Even patients who have lost decision-making capacity may still be able to participate in discussion and give their assent (i.e., an agreement to the proposed medical plan or procedure) (Ganzini et al., 2003, 2005).

Minors and Decision-Making Capacity

Adult patients of sound mind are presumed to have the ability to make decisions about their medical treatment. However, minors who are approaching the age of majority present a special challenge. Under state laws, minors of a specified age may consent for certain medical tests and procedures including treatment for sexually transmitted infections (STIs), including testing and treatment for HIV, and for drug and alcohol treatment. The age at which minors are able to consent to make these medical decisions may vary by state. Minors may also be able to consent to treatment for pregnancy, and in some states, may be able to obtain contraception or consent to an abortion.

Most states recognize "emancipated" minors, who may make their own decisions. These minors are deemed by statute as emancipated, sometimes by being married or they may just live apart from their parents and support themselves. Serving in the military may also confer decisional authority to the minor. Additionally, courts may recognize so-called mature minors who may make decisions concerning their medical care. For instance, these mature minors may be able to make organ donations.

In general, minors have a much stronger ability to consent to needed medical treatment without parental consent than to refuse life-sustaining medical treatment. However, there have been some cases in which mature minors have been able to refuse even life-sustaining medical treatment, when the risks or burdens of treatment are significant, and the likelihood of success is not great.

Case Discussion

In the case presented at the beginning of the chapter, the family physician evaluated the patient's decision-making capacity, including her ability to understand the risks and benefits of artificial nutrition and hydration, her ability to evaluate her choice in light of her long-standing values, and to express her choice consistently over time. The HEC considered the physician's assessment and the additional supporting information from her daughter and agreed that this was her mother's autonomous choice. The HEC agreed that, since the patient had decision-making capacity for this medical decision, the patient's wishes should be respected. Oral feedings were intermittently offered to the patient, though consistently refused, and supportive end-of-life care was provided to the patient at home until the patient died.

Conclusion

Many of the ethical issues that HECs and consultation teams face depend upon the patient's autonomous and informed choice with respect to the current medical condition. Because of the vital importance of decision-making capacity in the ability of a patient to exercise autonomy by accepting medical treatment – or refusing it, even if the treatment is life-sustaining – whether the patient is able to make this choice is a crucial determination that has important consequences. The determination of whether a patient has decision-making capacity is critical for the HEC member to be able to make the best ethical recommendations.

Questions for Discussion

1. Conceptual: How should determination of decision-making capacity be made? What are the common approaches used by your healthcare staff?
2. Pragmatic: When does patient decision-making capacity come into question? How is this addressed in your institution?
3. Strategic: When a patient loses decision-making capacity, who should make decisions for the patient and what standard should be used? What are the laws and policies that apply in your institution?

References

American Bar Association Commission on Law and Aging. (2021, April 20). Capacity Assessment. www.americanbar.org/groups/law_aging/resources/capacity_assessment

Appelbaum PS (2007). Assessment of patients' competence to consent to treatment. *New England Journal of Medicine*, 357(18): 1834–1840.

Brock DW, Wartman SA (1990). When competent patients make irrational choices.

New England Journal of Medicine, 322(22): 1595–1599.

Buchanan AE, Brock, DW (1989). *Deciding for Others: The Ethics of Surrogate Decision Making.* Cambridge University Press.

Cruzan v. Director of Missouri Department of Health. (1990), 497 US 261, 110 S.Ct. 2841, 111 L.Ed. 2d. 224.

Derse AR, Schiedermayer DL (2015). *Practical Ethics for Students, Interns & Residents*, 4th ed. Hagerstown, MD: University Publishing Group.

Ganzini L, Volicer L, Nelson W, Derse AR. (2003). Pitfalls in assessment of decision-making capacity. *Psychosomatics*, 44(3): 237–243.

Ganzini L, Volicer L, Nelson WA, Fox E, Derse AR (2005). Ten myths about decision-making capacity. *Journal of the American Medical Directors Association*, 6(3 Suppl.): S100–S104.

Folstein MF, Folstein SE, McHugh PR (1975). "Mini-mental state." A practical method for grading the cognitive state of patients for the clinician. *Journal of Psychiatric Research*, 12(3): 189–198.

Joint Centre for Bioethics. (n.d.). Aid to Capacity Evaluation (ACE). http://128.100 .72.105/tools/documents/ace.pdf

Nasreddine ZS, Phillips NA, Bédirian V, et al. (2005). The Montreal Cognitive Assessment, MoCA: A brief screening tool for mild cognitive impairment. *Journal of the American Geriatrics Society*, 53(4): 695–699.

President's Commission for the Study of Ethical Problems in Medicine and Biomedical and Behavioral Research. (1992). *Making Health Care Decisions*, Vol. 1. https://repository.library .georgetown.edu/handle/10822/559354

Roth LH, Meisel A, Lidz CW (1977). Tests of competency to consent to treatment. *American Journal of Psychiatry*, 134(3): 279–284.

Discharge Challenges
Shifting from Acute to Chronic Care

Wayne Shelton

Upon reading and considering the content of this chapter, the reader should be able to:

1. Anticipate the ethical challenges presented by discharging hospital patients with continuing chronic care needs.
2. Identify and convene relevant stakeholders in the discharge process to assess the needs of a particular patient and the continuing responsibilities of the facility and/or care team.
3. Assess how local or regional resources influence safe placement options.

Case 1

Joe is a 70-year old, alert man admitted for shortness of breath and diagnosed with aspiration pneumonia. Shortly after admission he went into alcohol withdrawal, which required intubation to protect his airway. Within a few days Joe was extubated but remained at risk of aspirating due to dysphagia from alcoholic myopathy. Joe has chronic obstructive pulmonary disease from smoking as well as severe alcohol use disorder. These comorbidities have required multiple admissions and intubations. During multiple admissions he has been determined to have capacity and refused offers to receive outpatient and inpatient treatment for his alcohol use disorder, instead insisting on returning home. Both the care team and his daughter believe nursing home placement would be the prudent option, but he refuses. Joe is determined to have capacity and states he wants to return home.

Case 2

Mary is an 83-year-old woman without capacity, due to advanced vascular dementia who was admitted from home with new onset-weakness and syncope thought to be the result of repeated urinary tract infections (UTI). While hospitalized, tests show the patient recently suffered a small stroke that most likely explains her new symptoms. Within a week she is medically stabilized and ready for discharge. The healthcare team believes she requires a higher level of care than is available living with her husband, Jim, also in his 80s and in declining health. Jim is her caregiver and surrogate decision maker, and he strenuously objects to her going to a rehabilitation facility and wants her to return home where he believes she would rather be. The care team is concerned that the husband may not be able to manage this patient's increasingly complex medical problems that they feel will eventually require full-time nursing care.

> **Case 3**
>
> Dan is a 39-year-old man with a prior medical history of uncontrolled hypertension, cardiomyopathy, and congestive heart failure, requiring an automated implantable cardioverter defibrillator and end-stage renal disease on hemodialysis. He is admitted with culture-negative endocarditis that requires a treatment regimen of 6 weeks of IV antibiotic therapy, twice daily. Dan came to the United States 2 years ago on a 10-year visa, which requires him to return to his home country every 6 months, which he has failed to do. Because he is not a United States citizen, he does not qualify under Federal regulation for free dialysis nor can he be a candidate for kidney transplantation. Dan has no healthcare insurance coverage; however, Emergency Medicaid will cover his dialysis treatments. Normally, a patient with his most recent diagnosis would be discharged to a skilled nursing facility. However, the only way Dan can receive his antibiotic therapy is to remain in the hospital for 6 weeks.

Introduction

An integral part of quality hospital care is the planning involved for the timely and safe discharge of patients once their course of medical treatment requiring hospitalization is complete. In the majority of cases, patients enter the hospital with a medical condition, for which medical goals are established, agreed upon, and accomplished, resulting in a successful discharge. However, in some cases sound discharge planning encounters difficult challenges, including ethical conflicts, particularly in the growing population of patients with complex chronic diseases. Lifestyle-related risk factors such as poor nutrition and lack of exercise, and alcohol and drug use disorders cause, or contribute to many of these illnesses, such as heart and lung disease, obesity, diabetes, and addiction. These patients frequently have difficulty managing their illness and adhering to therapeutic regimens. Other conditions, like various forms of dementia, progressively deprive the individual of the ability to self-manage or participate in treatment.

Regardless, when patients are hospitalized for acute exacerbations of their chronic illnesses, once they no longer need inpatient level of care, a discharge plan is developed. The plan generally includes a need for ongoing medical management, or rehabilitation that either the patient or their professional and personal caregivers provide, or care delivered in some type of nursing care facility. In recent years, ethics consultations have been more involved with discharge planning issues and can help bring to light system problems relating to policies and practices within an institution (Milliken et al., 2018). While these issues have received more attention from professionals and scholars, they remain relatively undeveloped compared to other areas in clinical bioethics (Swidler et al., 2007). This has left many healthcare ethics committees (HECs) to navigate the ethical issues without adequate resources.

Ethically Unproblematic, Yet Challenging Cases

A common type of discharge challenge in large hospitals is when the patient or the patient's surrogate refuses to give permission for the patient to leave the hospital. This is because either the patient does not feel ready to leave or the patient's surrogate simply prefers the patient remain in the hospital longer for various reasons such as convenience or lack of comfort level to leave the hospital. From an ethical and hospital policy perspective, patients do not have the right to remain in the hospital if there is no medical condition requiring hospitalization. However, forcing a patient to leave the hospital against their will or that of a surrogate, even after appeals, is not an easy process. Given the abundant evidence of nosocomial risks (Barnett et al., 2013), physicians have obligations both not to expose their patients to risks from unnecessary hospital days and at the same time to open up beds for a more appropriate patient in need of hospitalization. The former obligation is based on the principles of beneficence and nonmaleficence while the latter is based on the principle of justice. As such, in an era of growing concerns about cost and limited hospital beds, and also the best interest of the patient, there is appropriately less consideration accorded to patient and surrogate preferences in such situations today if the patient clearly is ready for discharge than in previous decades. When the HEC receives a request for ethical guidance on this type of case, in most cases the recommendation should be that patients have no right to remain in the hospital. Because this type of discharge case is relatively clear ethically, it will not be addressed further.

Ethically Problematic Types of Discharges

The focus of the rest of this chapter will be on a set of more ethically problematic discharge challenges that often lead to a request for a clinical ethics consultation. One type occurs when the patient and/or surrogate is not opposed to discharge, but the care team is concerned that the patient's or surrogate's preferred discharge option cannot ensure that the patient's medical management needs will be met satisfactorily. This results in an impasse in the care plan moving forward that both Cases 1 and 2 above demonstrate, albeit with somewhat different concerns. Another common impasse occurs when there are no viable options for placement within the regional healthcare system for an appropriate discharge, which is exemplified in Case 3. We can now move on to explore in greater detail and depth the ethical issues involved in these three cases, beginning with the persistent need to balance patient safety with the patient's (or their surrogate's) preferences and values.

Challenges to a Safe Discharge

Professional care providers have an obligation to ensure a safe discharge plan. Fortunately, most patients, upon discharge, return home where they receive the help and support of their families or other caregivers to meet their medical needs; others, because of lack of family support or more complex medical needs requiring a higher level of care, are more appropriate for a skilled nursing facility or an extended care facility (Alper et al., 2017). Care teams should promote shared decision making by taking into consideration the preferences of patients and/or surrogates about discharge, and make an effort to accommodate them if possible, before a final decision is made. This can be particularly challenging when caring for patients with chronic and comorbid conditions who are at considerable risk for readmission without proper medical management following hospitalization. When there is a failure to reach agreement, the result can be an impasse in the care plan, leading to a request to the HEC for ethical advice.

One persistent problem arises when the individual patient desires to pursue a discharge plan, which appears to the care providers as imprudent, even to the point of being life threatening. In such cases, the care provider obligations to beneficence and nonmaleficence, that is, to do good and do no harm, raise immediate care providers' concerns. But before those concerns can be addressed, care providers must first take into consideration the obligation to respect patient autonomy, which is a paramount principle when patients have decision-making capacity.

Problems with Individual Patients with Decisional Capacity

A common type of discharge planning challenge arises when the patient is generally presumed to have capacity, which implies the obligation to respect the patient's autonomous choices, but is refusing to follow the discharge recommendation of the care team. Instead, the patient prefers an alternative deemed by the team to be unacceptable because of apparent risks relating to the patient's physical inability to act on and carry out their stated goals for the discharge. In the course of doing ethics consultations, it is common to have extended discussions with patients with serious medical or physical conditions who seem very well oriented and generally reasonable, but are insisting on returning home to resume their former life prior to hospitalization. For example, frail elderly patients who are hospitalized because of a fall or a treatable medical condition, such as a UTI or a patient with diabetic ketoacidosis because of poorly managed diabetes, may be ready for discharge medically, but physical and occupational therapists document their inability to perform basic activities of daily living. When such a patient had been living independently prior to hospitalization, even with capacity they might refuse to acknowledge a declining baseline. The idea of going to a nursing home for long-term care may be unacceptable, including even going to a rehabilitation facility for two weeks. Even the prospects of having in-home aids to help provide support and ensure safety with transfers to the bathroom, make meals, etc. may be unacceptable because of the fear of it representing a step toward a loss of independence.

For those patients who continue to have keen mental capacity and can fully articulate the nature of the risks and why their personal goals are important to pursue, respect for patient autonomy must be balanced over and against prudence in the name of the principles of beneficence and nonmaleficence. Care providers, sometimes with the help of the HECs, may engage such patients in discussions and seek compromises. Family members may be particularly helpful in helping their high-risk loved ones come to terms with and accommodate changes in their lives. Still, in spite of everyone's best efforts to discuss and negotiate prudent discharge options, respect for patient autonomy in most cases should remain the guiding principle (Hill and Filer, 2015) because of the importance of individual personal freedom as a foundational value with the US ethical and legal tradition. The clear implication for care providers is that at times a discharge will proceed that the care team is very concerned about and would prefer not to happen.

In Case 1, the care teams at the hospital in charge of Joe's care likely got to know him and documented his declining condition with each admission due to his continuing habits and poor self-management of his medical needs. At each point, capacity was assessed and after excellent medical management by the care team of each acute hospitalization, within a couple of days, his medical condition improved and he was determined to have capacity. For care providers, managing patients with multiple admissions for the same acute problem is enormously challenging. As they bear witness to an individual's nonadherence to appropriate management of their chronic conditions and continual decline, sometimes leading to death, questions may arise about the value of their efforts and the goals they are attempting to accomplish. Given the prevailing ethical and legal requirement to respect the preferences of patients with capacity, when Joe is ready for discharge, care providers should view their efforts to provide him with opportunities to deal with his underlying problems, such as addiction treatments, utilizing more home care resources, and organizing family and community support, as an appropriate and valuable professional response to a complex problem. Finally, care providers also need support from each other and hospital resources, including HECs, so as to avoid moral distress and burnout.

Problems with Incapable Patients with Strong Dispositions

Many patients who are determined to lack capacity are unable to express any disposition to act cooperatively or not toward the recommended care plan, regarding either medical treatment or discharge planning options. However, some patients lacking capacity are alert and have strong dispositions against certain treatment or discharge planning options, which can create challenging situations for care teams. Generally speaking, care providers, surrogates, and family members of such patients should strive to gain cooperation and assent from such patients. But how to manage cases where all efforts to gain cooperation and assent have failed can become a difficult ethical problem, on which HECs and ethics consultants will likely be helpful.

When care providers and surrogates consider requiring patients without capacity to comply with a recommended discharge plan over their strong refusal, the guiding principle of respect for patient autonomy does not apply, at least not in a straightforward way. This should not mean that an ethical justification is not required to force the patient to adhere to the recommended plan. The patient is still a person who requires compassionate care and deserves a plan based on balancing the principles of beneficence and nonmaleficence in relation to the intensity of the patient's resistance against, and difficulty the care providers would have imposing, the recommended plan. Otherwise, the patient could be easily traumatized and harmed, emotionally and even physically. Specifically, it becomes necessary to do a benefit/harm analysis, which means considering the benefit or goal of patient adherence to the plan in relation to the anticipated harm caused by forcing adherence. It will be instructive to see how Case 1 might play out in the event that Joe's medical condition continued to deteriorate.

As was previously stated, patients like Joe may continue to decline. For example, let's assume Joe's condition deteriorates due to continued alcohol use and he is now diagnosed with Wernicke-Korsakoff Syndrome, which is a new level of physical and mental debilitation. Because he lacks capacity to make his own decisions for the foreseeable future and possibly permanently, his ability to self-govern, that is, to carry out his own life plan, has become considerably more diminished. This means that his surrogates will understandably have grave reservations about following their normal role responsibility to honor his prior wishes and allow him to care for himself and live independently. Doing so would no doubt lead the patient to experience considerable harm and possibly death. Concerns about the potential harm that would likely accrue from following his wishes would likely outweigh concerns about the moral harms of overriding his disposition against the recommended placement option. Therefore, a strong case can be made that the principles of beneficence and nonmaleficence should be given greater weight than respect for patient autonomy. Regardless, care providers and his surrogates should only force Joe to go to a facility over his refusal after all other support options for him to return home have been explored and failed. A patient's financial and insurance status will be significant factors in determining the available resources that would match his level of care needs.

Problems with Surrogate Decision Makers

When patients with chronic problems and who permanently lack capacity come to the hospital for acute medical problems, they require a surrogate decision maker to help make medical and discharge planning decisions. For diagnoses like Alzheimer's disease, a progressive, neurodegenerative disease, the prognosis is generally well known. The patient with this disease has a terminal illness and will continue to decline mentally and physically, eventually being unable to feed themselves and will require continual nursing care, including managing end-of-life comfort care and decision-making.

Turning to Case 2, the medical team learns during her hospitalization that Mary's overall health is deteriorating, as is evidenced by more frequent UTIs, increased general weakness, and a recent myocardial infarction. Mary is likely entering the final stages of Alzheimer's disease, which means her nursing care will grow more intense and constant, and will eventually include end-of-life, comfort care. This deterioration in Mary's condition will greatly shape the type of setting in which her medical needs can be adequately and safely met and the specific discharge planning recommendations her care team will make.

As we have already learned, surrogate decision makers can be the foci of discharge problems, for example insisting the patient remain in the hospital longer than their care providers deem appropriate, making unreasonable demands for the discharge to be within narrow geographic limits, or even undermining viable options (Jankowski et al., 2009). It can be assumed that when the surrogate decision maker acts to obstruct the timely and appropriate discharge of the patient, efforts should be taken to negotiate solutions and, if necessary, to take decisive action, such as to appoint another surrogate or discharge the patient over the surrogate's objections. HECs can be helpful both in the negotiation process and in the clarification of the ethical justification based on hospital policy, in cases of discharging the patient without the surrogate decision maker's agreement.

Since Mary cannot participate actively in the discharge planning decision, her husband, Jim, is the first choice to assume the role of her surrogate decision maker. Whatever decision is made about Mary's discharge, whether returning back home or to a nursing home, Jim's consent will be necessary.

As the care team learns more about Jim and his situation at home, they gain a clearer understanding of Jim's marginal ability to meet the daunting challenge of continuing to care for Mary. Jim's health is also declining, yet he understandably wants to maintain his independence and care for his wife, a plan they had often discussed and agreed upon. Like most elderly caregivers of individuals with dementia, Jim is at considerable risk himself for serious health problems, which could easily become debilitating. Though an ethical perspective must also consider the application of beneficence and nonmaleficence to Jim, he is a fully capable moral agent who is clearly expressing both his own and Mary's prior wish for her to return home so they can resume their previous life. He understands that he is getting old and there are risks associated with his plan, but, still, he wants to pursue it. Often in such situations the care team can involve family members and friends, to monitor the situation, engage additional community resources, and, depending on Jim's financial resources, recruit additional nursing support to ease the burden on him. In the end, if the care team has attempted to maximize safety and minimize harm for both Mary and Jim, they must respect Jim's decision to return Mary home under his care.

System Problems in Discharge Planning

Up to this point, discharge planning issues have focused exclusively on the rights and obligations of the actors (patients and surrogate decision makers) in individual cases. Now, attention will turn to a consideration of the complications created in individual cases due to the limitation of resources of the healthcare system in which discharge planning decisions must be made.

Increasingly, HECs will be asked for input on these systems issues at the level of policy and organizational ethics. The basic question is, are patients being given the care options they deserve and, some would say, they have a right to? Common problems include situations where the patient and/or the surrogate decision makers agree that discharge should happen as soon as possible but there are concerns about the available resources and options. For example, some patients or surrogates may have concerns over the quality of care in certain nursing homes and request another option that is not available. Even though the concerns being expressed about a certain facility may not be unreasonable, a patient's or surrogate's right to refuse to leave the hospital is limited. If the patient is ready for discharge and the patient or surrogate disagrees with the only available discharge plan, they may appeal; if they lose, as many do, they may be presented with a hospital-issued notice of noncoverage and become financially responsible for the patient's hospitalization.

Another problem that is also common is the concern being expressed by a surrogate decision maker or family member about the distance of a facility from their home and the difficulty involved in visiting the patient. If a patient needs a specialized service in the state in which the hospital is located, for example a facility that accepts chronically ill patients requiring long-term, ventilatory support or certain types of rehabilitation services for complex needs, the only available and viable discharge option may be well outside the geographical location of the patient's family and friends. In such cases, it should not be assumed that the patient or family is making unreasonable requests. Their concerns should be taken seriously and accommodated when possible, but any solution is almost always a matter of negotiation, which may be part of an ethics consultation. As is obvious, the root problem is the shortage of resources within the overall system, which impinges upon options in individual cases. The root problem of the shortage of resources within the overall system raises justice and fairness concerns that must be addressed at the public policy level (Schlairet, 2013).

Some of the complications created by limited resources within the healthcare system may become ethical crises for local hospitals, when there are no available resources to meet patient needs. No situation exemplifies this situation more poignantly than cases involving undocumented patients with complex and chronic medical problems (Parsi, 2012). In Case 3, Dan's current acute medical problem requires 6 weeks of IV antibiotic therapy, twice daily. Because he did not comply with his visa requirements to return to his home country every 6 months, he is not a candidate for kidney transplantation and healthcare insurance. The healthcare system does cover his dialysis, but he is not eligible to be discharged to a facility where his life-saving antibiotic therapy can be administered. The hospital is left with a highly vulnerable human being who will die if his acute medical problem resulting from his unmanaged chronic condition is not treated.

A basic ethical perspective of medical care is to show respect to all patients and promote access to health care, even in opposition to the public's unwillingness to support their healthcare needs (American Medical Association, 2021). Thus, notwithstanding Dan's lack of citizenship and medical coverage, the hospital hardly has any viable ethical option but to find a way to keep him in the hospital and administer the necessary antibiotic therapy. Hospitals that fulfill their ethical obligation to care for patients in such situations place themselves at financial and perhaps even legal risk, which may result in acts of civil disobedience (Essex and Isaacs, 2018). HECs consulting on these cases usually advise that all reasonable efforts be made to show respect for the patient and provide necessary medical care that benefits the patient. Yet, Dan's case raises many complex policy issues.

For example, a noncitizen patient with a terminal or untreatable condition may require extended hospitalization, which is one of many present-day burdens that challenge the hospital's capability to provide care to its service area. As healthcare costs are expected to increase and the future of the healthcare system in the United States remains uncertain, hospitals are in a precarious position. An ethical analysis at the policy level must balance the obligation to treat all patients with respect consistent with the proportional obligation to ensure that hospitals remain viable institutions able to fulfill their mission.

Conclusion

Ethical issues in discharge planning are common in today's healthcare system, and more so with patients with complex, chronic medical problems. Often requests for ethics consultations include discharge planning challenges. HECs and ethics consultation services must be prepared to grapple with the range of issues and questions they present.

Questions for Discussion

1. Conceptual: Discharge is often complicated when patients lack capacity or when they have long-term, chronic care issues that require higher levels of care than most home health and families can handle. As such, discharging patients poses many logistical challenges that might be better handled by case management, rather than HECs. What, then, are some ethical issues raised in challenging discharge cases?
2. Pragmatic: Given the ethical issues identified in answering the "conceptual" question, what practices or policies in your institution are implicated?
3. Strategic: In light of these practices and policies, what might the HEC suggest in order to mitigate proactively downstream ethical challenges to discharge?

References

Alper E, O'Malley TA, Greenwald J (2017). Hospital discharge and readmission. www .uptodate.com/contents/hospital-discharge- and-readmission

American Medical Association. (2021). AMA Principles of Medical Ethics. www.ama- assn.org/about/publications-newsletters/ ama-principles-medical-ethics

Barnett AG, Page K, Campbell M, et al. (2013). The increased risks of death and extra lengths of hospital and ICU stay from hospital-acquired bloodstream infections: A case–control study. *BMJ Open*, 3(10). doi .org/10.1136/bmjopen-2013-003587

Essex R, Isaacs D (2018). The ethics of discharging asylum seekers to harm: A case from Australia. *Bioethical Inquiry*, 15(1): 39–44.

Hill J, Filer W (2015). Safety and ethical considerations in discharging patients to suboptimal living situations. *AMA Journal of Ethics*, 17(6): 506–510.

Jankowski J, Seastrum T, Swidler RN, Shelton W (2009). For lack of a better plan: A framework for ethical, legal, and clinical challenges in complex inpatient discharge planning. *HEC Forum*, 21(4): 311–326.

Milliken A, Jurchak M, Sadovnikoff N (2018). When societal structural issues become patient problems: The role of clinical ethics consultation. *Hastings Center Report*, 48(5): 7–9.

Parsi K (2012). Complex discharges and undocumented patients: Growing ethical concerns. *The Journal of Clinical Ethics*, 23 (4): 299–307.

Schlairet MC (2013). Complex hospital discharges: Justice considered. *HEC Forum*, 26(1): 69–78.

Swidler RS, Seastrum T, Shelton W (2007). Difficult inpatient discharge decisions: Ethical, legal, and clinical practice issues. *The American Journal of Bioethics*, 7(3): 23–28.

Chapter 13

Surrogate Decision Making

Thomas V. Cunningham

Objectives

Upon reading and considering the content of this chapter, the reader should be able to:

1. Explain the foundations of surrogate decision-making for incapacitated, hospitalized patients.
2. Describe how healthcare ethics committees (HECs) can support surrogate decision-making through attention to organizational ethics, educational programming, and ethics consultation that includes quality review.
3. Identify who is responsible for determining surrogate decision makers and consider how understanding surrogates' experiences can improve practices involving surrogates.

Case

Mrs. McGuire is an 85-year-old woman with three adult children (Eric, Terry, and Marion) who lives in an assisted living facility (ALF). She was admitted to the hospital 8 days ago for worsening back pain and trouble walking. On clinical exam, she was diagnosed with a large right breast mass. Concerned that she may have a spinal tumor and that aggressive treatment may not benefit Mrs. McGuire, her physician requested a consult from a palliative care physician. The palliative care physician proposed a dobutamine stress echocardiogram to evaluate Mrs. McGuire for palliative spinal surgery. But when she was being moved to the operating room, Mrs. McGuire refused to be transferred while she was noted by a nurse to be "alert and oriented." So, the surgery was canceled. The palliative care physician is concerned that Mrs. McGuire can neither consent to nor refuse medical care. She is also unclear who would be responsible for making decisions for Mrs. McGuire if she cannot make her own decisions. Eric has visited his mother throughout her hospitalization. He often appears disheveled and angry, to an extent that he has been described as "confrontational" in the medical record. Social work notes indicate that Marion (daughter) interacts routinely with ALF staff, including paying for Mrs. McGuire's care, although she lives far away. Terry visits his mother once a year and also lives across the country from her.[1]

---

[1] Mrs. McGuire's case is abbreviated from the American Society for Bioethics and Humanities (ASBH)'s study guide (ASBH, 2017, 23–29; used with permission). Readers are encouraged to consult the full case there, because it provides a more nuanced description of a case of surrogate decision-making, complementing the information covered in this chapter.

Why Do We Need Surrogate Decision Makers and How Do We Choose Them?

Mrs. McGuire's situation is common. Estimates suggest about 40% of adult hospitalized patients and residential hospice patients lack decisional capacity, necessitating that someone be identified to make medical decisions for them (DeMartino et al., 2017). Choosing the right person for this job can be complicated. Healthcare providers (HCPs) will know what therapies or interventions may be possible for a given condition but are unlikely to know what the patient would choose based on their values, goals, and priorities. And in a case like Mrs. McGuire's, where there are multiple adult children variously involved in her care, it is also difficult to know whom to ask to get this information. This compounding of uncertainty – what the patient would choose and who should make decisions when they cannot – serves as the foundation for the concept of norms governing surrogate decision-making.

Conceptual Background

Our contemporary understanding of surrogate decision-making is based in legal precedent and bioethical theory. All state laws cover surrogate decision-making to some extent. Yet, crucially, terminology defining the surrogate role is routinely internally inconsistent (within a state) and externally inconsistent (compared with nearby states). There are no standard legal definitions of important concepts, like the qualities a person should exhibit when acting as a surrogate, whether an appointed surrogate's authority can be restricted by the hospital or courts, who can act as a surrogate when no qualified person can be identified (so called "unrepresented" patients), and how to mitigate conflict between potential surrogates. For example, over 30 states require that a surrogate be able to "engage in complex medical decision making" and that a surrogate be "willing to act" in the role; yet no states define how an HCP may assess the ability to engage in complex decision making or willingness to act (DeMartino et al., 2017, 1479). Furthermore, fewer than 40 states describe a *surrogacy hierarchy* delineating an ordered list of candidate surrogates to be reviewed when identifying and assessing potential surrogates. In most states this list includes spouses, adult children, and parents. Yet, while in some instances such a list includes a domestic partner or loved one who is not a relative by law or birth, other states omit statutory language recognizing such persons as qualified candidate surrogates.

Traditional bioethical theory regarding surrogate decision-making distinguishes among types of principles: intervention principles, authority principles, and guidance principles (Buchanan and Brock, 1989, 87–89). *Intervention principles* apply in situations where it is believed appropriate to remove or limit the authority of (candidate) surrogate decision makers and provide ethical constraints on interventions to challenge that authority, such as by the courts, representatives of government protection agencies, or HCPs. *Authority principles* provide means of specifying who is the appropriate authority to make decisions for incapacitated patients and on what grounds, prior to and independent from, any intervention to challenge the authority. What matters most for HEC members are the *guidance principles*, which provide a framework for determining how someone with decision-making authority should make decisions for an incapacitated patient.

The three guidance principles are often referred to as a hierarchy of *standards*: The *stated wishes standard* guides surrogates to make decisions based on the wishes the previously competent patient conveyed in a legally valid document, like an advance directive. The *substituted judgment standard* guides the surrogate to make a choice consistent with what the patient would choose, were the patient capable of making the decision, knowing what the surrogate knows about the patient's values, diagnosis, and prognosis. This standard guides the surrogate to imagine what the patient would choose and then to make that choice, regardless of whether the surrogate themself agrees with the values projected on to the patient and the choice following from them. The final standard is the *best interest* standard, which guides the surrogate to choose a treatment plan that is in the patient's best interests.

Determining which of the three guidance principles should be applied in practice requires assessing the amount of evidence available concerning the patient's healthcare values and preferences (Buchanan and Brock, 1989, 93–134). The stated wishes standard requires the most evidence, because it requires valid, documented evidence of the patient's stated values, either specifically about the treatments under consideration or about who the patient authorizes to speak for them if incapacitated. When such documentation is lacking, but where loved ones have credible information about the patient's values (such as from conversations with the patient prior to losing capacity), the substituted judgment standard should be used. Lastly, when there little or no testimonial evidence regarding the patient's values, the best interest standard is appropriate, and decisions should be made in accordance with what a "reasonable person" would want under the circumstances. When surrogates deviate from these standards, HCPs may guide them to perform their roles in ways more closely approximating them or consider intervening to shift authority to another decision maker.

Although the theory of a hierarchy of standards may be described concisely, the actual practice of decision-making for incapacitated patients is often more complicated than the concise picture lets on. For instance, it can be difficult to assess the validity of claims made by family members, surrogates, or healthcare professionals about patients' previously stated wishes. Some patients may complete multiple advance directives, living wills, or other documents that capture their values (such as a Physician Order for Life Sustaining Treatment, or POLST; see Chapter 14). Sometimes different HCPs will document different conversations in the medical record that suggest the patient's values have changed over time or were less clear or consistent than they appear in other documents. In these situations, it may be useful during an ethics consult to analyze the different documents and discern a narrative that, if attributed to the patient, forges agreement between these seemingly inconsistent interpretations of the patient's values. Another approach is instead to accept that the patient's stated wishes are inconsistent and then to move from utilizing the stated wishes standard to the substituted judgment standard, relying on the patient's designated or appointed surrogate to adjudicate the apparent conflicts between the patient's documented values.

Yet, evaluating how well surrogates are making substituted judgments may also be difficult in practice. While it might be expected that surrogates will make substituted judgments based on their knowledge of the patient's values, sometimes statements made by other people close to the patient or information in the medical record suggest that the surrogate believes the patient holds values that differ from those indicated by other information sources. In these situations, it can be difficult to distinguish whether this is because the surrogate harbors different beliefs about the patient's values than others do or that the surrogate is making decisions based on their own values, rather than on the patient's values.

Similarly, various difficulties arise when trying to make decisions for patients using the best interest standard. Since this standard presupposes little to no evidence is available to support claims about the patient's values, decision makers using this standard cannot refer to the patient's values to justify choosing one treatment pathway over another. In practice it can be hard to determine what is "best" or what a "reasonable person" would choose among available options without feeling like one is selecting the option that is preferred by the attending physician or medical team. One strategy for overcoming this predicament is to form a multidisciplinary group to support such decisions, and to involve HEC members who are community members in them (Pope et al., 2020). Ideally, including more perspectives in these decisions and a lay point of view increases the likelihood that different considerations of what is "best" for the patient in their circumstances will enter into the discussion, and that the procedural nature of those discussions will increase the chance that what is chosen as the "best" option is in fact best or at least one of the equally "best" options conceivable.

What Is It Like to Be a Surrogate Decision Maker?

As with all decision-making in health care, surrogates should engage with HCPs in *shared decision-making*: "[A] collaborative process that allows patients, or their surrogates, and clinicians to make healthcare decisions together, taking into account the best scientific evidence available, as well as the patient's values, goals, and preferences" (Kon et al., 2016, 190). A crucial component of shared decision-making for incapacitated patients is recognizing how profound the surrogate experience can be when supporting ethical medical decision-making. Scholarship on the surrogate experience indicates that being a family member or surrogate of a seriously ill patient is emotionally and cognitively demanding. Participating in surrogate decision-making is also burdensome, negatively impacting the way people think and interact with others (Wendler and Rid, 2011). Unlike healthcare professionals, surrogate decision makers are often unfamiliar with serious illness. In some cases, their loved one has been sick for some time, but has not disclosed the severity of their illness to their loved ones. Surrogates often also have not discussed their loved one's healthcare values with them. And even if they are informed, this may be the first time someone so close to them has been so ill. For this reason, surrogates may be confused, have trouble processing the information they receive, or show signs of not remembering or being in denial, as they are working through their surprise and grief over their loved one's predicament while also learning how to be a decision maker.

Thinking like a surrogate decision maker is also difficult and strange. In real time, a surrogate is undergoing their own experience, responding to her loved one's hospitalization. Yet, when participating in decision-making according to the substituted judgment standard, they also must think about how the patient would make decisions and separate the patient's point of view from their own. A surrogate decision maker is asked to *think for someone else* while at the same time reacting to all of the difficult information that comes along with having someone you love hospitalized and incapacitated. This cognitive distancing – thinking *for* an incapacitated person – is an inherently difficult thing to do, especially if the surrogate has not been educated about how to play the surrogate role by an HCP. Surrogates may struggle to understand this task and perform it well, causing them to assume patients have values they do not have and to make decisions that are not supported by patients' actual preferences (Shalowitz et al., 2006).

Additionally, surrogates may experience poor communication with members of the medical team, which research shows is exacerbated for Black patients and families (Welch et al., 2005) and likely other people of color. When poor communication occurs, surrogates can feel like they must make profound choices based on communications that are perceived as unsatisfying or suspect. National guidelines suggest ways to overcome this problem, including intentionally supporting family members during communication with them, using structured approaches to communication, and involving HCPs specially trained to improve communication, such as ethics consultants (Davidson et al., 2017).

Surrogates are also often involved in uncomfortable family dynamics when making medical decisions. Even in healthy family relationships, surrogates are often identified as spokespersons for a family, meaning they become responsible for communicating to family members what happens in the hospital. This is a position of familial authority that brings along expectations of attentiveness to other family members' emotional experiences. In situations where there is family conflict regarding the decision, or where some family members are estranged, the burdens of being a surrogate decision maker increase tremendously. These dynamics may lead surrogates to experience symptoms associated with post-traumatic stress disorder (Wendler and Rid, 2011).

How Can Ethics Committees Support Surrogate Decision-Making?

There is considerable room for creativity and ingenuity for the enterprising HEC chair or member to increase attention to surrogate decision-making, especially coupled with a patient-centered approach to care or organizational ethics. Here we cover three broad areas that often overlap in practice.

Organizational Priorities

A practical approach to organizational prioritization conversations is to begin by discussing surrogate decision-making at a regular HEC meeting. The committee could review a case from the hospital's ethics consult service or published in the literature, discuss hospital policies or state laws concerning surrogate decision-making, or all of these things. The point is to initiate a sustained dialogue about the topic, so that the committee can assess whether there are any needs for improving hospital practices. This "needs assessment" may span multiple HEC meetings. Once the committee better understands the hospital's needs regarding surrogate decision-making, then hospital administrators can be invited to an HEC meeting for a presentation on the hospital's needs, allowing the HEC to influence priority setting.

A similar opportunity for influencing hospital priorities may arise if hospitals leaders identify advance care planning (see Chapter 14) as a priority. For example, if they prioritize advance care planning, hospital leaders may use measures to assess whether advance care planning is improving, such as the number of advance directives completed monthly or annually. In this type of situation, the HEC can contribute to priority setting by thinking critically about the relationship between completing advance directives and supporting surrogate decision-making. Good decisions are aided by high quality advance directives when the patient's actual values and preferences are recorded in an unbiased way, the patient authentically selects and records who their agent(s) should be, and the legal document is validly authorized by a notary public or witnesses. Such advance directives support surrogates and members of the medical team by aiding them in identifying and agreeing on the patient's values and preferences, clarifying who the patient chose as their agent(s) if they became incapacitated, and confirming that these choices were recorded in a legally authoritative way. Lower quality advance directives, lacking one or more of these criteria, are more likely to generate or sustain decision-making conflict and uncertainty over whether ethical medical decision-making is occurring. When advance directives lack one or more of the elements of 'high quality' noted above, they are more likely to generate conflicts and uncertainty about end-of-life decisions needing to be made for the patient. Through explaining this concern to hospital leaders, HECs could play a role in improving organizational ethics.

Educational Programming

Either in concert with efforts to influence organizational priorities or independent from them, another approach to supporting surrogate decision-making for incapacitated, hospitalized patients is through educational programming across the hospital (see Chapter 28). Many topics relate to surrogate decision-making, including capacity assessment, documentation of surrogate selection, advance care planning, conflict resolution, ethics consultation, legal guidance, and bioethical theory. Depending upon the frequency of HEC educational programming, these can serve as a foundation for a series of presentations over time or can be combined into a single, longer educational program. Once the curriculum is developed, it may also be given to departments piecemeal or in groups.

The topic of surrogate decision-making is also well suited to a journal club for the HEC or other groups that meet regularly, such as a critical care committee. For advanced audiences, the HEC should consider performing ongoing literature reviews as there continue to be new developments in clinical practices and occasional changes in local laws. Professional bodies in medicine routinely update their guidance on topics that bear on surrogate decision-making. Scholars continue to improve our understanding of the surrogate experience and how HCPs can change practices to improve it. A journal club format creates a means for regularly reviewing such changes in professional recommendations or improvements in practices, which then creates organizational momentum for reviewing and optimizing hospital policies and procedures for surrogate decision-making to increase alignment with them.

Ethics Consultation and Quality Review

A primary responsibility of HECs is to support ethics consultation (see Chapters 7 and 8). Although limited data are available, what we know suggests that issues surrounding surrogate decision-making lay behind a significant proportion of requests for ethics consultations. In a study of 372 consults in one health system over 3 years, the author found that about 36% of consults arose from concerns about surrogate decision-making (19.1%) or decisional capacity (17.1%; Homan, 2018, 86). Another study, looking at

703 consults at two separate institutions over 2 years, found that about 28% of their consults stemmed from issues regarding surrogate decision-making (Harris et al., 2020). Therefore, it is reasonable for HECs that are responsible for clinical ethics consultation to be prepared for consults regarding surrogate decision-making and related issues.

In addition to being ready to perform ethics consultation concerning issues associated with surrogate decision-making, HECs should also undertake some type of quality assessment of ethics consultations they provide (Cunningham et al., 2019; see Chapter 30). In doing this, the HEC could assess how well the ethics consultant (or team) described the different standards for surrogate decision-making and recommended that the correct standard be applied, given the amount of evidence for the patient's values and preferences that was available at the time of the consult. The HEC could also review how well the surrogate experience was considered and documented during the shared decision-making process. Other ethical issues commonly related to surrogate decision-making could also be focused on during quality assessment of ethics consults, as they arise, such as capacity assessment, whether a patient is unrepresented, the potential for implicit bias in decision-making, the validity or applicability of advanced care planning documents, and family or provider conflict. Once quality assessment of ethics consultation activities is complete, it can be used for setting priorities within the ethics committee or at the organizational level.

Conclusion

The concepts defined in this chapter provide a means for understanding Mrs. McGuire's circumstances in terms of surrogate decision-making. First, knowing the conceptual background helps us see that a central issue in Mrs. McGuire's case is that the HCPs involved have not assessed her capacity and have not determined who is the appropriate decision-making authority. Second, knowing this, an ethics consultant or HEC member involved in a consult could aid the medical team in recognizing who has what responsibilities for assessing capacity, appointing a surrogate, communicating with the family and surrogate, and supporting the surrogate as they make decisions. Third, understanding the surrogate's experience helps a consultant or HEC member frame the work to be done when supporting shared decision-making with surrogates for incapacitated patients.

Questions for Discussion

1. Conceptual: What framework (e.g., ethical, legal, practical) should we use to characterize how to involve surrogates in ethical medical decisions?
2. Pragmatic: Considering the relationships between Mrs. McGuire's children and the healthcare team as an example, how should we determine those conflict pertaining to surrogate decision-making and begin working toward its resolution?
3. Strategic: What can the HEC do to evaluate whether the organization is sufficiently aware of and responsive to issues regarding surrogate decision-making?

References

American Society for Bioethics and Humanities [ASBH], Clinical Ethics Consultation Affairs Committee. (2017). *Addressing Patient-Centered Ethical Issues in Health Care: A Case-Based Study Guide.* Chicago: ASBH.

Buchanan AE, Brock DW (1989). *Deciding for Others: The Ethics of Surrogate Decision Making.* Cambridge University Press.

Cunningham TV, Chatburn A, Coleman C, et al. (2019). Comprehensive quality assessment in clinical ethics. *The Journal of Clinical Ethics,* 30(3): 284–296.

Davidson JE, Aslakson RA, Long AC, et al. (2017). Guidelines for family-centered care in the neonatal, pediatric, and adult ICU. *Critical Care Medicine,* 45(1): 103–128.

DeMartino ES, Dudzinkski D, Doyle CK, et al. (2017). Who decides when a patient can't? Statutes on alternate decision makers. *New England Journal of Medicine,* 376(15): 1478–1482.

Harris KW, Cunningham TV, Hester DM, et al. (2020, November). Comparison is not a zero-sum game: Exploring advanced measures of healthcare ethics consultation. *AJOB Empirical Bioethics E-pub.*

Homan ME (2018). Factors associated with the timing and patient outcomes of clinical ethics consultation in a Catholic health care system. *The National Catholic Bioethics Quarterly,* 18(1): 71–92.

Kon AA, Davidson JE, Morrison W, Danis M, White DB. (2016). Shared decision making in intensive care units: An American college of critical care medicine and American Thoracic Society policy statement. *Critical Care Medicine,* 44(1): 188–201.

Pope TM, Bennett J, Carson SS, et al. (2020). Making medical treatment decisions for unrepresented patients in the ICU: An official American Thoracic Society/American Geriatrics Society policy statement. *American Journal of Respiratory and Critical Care Medicine,* 201(10): 1182–1192.

Shalowitz DI, Garrett-Mayer E, Wendler D. (2006). The accuracy of surrogate decision makers: A systematic review. *Archives of Internal Medicine,* 166(5): 493–497.

Welch LC, Teno JM, Mor V (2005). End-of-life care in black and white: Race matters for medical care of dying patients and their families. *Journal of the American Geriatrics Society,* 53(7): 1145–1153.

Wendler D, Rid A (2011). Systematic review: The effect on surrogates of making treatment decisions for others. *Annals of Internal Medicine,* 154(5): 336–346.

Chapter

14
Advance Care Planning and End-of-Life Decision-Making

Nancy M. P. King and John C. Moskop

Objectives

Upon reading and considering the content of this chapter, the reader should be able to:

1. Identify key moral concepts in the care of patients near the end of life.
2. Describe the process of advance care planning and explain how it helps prevent moral conflicts in end-of-life care.
3. Examine the main types of advance directives and portable medical orders for end-of-life care, and understand how they help guide treatment decisions.
4. Identify continuing challenges in making and implementing end-of-life treatment decisions.

Case

Joan Thompson, a nurse in the cardiology unit, requests an ethics consultation regarding the care of her patient, Mrs. Mary Wilson. Seventy-eight-year-old Mrs. Wilson was diagnosed with congestive heart failure 4 years ago; her condition has worsened gradually since then. She was admitted to the hospital 2 days ago with symptoms of shortness of breath, recurrent chest pain, fatigue, and confusion. This is her third hospitalization in the past 6 months. Mrs. Wilson's difficulty in breathing has persisted despite drug therapy, and Dr. Kelly, Mrs. Wilson's cardiologist, is preparing to intubate her and provide mechanical ventilation. Mrs. Wilson has confided to Ms. Thompson, however, that she does not want to be on a ventilator again, and wants only treatments to relieve her pain and allow her to rest. Ms. Thompson has observed that Dr. Kelly is reluctant to discuss palliative care with his patients and to write do-not-attempt-resuscitation (DNAR) orders. She is concerned that Mrs. Wilson's wishes are not being respected.

Introduction

Mrs. Wilson's case exemplifies one kind of disagreement about treatment near the end of life that occurs frequently in hospitals and often prompts a request for ethics consultation. There are several reasons for the frequent resort to ethics consultation in these situations. The values at stake, including freedom from suffering and disability and prolongation of life, are significant. In addition, treatment choices are often complex, offering uncertain benefits and burdens. Finally, as the long, public, and bitter legal battle over the care of Terri Schiavo made clear, Americans hold strong and divergent views about which life-sustaining treatments should, and should not, be pursued (Gostin, 2005). In this chapter, we explain that advance care planning and attention to goals of

121

care can prevent or ameliorate much uncertainty and conflict over treatment decisions near the end of life.

Advance Care Planning

As the introductory case suggests, there is significant potential for uncertainty and disagreement about treatment decisions near the end of life. People who recognize the moral significance of these decisions can be encouraged to reflect on them in advance, to formulate preferences, and to communicate those preferences to others. This approach, called advance care planning, provides guidance for end-of-life treatment decisions and may help prevent confusion and conflict about them.

A highly effective advance care planning process should include the following six steps:

1. People engaged in advance care planning ("planners") must *recognize* that there are important treatment choices to be made as they approach the end of life and that they can express treatment preferences in advance.
2. Planners must *learn* about these end-of-life treatment options and about available methods for communicating their treatment preferences.
3. Planners can *discuss* these treatment options with others and *reflect* on what options embody their own values and goals.
4.. As a result of this discussion and reflection, planners can *make decisions* about their preferences for end-of-life care.
5. Planners can *communicate* these decisions to loved ones and healthcare providers, so that they are known. Planners can use several types of documents for this communication, including *advance directives* and *portable physician orders for life-sustaining treatment.*
6. Planners can *review* their decisions periodically and, if desired, change their plans for end-of-life care (Moskop, 2016, 216–217).

When patients have questions about advance care planning or end-of-life care options, healthcare ethics committee (HEC) members may be called upon to assist in any of these steps.

Advance care planning can improve treatment decisions near the end of life in several ways. It can help people overcome initial barriers of ignorance and avoidance of end-of-life issues, formulate clear preferences for care, and communicate those preferences to others. Clear evidence of a person's treatment preferences can minimize uncertainty and disagreement about what treatment plan to pursue. HECs can then help surrogate decision makers and healthcare professionals honor the patient's preferences even after the patient has lost decision-making capacity.

General Considerations for Ethics Committees

Many features of end-of-life decision making raise moral questions for patients, families, and healthcare providers. Because decisions about treatments for patients approaching the end of life fall within the broader domain of healthcare decision-making, many concepts and issues in healthcare ethics have special relevance near the end of life. First, the moral and legal concept of *informed consent* (see Chapter 7) is central to end-of-life treatment. The duty to obtain the patient's informed consent to treatment emerged in the latter half of the twentieth century as the primary mechanism to enable patients to participate more actively in decisions about their care, thereby respecting their autonomy as moral agents and also promoting their well-being. Court decisions in the USA from Quinlan (1976) to Cruzan (1990) applied the concept of informed consent and its corollary, *informed refusal of treatment*, to the care of critically ill and profoundly disabled patients; these decisions established a clear precedent that the right to refuse treatment extends to life-sustaining (or life-prolonging) treatment. To exercise this right, patients must have decision-making *capacity*, that is, the ability to understand and appreciate relevant information and to use that information in a reasoning process to reach a treatment decision (see Chapter 11); otherwise, a *surrogate* must make these decisions (see Chapter 13).

If patients have a right to consent to, or refuse, life-sustaining treatment when it is offered, should they also have a right to receive life-sustaining treatment upon request or demand? One might assert a right to receive life-sustaining treatment in particular, or one might affirm a right to life-sustaining treatment as part of a general *right to health care*. Either way, it would seem that any recognition of a right to health care, including life-sustaining treatment, is necessarily constrained by its cost. Thus, citizens of the world's poorest nations have very limited access to health care of any kind, while citizens of many industrialized nations have guaranteed access to a wide variety of health services, including life-sustaining treatment. In the United States, a federal statute enacted in 1986, the Emergency Medical Treatment and Labor Act (EMTALA), requires hospitals to provide evaluation and stabilizing treatment for all patients who present to emergency departments with an emergency medical condition. This amounts to a very limited right to receive life-sustaining treatment in that particular setting.

In addition to its costs, several other reasons for limiting access to life-sustaining treatment have been widely discussed. Most prominent among these is the claim that provision of life-sustaining care in some circumstances is *futile*, or *medically inappropriate* (see Chapter 12). Proponents of the appeal to futility argue that provision of futile treatment provides no benefit to patients and therefore wastes valuable resources; opponents respond that we lack consensus about when treatment is futile, and that prognostic tools are not precise enough to enable accurate prediction of treatment outcomes. Providing treatment that is futile or harmful is also claimed to be a violation of professional integrity, and healthcare professionals may assert a right of *conscientious refusal* to comply with some requests for life-sustaining treatment.

Whether or not they choose to pursue life-sustaining treatments, patients with serious illness may also benefit from *palliative care*, with its emphasis on pain and symptom control and on psychosocial well-being. Many patients with terminal illness forgo aggressive efforts to prolong life in order to embrace *hospice care*, an organized approach to providing physical, emotional, spiritual, and social support for patients near the end of life. A small number of patients with severe or terminal illness request assistance in ending their lives via ingestion of a lethal medication prescribed for them by a physician. This type of *physician aid in dying*, or *physician-assisted suicide*, is a legal option in 10 US states and the District of Columbia (Compassion and Choices, as of Fall 2021).

All these options for care near the end of life may prompt requests to ethics committees for ethics consultation. Ethics committee members should be able to engage in careful consideration of the issues and questions brought to them, and should be familiar with tools and concepts that can help ameliorate tensions and disagreements and improve communication and understanding at an especially sensitive time for patients, families, and healthcare teams.

Advance Directives and Portable Medical Orders

Since its enactment in 1990, the federal Patient Self-Determination Act has required hospitals to ask patients upon admission if they have an advance directive or would like to complete one. How this duty is fulfilled varies across hospitals. Who asks the question, and when? How much help is offered to patients? Each ethics committee should know how its own process works, in order to follow up as needed. Advance directives can help both the treatment team and the ethics committee understand a patient's end-of-life care choices, even though these documents do not become effective until the patient loses decision-making capacity. If patients retain decision-making capacity, they can and should participate directly in decisions about treatment.

The introductory case does not mention an advance directive, but Mrs. Wilson may have prepared one, perhaps during a previous admission or at the suggestion of another of her physicians. If Ms. Thompson has not done so already, she should ask Mrs. Wilson if she has an advance directive or would like to complete one. If Mrs. Wilson does have an advance directive, it may have been added to her medical record during a previous hospitalization. The hospital's electronic medical record should make it easy to record, locate, and update an advance directive, and to record and read narrative information about patients' treatment preferences; this could help Dr. Kelly learn more about Mrs. Wilson and her choices (Lehmann et al., 2019).

In their broadest sense, advance directives are people's expression of their wishes for future health care if they have lost the capacity to make those decisions. In this broad sense, advance directives can be oral or written, and can be expressed more or less formally. We believe that there are good reasons to communicate one's healthcare preferences both orally and in writing as part of the process of advance care planning described above. In what follows, however, we focus on the most widely recognized forms of written advance directives. Documents acceptable in each of the 50 states are widely available (National Hospice and Palliative Care Organization, n.d.), and comprehensive advance care planning programs can help large numbers of people to complete them (Hammes et al., 2010).

The living will, so named because it was originally modeled on a standard will, is the oldest type of advance directive document. Living wills usually enable a person to express a general preference to receive or forgo medical interventions commonly employed near the end of life (e.g., artificial nutrition and hydration). The form and content of living wills have changed considerably since their introduction in the 1970s, but their principal characteristic – often deemed a characteristic weakness – is their attempt to describe in advance a person's treatment preferences for different medical conditions without naming a surrogate decision maker to communicate with the healthcare team and make complex treatment decisions, at the time they are needed, on behalf of a patient who has lost decision-making capacity.

The second major type of advance directive, the healthcare power of attorney, was designed in part to remedy weaknesses of the living will. In a healthcare power of attorney, a person names someone else to serve as healthcare agent and gives that agent broad authority to make healthcare decisions, including but not limited to end-of-life decisions, at any time the patient lacks decision-making capacity. Healthcare powers of attorney also allow preparers to limit the authority of their healthcare agents if they desire, and to give their agents specific instructions about their treatment preferences.

Healthcare powers of attorney have several significant advantages over living wills. They enable preparers to appoint as agent a trusted relative or friend with whom they have discussed their treatment preferences. Healthcare powers of attorney are also more versatile than living wills. Living wills are typically limited to treatment choices about only a few medical conditions, but healthcare agents can make all medical decisions for a patient who has lost decision-making capacity. Healthcare powers of attorney cannot, however, help patients who lack a trusted friend or relative to name as healthcare agent.

A newer kind of document, the portable medical order for end-of-life care, is a hybrid of advance directive and physician order. Portable DNAR orders were designed to direct and enable emergency medical technicians to refrain from initiating CPR in any setting (e.g., for patients at home or in nursing homes, or even seriously ill children attending school). More recently, portable medical orders have been expanded to address other end-of-life treatment choices, including the use of antibiotics, medically provided nutrition and hydration, and comfort care. Oregon was the first state to implement these broad portable orders for life-sustaining treatment (Physician Orders for Life Sustaining Treatment; POLST) in 1995; by 2019, all US states had established portable medical orders for end-of-life care (POLST: Portable Medical Orders, n.d.). POLST-type documents are medical orders, intended to be portable and effective in many settings and to be binding on nonphysician healthcare providers; they have also been embraced by hospitals as useful guidance when patients are transferred from nursing facilities or present to emergency departments. Because POLST-type documents are medical orders, not just patients' statements about their healthcare preferences, they are, strictly speaking, not advance directives. Unlike other medical orders, however, POLST-type orders require the signature of the patient or the patient's legally authorized representative; for this reason, and because they address treatment preferences near the end of life, they closely resemble advance directives.

Despite generally expressed public preferences for avoiding intrusive and ineffective interventions near the end of life, a systematic review of 150 studies published between 2011 and 2016 estimated that only about 37% of US adults have completed an advance directive (Yadav et al., 2017). To aid decision-making for patients without advance directives, many states have enacted statutes designating a hierarchy of surrogate decision makers for patients who lack decision-making capacity. These statutes help physicians to identify authorized surrogates and, with their participation, to make timely treatment decisions. Their obvious weakness is that the statutory surrogate may not know or share the patient's preferences.

Treatment Choices and the Goals of Care

Advance directives and portable orders provide valuable guidance when used well. It is not always clear how to use them well, however, because they often focus on choosing or refusing particular interventions. This approach portrays end-of-life decision-making as a series of autonomous choices to refuse (or accept) a variety of specific interventions. Yet a procedure-based decision-making approach may be significantly less useful than one that addresses the goals of treatment. If the ethics committee helps the healthcare team and the patient or the patient's surrogate to discuss the broader goals they seek to achieve through treatment, they can go on to discuss whether and how those goals can be achieved through available treatments, and to choose particular interventions in light of the patient's goals. Decisions about common interventions near the end of life – artificial nutrition and hydration, mechanical ventilation, hospice care, etc. – have little meaning if the goals of using them, and the likelihood of their achieving those goals, are not considered. A patient whose goal is to continue living as long as possible is likely to make different choices about particular interventions than one who seeks the best possible quality of remaining life. Goal-focused discussion can enable the healthcare team to advise the patient or surrogate in ways that go beyond choosing or refusing a list of specific interventions.

As we have discussed, advance care planning and advance directives have three related but distinct goals: to facilitate *making*, *communicating*, and *honoring* the choices patients make about end-of-life care. While making and honoring end-of-life decisions have their own challenges, ethics committees and consultants may often find it necessary to redirect communications that have, even with the best of intentions, gone awry. A common example serves as an illustration. Some healthcare providers may focus discussion and decision-making on life-prolonging interventions alone, and begin a discussion by saying, "There is nothing more we can do..." Such a beginning may then be followed by a series of procedure-focused questions: "So, if your heart stopped, would you like us to do CPR? Do you want IV fluids or tube feeding? What about a ventilator, to assist your breathing?" To all this, a confused patient is likely to respond, "But doctor, I don't understand; I thought you said there was nothing more that could be done. If you can do all these things to help me, you should!" Redirecting communication to focus on treatment goals can help alleviate this type of confusion.

When advance directives were first introduced, they were based on a vision of the dying process that probably fit best with just a few types of cases: the highly predictable decline of advanced cancer, the unchanging unawareness of the chronic vegetative state, and the sudden collapse of a cardiopulmonary arrest. It soon became apparent, however, that the end of life has many variations that can make both prognosis and decision-making extremely difficult. A few examples may be instructive. The POLST paradigm came about in part as a response to the challenges of determining how to make treatment decisions for patients with DNAR orders before a cardiopulmonary arrest occurs. What should be done for patients if their heart rate slows, or if a patient has difficulty breathing, but there is no immediate need for resuscitation? Should a patient in a chronic vegetative state be prescribed antibiotics, or placed on dialysis? A second example comes from recent developments in imaging technology. It is now possible to distinguish between a chronic vegetative state and a "minimally conscious state." The cognitive experience and prognosis of patients in a minimally conscious state are more ambiguous than those of patients in a chronic vegetative state. Thus, it may be more difficult to determine appropriate goals of care for these patients. Finally, much more has been learned about the disease course for patients with some diagnoses, including congestive heart failure like Mrs. Wilson's. Congestive heart failure, unlike advanced cancer, can have a highly unpredictable course, at times appearing more like a rollercoaster ride than a gradual decline. The resulting increase in uncertainty makes it both more important and more difficult to focus on the goals of treatment and consider whether they can be achieved through available medical interventions.

Continuing Controversies and Challenges

We have argued that advance care planning and attention to goals of care can prevent or ameliorate much uncertainty and conflict over treatment decisions near the end of life. As we have also noted, however, neither of these strategies can resolve all end-of-life problems. Despite the considerable progress made in advance care planning and end-of-life decision-making over the last 40 years, facing the end of life understandably is, and will continue to be, difficult for patients, families, surrogates, and healthcare providers alike (Wolf et al., 2015). Mrs. Wilson's disagreement with her cardiologist is a divergence of goals that illustrates the very controversy that launched the "death with dignity" movement and that remains perhaps the most common type of end-of-life conflict. Goal divergence between the healthcare team and the patient is only one species of such disagreements; ethics committees and consultants may need to help manage disagreements about whether the patient's goals are achievable, about the interpretation of medical information, or about what the patient's best interests are, while reminding everyone that the goals sought by the patient should generally take precedence.

A particularly challenging type of disagreement arises when there are divergent views about the value of a chance. Mrs. Wilson and Dr. Kelly may disagree about the likelihood that ventilatory support will be both helpful and temporary; this is an essential inquiry and discussion for an ethics committee or consultant to initiate. When there is uncertainty, decision makers can easily diverge in their assessment of what likelihood of success represents a chance worth taking – an obviously value-laden judgment. The healthcare team's assessment may be based on outcomes data, the family's assessment may be based on its sense of responsibility to the patient, and the patient's own assessment, when available, may be based on direct experience of illness, or on fear of death. Here too, the ethics committee or consultant should help ensure that the patient's assessment takes priority. The patient's perspective should not simply override all others, but the patient's experience and evaluation must be focal points for consideration and discussion of the decisions that are needed.

Finally, cultural and religious values and perspectives may also give rise to, or contribute to, disagreements in end-of-life treatment decision-making. Religion and culture are often cited as significant reasons for the reluctance of patients and families to discuss end-of-life decisions or to forgo life-sustaining treatments, and training in "cultural competence" is often considered a primary tool for overcoming that reluctance. In our experience, "cultural sensitivity" and "cultural humility" are concepts that ethics committees can better employ to help healthcare providers avoid overgeneralization, recognize that medicine too is a culture, learn from patients and families how their beliefs and values influence their end-of-life choices, and acknowledge those beliefs and values in the decision-making process (Hunt, 2019; see Chapter 5, also).

In the introductory case, consultation with the ethics committee should have the goal of helping Mrs. Wilson make some choices now, identify a healthcare agent if possible, and record those decisions by completing an advance directive and/or a POLST-type document. Ethics consultation should also help Dr. Kelly understand better how to treat Mrs. Wilson in light of her chosen goals of care. The discussion questions below are just the beginning of the ethics committee's work in cases like this; readers should answer them expansively.

Questions for Discussion

1. Conceptual: How do the different forms for advance care planning differ, and in what contexts are each of them most useful?
2. Pragmatic: How do your state's statutes on informed consent and end-of-life treatment decisions and documentation address Mrs. Wilson's circumstances? Do your hospital's end-of-life care policies provide flexibility and promote respect for patients?
3. Strategic: How would you talk with Ms. Thompson? What else would you do? What can you do, as a matter of preventive ethics, to avoid similar situations in the future?

References

Compassion and Choices. (n.d.). *In Your State.* https://compassionandchoices.org/take-action/in-your-state/.

Cruzan v. *Director, Missouri Department of Health.* (1990). 110 S.Ct. 2841.

Gostin LO (2005). Ethics, the constitution, and the dying process: The case of Theresa Marie Schiavo. *Journal of the American Medical Association*, 293(19): 2403–2407.

Hammes BJ, Rooney BL, Gundrun JD (2010). A comparative, retrospective, observational study of the prevalence, availability, and specificity of advance care plans in a county that implemented an advance care planning microsystem. *Journal of the American Geriatrics Society*, 58(7): 1249–1255.

Hunt LM (2019). Beyond cultural competence: Applying humility to clinical settings. In Oberlander J et al., eds., *The Social Medicine Reader*, 3rd ed., vol. II. Durham, NC: Duke University Press, 127–131.

Lehmann CU, Petersen P, Bhatia H, Berner ES, Goodman KW (2019). Advance directives and code status information exchange: A consensus proposal for a minimum set of attributes. *Cambridge Quarterly of Healthcare Ethics*, 28(1): 178–185.

Moskop JC (2016). *Ethics and Health Care: An Introduction.* Cambridge University Press.

National Hospice and Palliative Care Organization. (n.d.). Caring Connections. www.caringinfo.org/.

POLST: Portable Medical Orders. (n.d.). *POLST State Programs.* https://polst.org/state-programs/.

In re Quinlan (1976). 70 N.J. 10, 355 A.2d 647.

Wolf SM, Berlinger N, Jennings B (2015). Forty years of work on end of life care – from patients' rights to systemic reform. *New England Journal of Medicine*, 372(7): 678–682.

Yadav KN, Gabler NB, Cooney E, et al. (2017). Approximately one in three US adults completes any type of advance directive for end-of-life care. *Health Affairs (Millwood)*, 36(7): 1244–1251.

Chapter 15

Potentially Inappropriate Treatment and Medical Futility

Thaddeus Mason Pope

Objectives

After reading this chapter, the reader will be able to:

1. Distinguish "potentially inappropriate treatment" from "futile treatment".
2. Describe how different conceptions of what is beneficial or desired lead to disagreements in medical decision-making.
3. Distinguish six strategies that ethics committees can use to prevent and to resolve potentially inappropriate treatment disputes.

Case

One year ago, 73-year-old Mr. B came to the hospital for surgery on a thymus gland tumor. While the surgery was successful, during his postoperative recovery, Mr. B's endotracheal tube became dislodged. This resulted in severe, irreversible brain damage. Mr. B was subsequently discharged to other facilities. But, 6 months ago, he was readmitted to your hospital with a diagnosis of renal failure. He has remained there ever since, in a persistent vegetative state, dependent for survival on mechanical ventilation, hemodialysis, and tube feedings. Mr. B has developed increasingly severe decubitus ulcers and recurrent infections. He remains a full code.

Because of his deteriorating status, Mr. B's physicians determined that he is beyond medical rescue. They think that it is medically inappropriate, nonbeneficial, and outside the standard of care to continue his life-sustaining treatment. Indeed, they think it is ethically inappropriate, inhumane, and even torture to sustain Mr. B artificially while his body is decomposing.

The treatment team wants to discontinue dialysis and issue a do-not-attempt-resuscitation (DNAR) order. They have carefully explained this proposed treatment plan to Mr. B's surrogate, his daughter. But, even after many conferences, she will not provide consent. Mr. B's family is very close. Discussion with his wife and sons confirms that the surrogate is acting in accordance with Mr. B's consistent, considered, and deliberated preferences. The hospital attempted to find another facility to accept Mr. B as a transfer patient, but none could be found. Mr. B's attending physician has sought guidance from the ethics committee.

Introduction to Potentially Inappropriate Treatment

Like Mr. B, hospitalized patients at the end of life frequently lack decision-making capacity. So, decisions regarding their treatment are usually made by surrogate decision makers (Chapter 13). A potentially inappropriate treatment (PIT) dispute is typically described as a situation in which a surrogate wants to continue the patient's nonpalliative treatment (usually life-sustaining treatment) but the healthcare provider wants to stop (Bosslet et al., 2015). Providers normally need consent to withhold or withdraw treatment. Therefore, to resolve PIT disputes, providers must: (1) accede to the surrogate, (2) obtain consent, or (3) find a legitimate basis to withhold or withdraw treatment without consent.[1]

PIT is one of the most common reasons for ethics consultation and ethics committee review. This chapter serves as a basic primer to PIT disputes. It first provides some essential context and background, including the leading terminology and definitions. Then it reviews the primary factors that cause PIT disputes. After providing this conceptual and sociological background, this chapter then addresses how PIT disputes can be avoided and resolved. Included is a discussion of preventative ethics, leading mechanisms for resolving PIT conflicts, and questions for further discussion to motivate healthcare ethics committee (HEC) members' thinking on the issues surrounding PIT.

Terminology and Definitions Regarding PIT

For decades, bioethicists have warned that there is a temptation and tendency to use the seemingly objective and scientific term "medical futility" to mask heavily value-laden judgments (Truog et al., 1992; Luce, 2010; Wilkinson and Savulescu, 2011). Indeed, many healthcare providers, and even ethics committee members, employ this term as an excuse to stop treatment without devoting sufficient attention to the underlying rationale for refusing or wanting to refuse treatment.

To avoid this danger, some have suggested that rather than describing treatment as "futile," it should instead be described as "nonbeneficial" or "inappropriate." But replacing the adjective does not solve the problem. The proposition that clinicians need not offer or provide inappropriate treatment seems uncontroversial. But it is also vacuous. Applying that proposition to any situation requires more than affixing a label. It requires an argument and plan.

The most widely recognized guidance is a 2015 policy statement by five major critical care societies (Bosslet et al., 2015). This statement distinguishes four types of treatment: (1) futile treatment, (2) legally proscribed treatment, (3) legally discretionary treatment, and (4) potentially inappropriate treatment.

Futile Treatment

The narrowest and most clearly defined category is "futile treatment." This is also known as "physiological futility" (Pope, 2007). Futile interventions are considered inappropriate because they have no chance of being effective. Commentators have offered a multitude of colorful examples, including prescribing antibiotics for a viral illness, performing CPR in the presence of cardiac rupture or severe outflow obstruction, and offering chemotherapy for an ulcer.

---

[1] While PIT disputes are paradigmatically between the responsible physician and the surrogate, there are three other types. First, there is intra-professional conflict, between members of the treatment team. Second, there is intra-familial conflict, between members of the patient's family. Third, there are questions regarding unrepresented patients without proxies.

When treatment is futile, the ethics committee member does not make any evaluative assessment that the treatment's effect is too unlikely, too small, or not worthwhile. There is no normative disagreement. Instead, the basis for refusing treatment is an empirical one: The treatment simply will not work.

However, this objectivity comes at a steep price. Futility, understood in this narrow way, has a very limited applicability. Decisions about withholding and withdrawing treatment are usually based on probabilities as opposed to certainties. Providers can rarely be certain that there is a 100% probability that a given intervention will have zero effect. In the case of Mr. B, for example, neither ventilation nor dialysis are futile. They have been working successfully for months.

Legally Proscribed Treatment

Unlike "futile" treatment, "legally proscribed" treatment might accomplish an effect desired by the patient. But the treatment is prohibited by applicable laws, judicial precedent, or widely accepted public policies. For example, a critically ill patient may ask a physician to circumvent organ allocation policy to get faster access to an organ for transplantation. Clinicians should explain the situation and provide emotional support, but they need not provide this treatment.

Legally Discretionary Treatment

"Legally discretionary" treatments are those for which there are specific laws, judicial precedent, or policies that give physicians permission to refuse to administer them. For example, clinicians have no duty to provide ongoing physiologic support for a patient correctly declared dead by neurological criteria (aka, "brain dead") who is not an organ donor (Chapter 16). Clinicians should explain the situation and provide emotional support, but they need not provide this treatment.

Potentially Inappropriate Treatment

Unfortunately, few ethics cases involve treatment that is futile, proscribed, or discretionary. Treatment in most cases, when clinicians believe that competing ethical considerations justify not providing requested interventions, fall under the concept of "potentially inappropriate treatment" (PIT). While clinicians should communicate and advocate for the treatment plan they believe is appropriate, requests for PIT that remain intractable despite intensive communication and negotiation should be managed by a fair process of dispute resolution.

Quantitative Futility

To operationalize PIT, two other concepts may be useful: quantitative futility and qualitative futility. Proponents of quantitative futility note that clinical studies and scoring systems can provide enough information to provide an empirical basis for establishing thresholds based on clinical experience and percentages (Schneiderman and Jecker, 2011).

However, quantitative futility suffers from two serious problems. First, setting the threshold of probability is a value judgment about which there is considerable variability. Second, even if healthcare providers and society could settle upon a threshold percentage, available measures from population-level studies are imprecise when applied to particular patients.

Qualitative Futility

Qualitative futility has two forms. The first form asserts that treatment is inappropriate when its prospective benefits are outweighed by its associated burdens to the patient. For example, performing CPR on a patient with metastatic cancer is arguably disproportionately burdensome. It cannot restore the patient but, by causing multiple rib fractures, would serve to increase the patient's suffering.

The second form of qualitative futility asserts that treatment is inappropriate when it simply cannot provide the patient a minimum quality of life worth living. The expected outcome is of little or no value given the patient's extremely poor condition or prognosis. While providing the disputed treatment might not cause the patient to suffer, it does not offer the patient any reasonable benefit. But be careful about judging the patient's quality of life to be far less than the patient would. For example, people with physical and cognitive disabilities obtain many satisfactions and rewards in their lives that others may not recognize.

Summary

Except in the rare cases in which treatment is futile, proscribed, or discretionary, the ethics committee member has no simple algorithm to determine when requested treatment is inappropriate. Nevertheless, the concepts of "quantitative futility" and "qualitative futility" provide a useful framework to guide thinking and analysis.

Causes of PIT Disputes

PIT disputes typically result from surrogates requesting treatment that clinicians do not want to provide. To understand the causes of these disputes, it is useful to examine why surrogates insist and why clinicians resist. First, this section summarizes the main reasons that surrogates demand nonrecommended treatment. Second, this section summarizes the main reasons that clinicians are unwilling to provide the desired treatment.

Reasons for Surrogate Requests

Repeated surveys demonstrate that the public is far more likely than healthcare providers to believe that patients have a right to demand treatment that doctors think will not help. The reasons that surrogates request PIT can be grouped into four categories: (1) distrust, (2) cognitive issues, (3) psychological and emotional issues, and (4) values, religion, and miracles (Pope, 2007).

Distrust

Surrogates are aware of the limits of prognostication, sometimes because of a prior error in the patient's treatment. Accordingly, they may doubt that things are as bad as physicians represent. Moreover, with greater access to medical information, surrogates are more confident in challenging healthcare providers.

Distrust is especially prevalent among African Americans and Hispanics. There is substantial evidence that these patients and surrogates are more likely to request unconditional prolongation of life-sustaining treatment and are less likely to agree with a recommendation to withdraw or withhold. Furthermore, even nonminorities are increasingly distrustful, due to growing attention on providers' economic incentives, conflicts of interest, and biases (Rosoff, 2013).

Cognitive Issues

Unfortunately, surrogates frequently do not understand the clinical status of the patients whom they represent. Some studies have shown that less than half of surrogates, regardless of educational level, had adequate knowledge of what was going on and what would happen to the patient (Chapter 13). Sometimes, the surrogate lacks capacity to make the relevant decisions. But even when the surrogate has capacity, there are three key iatrogenic causes of surrogate misunderstanding. First, providers often fail to explain clearly the patient's condition and prognosis with clear, jargon-free language. Second, providers may place undue pressure on the surrogate and fail to allow enough time to process information. Third, different specialists often supply the surrogate with uncoordinated, even conflicting information.

Psychological and Emotional Issues

In addition to cognitive issues, many surrogates have clinically diagnosable conditions such as stress, depression, and anxiety. These psychological problems may impair the surrogate's decision-making capacity (Chapter 13). But even if the surrogate has capacity, they may not understand that their role is to exercise substituted judgment or act in the patient's best interest. Furthermore, even when they understand their responsibility, some surrogates find it difficult to carry out their fiduciary duties, because of loyalty, guilt, or uncertainty about the patient's wishes, or because of other family dynamics. Furthermore, some surrogates may have "dubious motives" in that they are looking out for their own interests rather than the patient's interests.

Values, Religion, and Miracles

While some requests for PIT can be explained by the surrogate's distrust or by cognitive or psychological impairment, the most intractable futility disputes tend to be those in which the surrogate's decision is based on a value difference over "odds and ends," over what is a worthwhile chance or what is a worthwhile outcome.

Religion is at the bottom of the most intractable futility disputes (Zier et al., 2009). For example, in the Samuel Golubchuk case, physicians determined that their patient had minimal brain function and that his chances for recovery were slim. Mr. Golubchuk's insurmountable problem with wound infections required providers to repeatedly surgically debride his skin ulcers. Several physicians resigned because they thought this was tantamount to "torture." Still, Mr. Golubchuk's adult children argued that taking their father off life support would be a sin under their Orthodox Jewish faith.

Even apart from religion, many surrogates request treatment with very low odds of success, because they think that *any* chance is worth taking when the stakes are life and death. Indeed, most Americans believes in miracles. They believe that even if doctors said futility had been reached, divine intervention by God could save their family member. Increasingly, surrogates request treatment even after the patient has been determined dead on neurological criteria (Pope, 2017).

Reasons for Provider Resistance

Since the surrogate speaks for the patient, respect for autonomy typically means that providers should generally follow surrogate decisions. But PIT concerns the "limits" of autonomy. There are five main reasons that providers resist surrogate treatment requests.[2] They want to: (1) avoid patient suffering, (2) respect patient autonomy, (3) protect the integrity of the medical profession, (4) avoid moral distress, and (5) promote good stewardship.

Avoid Patient Suffering

Perhaps the most significant reason that providers resist surrogate requests is the desire to avoid being engaged in causing suffering. In the Golubchuk case, one physician described the surrogate-requested treatment as an "abomination," "immoral," and "tantamount to torture." In another case from Boston, a staff member said: "This is the Massachusetts General Hospital, not Auschwitz."

Of course, healthcare providers are willing to inflict things that cause pain and discomfort (e.g., chemotherapy). But they are willing to do this only because such side effects are outweighed by some benefit. In other words, providers are not really opposed to being complicit in causing patient suffering per se. They are opposed to participating in "unwarranted suffering."

Respect Patient Autonomy

Providers want to do what they think the patient would have wanted. They often doubt that the surrogate's decision accurately reflects the patient's wishes, preferences, or best interest. Indeed, significant empirical evidence shows that surrogates frequently do not make the same treatment decision that the patient would have made for themself. Significant evidence shows that most patients prefer less aggressive medicine at the end of life (Pope, 2010).

Protect the Integrity of the Medical Profession

Physicians want to defend the integrity of the medical profession. They do not want to be beholden to provide whatever treatment patients or surrogates want. Physicians are not "indentured servants," "reflexive automatons," or "vending machines." The medical profession is a self-governing one with its own standards of professional practice.

Avoid Moral Distress

Medical futility is the leading cause of moral distress among nurses. Nurses "know the right thing to do" but institutional constraints make it nearly impossible to pursue that right course of action. Moral distress can drive people from the profession and thus reduce access. It can also reduce staffing levels and make people operate less well, thus adversely impacting other patients' quality of care (Chapter 6).

---

[2] These are *professional* reasons for wanting to refuse a surrogate's request for life-sustaining treatment. Increasingly, healthcare providers are also asserting *personal*, conscience-based objections to patient treatment requests (Chapter 24).

Promote Good Stewardship

Finally, providers want to be good stewards of healthcare resources. In most PIT disputes they balance respecting autonomy against beneficence or nonmaleficence. But sometimes, autonomy must be balanced against justice (Chapter 27). While end-of-life costs have been a major subject of health policy debates, they have not played, and generally should not play, a role at the bedside. On the other hand, physicians do want to be careful with the allocation of scarce "hard" resources like ICU beds, particularly in true triage situations like those confronted during the COVID-19 pandemic.

Summary

Identifying and understanding the causes of PIT disputes is important for their successful collaborative resolution. In particular, with a better understanding of surrogates' motivations and rationales for resisting provider recommendations to discontinue life support, the ethics committee can better develop empirically derived interventions. The committee can incorporate targeted interventions into its dispute resolution mechanisms and deploy them according to the precise basis for surrogate dissent. For example, if the basis for disagreement is prognostic distrust, it might be most effective to offer an independent second opinion or a time-limited trial of the disputed therapy.

Preventative Ethics

If possible, it is preferable to prevent PIT disputes from arising in the first place, rather than to attempt resolution after they have arisen. There are four main mechanisms by which an ethics committee can engage in preventative ethics: (1) advance care planning, (2) surrogate training, (3) staff education, and (4) mandatory consults.

Advance Care Planning

Most patients do not want aggressive interventions with heavy burdens and minimal benefits. These patients can avoid PIT disputes with better advance care planning (Chapter 14). By discussing or recording their treatment preferences before losing capacity, patients can better assure agreement between their clinicians and surrogates.

Surrogate Training

Surrogates find themselves performing a new role, for the first time, under difficult circumstances. Therefore, healthcare providers should advise the surrogate of the duties of a good substitute decision maker and provide statistical information on patient preferences (Cunningham et al., 2018). The ethics committee can help by making resources available like the American Bar Association's booklet, *Making Medical Decisions for Someone Else: A How-To Guide*.

Staff Education and Good Communication

Most conflict over end-of-life treatment is due to communication failures. The ethics committee can preemptively address these deficiencies by arranging for staff education and training. Importantly, providers must establish goals of care early and evaluate them routinely. They must foster realistic expectations. And they must reassure surrogates that the patient will never be abandoned. Palliative care is always appropriate. The patient's comfort and dignity must always be maintained.

Mandatory Consults

Most of the PIT literature focuses on surrogate demands for therapy that the provider judges nonbeneficial. But surrogates are not always the problem. Many healthcare providers recommend or insist on overly aggressive treatment at the end of life. There are many causes for this, including: (1) the physician's anti-death attitude, (2) the physician's desire to maintain hope, (3) the physician's need to avoid failure and shame, (4) the physician's religion, (5) the physician's reimbursement incentives, and (6) the physician's sense of the goals and ends of medicine.

These situations rarely mature into conflict. Sometimes the physician accedes to the surrogate's demands to avoid the potential time and stress of litigation or institutional dispute resolution processes. Usually there is no conflict because the surrogate is unaware of the treatment's low chances, side effects, or alternatives. In response, some states, like New York and California, have enacted "right to know" laws that require providers to tell terminally ill patients their end-of-life options, including palliative care and hospice.

There are at least two ways that an ethics committee can check physician-driven overtreatment. First, it can permit not only physicians but also nurses, consultants, and family members to refer cases to the ethics committee. Second, the committee can institute mandatory ethics or palliative care consultation for certain populations of patients. For example, some facilities automatically trigger a consult for all ICU patients after a defined number of hours or days.

Dispute Resolution

While good preventative ethics can reduce the number of PIT disputes, it will not eliminate them altogether. Procedurally, there are six things that an ethics committee can do to resolve conflict. First, the committee can draft and implement an institutional policy. Second, the committee can serve as a mediator. Third, the committee can recommend accommodation. Fourth, the committee can facilitate surrogate selection. Fifth, the committee can recommend the patient's transfer. Sixth, the committee can support or authorize unilateral refusal of treatment.

Institutional Policy

In 1996, the American Medical Association recommended that all hospitals adopt a medical futility policy (AMA, 1999). Over the past quarter-century, more hospitals have been drafting and implementing medical futility policies. Sometimes, these are stand-alone policies and sometimes they are amendments to a DNAR or other policy.

Having an institutional policy can provide significant benefits (Chapter 26). It can assist providers in decision-making about inappropriate interventions. It can provide mechanisms for clarifying values and goals. And a futility policy can offer guidelines that ensure a fair and transparent process for resolving conflict (Joseph, 2011).

The more recent five-society policy statement recommends following a "due process" approach (Bosslet et al., 2015). Since there are no accepted substantive criteria or formulas for medical futility, the ethics committee member must resort to procedural criteria. If we cannot identify *what* is a right decision, we can at least address *how* to reach it.[3]

Goal Clarification and Mediation

Most PIT disputes are resolved informally and internally. In cases of misunderstanding or mistrust, it is effective to get an independent medical opinion. In other cases, ethics consultants, social workers, chaplains, ethics committees, legal counsel, ombudspersons, and other hospital resources are quite effective at achieving consensus. Only around 5% of medical futility disputes prove intractable.

Accommodation

Even when treatment is deemed nonbeneficial, it may be appropriate to make a short-term accommodation. This provides the family with time: to resolve personal matters, to say goodbye, and to grieve. Even brain-dead patients are often maintained on life support for several hours or days as a matter of sensitivity to religious, cultural, or moral values (Pope, 2017).

Surrogate Selection

Only rarely do disputes remain intractable. In such cases, surrogate selection may be appropriate. A surrogate is the patient's agent and, as such, must act according to the patient's instructions, known preferences, and best interests. When a surrogate exceeds the scope of their authority, they can and should be replaced (Pope, 2010).

While an effective mechanism for many disputes, surrogate selection cannot resolve some categories of conflict. In some cases, it will be difficult to demonstrate surrogate deviation. Since too few individuals engage in adequate advance care planning, applicable instructions and other evidence regarding patient preferences are rarely available. Other times, as in the Golubchuk case, the available evidence shows that the surrogate is acting faithfully and making decisions consistent with the patient's instructions, preferences, and values.

Transfer

When surrogate selection is not available and efforts at reaching consensus have failed, the ethics committee may transition from a mediation role to an adjudication role. The five-society policy statement provides that if the committee (or, ideally, a separate medical appropriateness review committee) supports the surrogate's position and the physician remains unpersuaded, transfer of care to another physician within the institution may be arranged (Bosslet et al., 2015). If the committee supports the physician's position and the surrogate remains unpersuaded, the patient's transfer to another

---

[3] The five-society statement recognizes that time pressures may sometimes make it infeasible to complete all steps of a due process approach. In these cases, clinicians may refuse to provide the disputed treatment if they (1) have a high degree of certainty that the requested treatment is outside accepted practice and (2) if they complete as much of the process as possible.

institution may be sought. The disputed treatment should continue pending transfer. In practice, such transfers are difficult to find.

Unilateral Refusal

The final step of the due process approach provides that if transfer is not possible, then the intervention need not be offered. This should not happen without giving the surrogate reasonable notice and time to seek extramural appeal or judicial intervention. The "legal ramifications of this course of action are uncertain" (AMA, 1999, 940). Unilateral refusal is prohibited in some states. Only in California, Texas, and Virginia do decisions of the ethics committee clearly confer legal immunity on healthcare providers who withhold or withdraw life-sustaining treatment without consent. Nevertheless, the ethics committee can still serve a useful role even in states where it has no special legal authority. The process itself usually helps all stakeholders reach consensus.

Questions for Discussion

1. Conceptual: How clear and useful are the five societies' distinctions among treatments that are: (a) futile, (b) legally proscribed, (c) legally discretionary, and (d) potentially inappropriate?
2. Pragmatic: Dispute resolution procedures with too much vetting and oversight may be too cumbersome and time-consuming. How should an institutional futility policy balance efficiency and due process?
3. Strategic: How might an HEC proactively address the causes of PIT disputes?

References

American Medical Association. (1999). Medical futility in end-of-life care: Report of the Council on Ethical and Judicial Affairs. *JAMA*, 281(10): 937–941.

Bosslet GT, Pope TM, Rubenfeld GD, et al. (2015). An official ATS/AACN/ACCP/ESICM/SCCM policy statement: Responding to requests for potentially inappropriate treatments in intensive care units. *American Journal of Respiratory and Critical Care Medicine*, 191(11): 1318–1330.

Cunningham TV, Scheunemann LP, Arnold RM, White D (2018). How do clinicians prepare family members for the role of surrogate decision-maker? *Journal of Medical Ethics*, 44(1): 21–26.

Joseph R (2011). Hospital policy on medical futility: Does it help in conflict resolution and ensuring good end-of-life care? *Annals of the Academy of Medicine, Singapore*, 40(1): 19–25.

Luce JM (2010). A history of resolving conflicts over end-of-life care in intensive care units in the United States. *Critical Care Medicine*, 38(8): 1623–1629.

Pope TM (2007). Medical futility statutes: No safe harbor to unilaterally refuse life-sustaining medical treatment. *Tennessee Law Review*, 75(1): 1–81.

Pope TM (2010). Surrogate selection: An increasingly viable, but limited, solution to intractable futility disputes. *St. Louis University Journal of Health Law and Policy*, 3(2): 183–252.

Pope TM (2017). Brain death forsaken: Growing conflict and new legal challenges. *Journal of Legal Medicine*, 37(3–4): 265–324.

Rosoff PM (2013). Institutional futility policies are inherently unfair. *HEC Forum*, 25(3): 191–209.

Schneiderman LJ, Jecker NS (2011). *Wrong Medicine: Doctors, Patients, and Futile Treatment*, 2nd ed. Baltimore, MD: Johns Hopkins University Press.

Truog R, Brett AS, Frader J (1992). The problem with futility. *New England Journal of Medicine*, 326(23): 1560–1564.

Wilkinson DJ, Savulescu J (2011). Knowing when to stop: Futility in the ICU. *Current Opinions in Anaesthesiology*, 24(2): 160–165.

Zier LS, Burack JH, Micco G, Chipman AK, Frank JA, White DB (2009). Surrogate decision makers' responses to physicians' predictions of medical futility. *Chest*, 136(1): 110–117.

Cognitive Dissonance and the Care of Patients with Disorders of Consciousness

Joseph J. Fins

Objectives

Upon reading and considering the content of this chapter, the reader should be able to:

1. Recognize the diagnostic, therapeutic, and ethical challenges in referring to and categorizing disorders of consciousness and neurological death.
2. Apply strategies to address the prognostic uncertainty of disorders of consciousness with families.
3. Discuss responsibilities to vulnerable persons with liminal or covert consciousness.
4. Identify rehabilitation and palliation as ethically sound options under certain clinical circumstances when these meet with patient and family preferences.

Case

Devon Chester, a 37-year-old father of two, sustained a severe brain injury after being struck by a drunk driver. For 5 days he was in the ICU, unconscious. The family was so distressed by his circumstances that they wanted the team to take him off the ventilator.

Dr. Longwood, the pulmonologist who ran the ICU, told the family that Mr. Chester was in a comatose state and painted a grim prognosis for Mrs. Chester. He told her that while her husband would certainly survive the accident and come off the ventilator – because he wasn't brain dead – he would never "be himself," that he would essentially be a "vegetable," that is, be in the vegetative state.

Dr. Longwood said he had lots of experience with such cases. The best thing would be to let him go and make him an organ donor, "so that others might live and some good can come out of this tragedy." Agreeing with Dr. Longwood, one social worker commented, "We needed to let her know he has a right to die and that the life ahead of him is no life at all."

The next morning Mrs. Chester spoke to the charge nurse, agitated and eager to talk to the doctor. "I just saw him open his eyes and look at me. He's suffering in there. I can tell. He wouldn't want to be this way, ever. Please, turn off that machine, right now, before it's too late. He just can't go through life this way."

The nurse asked the resident, Dr. Battenfeld, to speak to Mrs. Chester. When Dr. Battenfeld did, Mrs. Chester said, "It's time, time for him to go, and be at peace. He is suffering so." While Dr. Battenfeld reassured Mrs. Chester that her husband wasn't suffering, he didn't know whether the opening of his eyes signified awareness or something else. In fact, he became concerned that the family was jumping to conclusions and not getting the information they needed for an informed choice, one way or another.

He told Dr. Longwood about his conversation with Mrs. Chester and suggested a follow-up neurology consult. He also thought an ethics consult might be helpful. Dr. Longwood agreed with both ideas.

Introduction

Although there is a substantial and growing scholarship on disorders of consciousness – conditions spanning coma, brain death, the vegetative state, and the minimally conscious state – when these cases occur in clinical practice, the degree of clinician ignorance can make it seem as if these scenarios were occurring for the very first time (Giacino et al., 2014). Care can be marked by improvisation and ignorance to the detriment of patients and families as well as to staff whose resilience can be tested by the challenges posed by severe brain injury.

This is troubling given the copious work that has been produced just in the last two decades. Most notably, in 2018, the American Academy of Neurology (AAN), the American College of Rehabilitation Medicine (ACRM), and the National Institute of Disability and Independent Living Research and Rehabilitation (NIDILRR) completed landmark evidence-based practice reviews of the diagnosis and treatment of these conditions, practice guidelines based on these data, and accompanying commentary addressing the ethical, legal, and clinical implications of these developments (Fins and Bernat, 2018; Giacino et al., 2018).

To make sense of the entire landscape of disorders of consciousness as well as the 2018 recommendations, it is important to distinguish different disorders of consciousness in order to address unique concerns each may raise. While it is not uncommon to hear comments that suggest that these patients "are all basically brain dead," each of these brain states is distinct, with its own physiology, physical findings, and prognoses. These distinctions inform clinical, legal, and normative considerations.

Coma

Coma Defined: Coma is an eyes-closed state of unresponsiveness. Coma is a more prolonged loss of consciousness than syncope, when a patient has a fainting spell, and is the gateway condition to disorders of consciousness. On one extreme coma may lead to brain death (see next section), and on the other, it can lead to recovery as when a patient is placed under anesthesia and put into a comatose state.

Physiologically coma is marked by low metabolic activity in all parts of the brain, including the autonomic structures of the brain stem and the higher cortical areas responsible for thought and sensation. There are multiple causes of coma including anoxic brain injury (as from the severe and prolonged deprivation of oxygen following prolonged cardiac arrest), traumatic brain injury, metabolic derangement like hypoglycemia (low blood sugar), or general anesthesia. At the bedside comatose patients appear to be asleep and unarousable. Unless coma is medically induced and thus prolonged by sedative agents, it is self-limited, lasting around 2 weeks. Coma can progress to brain death, the vegetative state, the minimally conscious state, or full recovery.

Considerations: Of course, it is quite common to hear not only laypeople but healthcare providers themselves use the term "coma" quite loosely to refer to a range of states of unconsciousness. This kind of sloppiness leads not just to ambiguity but to confusion among practitioners and between the team and the family.

Brain Death

Brain Death Defined: Brain death (or, more precisely, "death according to neurological criteria") was defined in 1968 by the Ad Hoc Committee of the Harvard Medical School as "irreversible cessation of functioning" of the whole brain including the brain stem and higher cortical structures (this definition was later taken up by the President's Commission in 1981 and codified, sometimes with modifications, in all state laws).

Because brain-dead patients do not have a functioning brain stem, they have lost the autonomic ability to breathe without assistance of a ventilator (Schiff and Fins, 2016). Brain death is determined through a specific set of examinations that includes a complete history, physical and neurological exam, as well as laboratory tests. The history helps to identify a predicate cause for brain death and, more importantly, exclude causes that might confound assessment of brain death testing. For example, patients who have high levels of barbiturates in their blood might appear brain dead when they are very heavily sedated. Another confounder is hypothermia as might occur after a winter drowning; in that case, patients have to be warmed before they can be assessed.

In addition to a physical exam, the neurological exam is performed specifically to determine the complete absence of brain stem function as assessed by the inability to elicit any response from the cranial nerves. The final confirmatory test is the apnea test that assesses the ability of the brain stem to drive respiration when CO_2 has accumulated. To do an apnea test, patients are detached from the ventilator and placed on 100% oxygen to see whether they can generate respiration without mechanical assistance. A patient who does not breathe once CO_2 levels have accumulated 20 mm Hg above baseline is brain dead; that is, even when the brain stem is exposed to extreme hyper-capnic (high CO_2 levels) conditions it was not prompted to initiate respiration.

There are other tests to assess brain death, but its assessment is a fundamentally clinical one. Ancillary tests like imaging studies can be useful when a patient is too unstable to undergo an apnea test or when facial disfigurement makes it impossible to do a neurological exam. A nuclear perfusion study will demonstrate the complete lack of radioactive tracer within the brain, illuminating only surrounding areas like the skull and sinuses. More recently single photon emission computerized tomography has been used to clarify ambiguous assessments. EEG testing is contraindicated because of false positive results due to ambient electrical noise.

Concerns: Understandably, death pronounced using neurological criteria can be quite challenging for families and for staff. While it is the general consensus of the neurology community that brain death is a scientifically informed diagnosis, there are ethical challenges to this concept. Some families may feel that they are violating core beliefs by acceding to brain death determinations. Recent cases like that of Jahi McMath have raised questions about the rights of families to object to the diagnosis. Even though brain death is legally equivalent to cardiac death in most states and consistent with the criteria used by the United Network for Organ Sharing, one state (New Jersey) allows for religious exemptions while another (New York) allows for "reasonable accommodation" to family dissent to brain death. As a result, professional staff may be tested when they are compelled to treat a patient whom they might characterize as a "corpse."

While conscientious objection to caring for such patients (or "bodies") is an option for staff as long as the ethical mandate of nonabandonment is upheld, a better course of action may be to attempt mediation. Mediation can be helpful to frame the dilemma within the patient's religious tradition. Seen this way, there are two competing mandates: preserving life and not prolonging the dying process when one is imminently dying. Instead of attempting to impose a secular definition of life or death, the ethical challenge can be reframed within a culturally sensitive context. Although this approach does not always decrease conflict, it can be helpful working with cultural intermediaries and clergy.

Vegetative State

Vegetative State Defined: While both comatose and brain-dead patients are characterized by a sleep-like state, there are other tragic and significant neurological conditions that can be distinguished from these states if properly assessed. One of these is the vegetative state, first described by Bryan Jennett and Fred Plum (Jennett and Plum, 1972; Fins, 2019b). Patients who are in the vegetative state are in a state of wakeful unresponsiveness, and in contrast to coma in an eyes-open state. Nonetheless, there is no awareness self, others, or the environment. They have sleep–wake cycles, can grimace in response to pain, and evince a startle reflex. At times a temporal adjective is added before "vegetative" to convey its likely duration. When first described by Jennett and Plum the designator was "persistent." By 1994, the Multi-Society Task Force (MSTF) decided that a vegetative state became persistent if it lasted 1 month after the inciting event, usually traumatic or anoxic brain injury, and "permanent" 3 months after anoxic injury or 12 months after traumatic injury. In 2018, as we will see, the "permanent" designation was replaced by "chronic."

Concerns: A vegetative state diagnosis can be disquieting to families who see the patient emerge from coma and open their eyes. Some find it hard to realize that those eyes are unseeing and unfeeling as it is only natural to expect that eye-opening heralds the return of sentience. To appreciate that it is otherwise can be emotionally devastating.

A good example of this emotional challenge is seen in the words of Julia Quinlan, the mother of Karen of the landmark legal case. In her memoir Mrs. Quinlan writes of her joy when her daughter opened her eyes. She shouted Karen's name and leaned over to kiss her. The nurses "came hurrying over, and there was all kinds of excitement. For just a few minutes we thought it was all over and that she had come back. . ." (Fins, 2015). But soon she realized Karen was unaware. As she put it, "that was the most disheartening development of all, watching her eyes look into space." While the vegetative state gained national prominence in the 1976 Quinlan case, it has also been at the center of the culture wars pitting such substantive norms as the sanctity of life against self-determination and choice. The debates over Nancy Beth Cruzan and Terri Schiavo, two other women in the vegetative state, continued this national debate. *Cruzan v. Missouri Department of Health* reached the US Supreme Court in 1990 (Fins, 2020). The battle over the fate of Ms. Schiavo influenced Florida politics in 2003 and prompted debates in Congress and the attention of the White House in 2005, with some disputing her diagnosis. Even the term "vegetative" has been the object of critique.[1]

---

[1] Some European neurologists have recently advanced a new name for the vegetative state that relies on behavioral findings. Concerned that the "vegetative" adjective was pejorative, these

Minimally Conscious State and Covert Consciousness

Minimally Conscious State Defined: In contrast to the vegetative state, a minimally conscious state (MCS) is a state of consciousness in which a patient has awareness of self, others, and the environment (Giacino et al., 2002). They may look up when a loved one comes into the room, reach for a cup, or even say their name. The challenge is that these behaviors happen sporadically and may not be reliably reproduced. When patients are not exhibiting these kinds of purposive behaviors, they can be mistaken to be vegetative.

Biologically, MCS is distinct from the vegetative state. MCS patients have widely distributed neural networks in the brain, unlike vegetative patients who *lack* integrative function. These network connections sustain consciousness for patients in MCS. Sometimes network activations can be present in the *absence* of behavioral responsiveness that would indicate an awareness of the environment. These patients have a discordance between their inner brain state and overt behaviors and are said to have cognitive motor dissociation (CMD) (Schiff, 2015). For example, CMD patients do not respond to commands with behavioral responses but when placed in a functional MRI and asked to imagine performing a volitional task –like walking around their house, playing tennis, or distinguishing similar words – the areas in the brain responsible for spatial, motor, or linguistic tasks will be activated.

Assessment of *covert* consciousness done in patients in chronic care has now been introduced into the acute care setting (Edlow and Fins, 2018; Classen et al., 2019). Using functional neuroimaging and EEG studies, covert consciousness has been detected in seemingly unresponsive ICU patients. These patients, when followed longitudinally, have better outcomes at 1 year than similarly appearing patients who do not have CMD. Given these prognostic implications, the search for covert consciousness likely will become the standard of care for unresponsive patients during their acute hospitalization.

Concerns: In the years after the 1994 MSTF Report, presumptions about the permanence of the vegetative state began to erode because of a number of unsettling reports of the recovery of consciousness in patients presumed to have been vegetative for years, and even decades. These "recoveries" came as a surprise to clinicians and generated international media attention.

Most notable of these cases was Terry Wallis, an Arkansan who spoke spontaneously 19 years after a car accident that seemed to have left him in the vegetative state in 1984. The operative word is "seemed" because unbeknownst to medical science, Wallis had

---

clinicians suggested that it be renamed Unresponsive Wakefulness Syndrome (UWS), echoing the original language of Jennett and Plum. This redesignation is confusing and should be avoided for three reasons. First, even though the language of unresponsive wakefulness harkens back to Jennett and Plum's *Lancet* article, it is not a fiducial use of language. Notably, Jennett and Plum were careful to note of the vegetative state that, "it *seems* wakefulness without awareness" (italics added) leaving open the possibility of consciousness in patients who did not have behavioral evidence of awareness. Second, the etymology of the vegetative state is steeped in the history of philosophy and science. It was never intended to be pejorative. Its origins date to Aristotle's *De Anima* (see Adams and Fins, 2017). In the modern era, this designation has become central to clinical ethics and jurisprudence. But finally, and most importantly, as a behavioral category, UWS does not account for the possibility of covert consciousness in patients who might present at the bedside as unresponsive and wakeful. As such, this problematically equates those who are in the vegetative state with those who may, in fact, have *covert* consciousness.

entered into MCS, a diagnostic category that was not formalized until 2002, a year after he regained fluent speech. In fact, an international study found that 41% of vegetative patients in chronic care following traumatic brain injury were actually in MCS when assessed with the Coma Recovery Scale-Revised, a validated neuropsychological test designed to assess disorders of consciousness.

Whatever the designation, though, the critical task is to distinguish patients who are conscious from those who are not. Differentiating the vegetative state from MCS (or CMD) (Schiff, 2015), has *significant* clinical implications. Using functional neuroimaging, MCS or CMD patients have been shown to activate pain networks and process language in contrast to vegetative patients. As such, MCS and CMD patients have the neural circuitry to perceive pain and potentially hear what is said in their room. Given this, an important implication is that patients should be presumed to be sensate, and thus, providers should engage *universal pain precautions*. These patients should receive pain and symptom relief as would any other patient. Because the experience of pain may be masked by a paucity of behavioral output, clinicians should be particularly attentive to autonomic signs of untreated pain and treat accordingly. Similarly, because these patients may hear what is said at the bedside, good counsel would be to take conversations outside the room unless the offering are words of encouragement.

Importantly, because MCS and CMD patients have widely distributed neural networks, they are more responsive to emerging therapeutic interventions that are able to activate dormant networks. Over the past decade various neuromodulation techniques – including deep brain stimulation, transcranial magnet stimulation, vagal nerve stimulation, and ultrasound – have been shown to activate circuitry that undergirds consciousness investigational studies. While these techniques are still under study and not established therapies, pharmacologic approaches like amantadine hydrochloride have been shown to be effective in a randomized clinical trial and have become the standard of care in neurology and rehabilitation medicine.

Current Practice Guidelines

Having distinguished different states of consciousness and provided some historical context about this evolving diagnostic framework, we can now return to the 2018 AAN/ACRM/NIDILRR 2018 evidence-based practice guideline. A great deal has been learned since the 1994 MSTF Statement on the vegetative state, and these newer guidelines reflect much of that knowledge, resulting in important changes to terminology to capture the nuances of each of these conditions. As noted, the permanent vegetative state has been redesignated as the *chronic* vegetative state, noting that 20% of patients thought to be permanently vegetative migrated out of the vegetative state. Upwards of half of these patients were misdiagnosed as vegetative and, in MCS, some were in CMD and others had late structural changes in their brain that made consciousness possible (Fins and Bernat, 2018).

This redesignation is a meaningful development for bioethics and the law because the futility of the vegetative state was central to establishing the right to die. This development prompts the question: If the vegetative is not as permanent as once thought, is withdrawal of life-sustaining therapies ethically and legally permissible? In response, it is important to note that decisions to withhold or withdraw life-sustaining therapy are now made routinely for upwards of 75% of patients in American hospitals. One does not need to be in the vegetative state to make these choices. Moreover, it is important not to overestimate the 20% who might recover above the vegetative state, recalling that 80% will not (Fins, 2015).

Of course, the ethical acceptability of foregoing life-sustaining therapies in these patients is predicated on careful and evidence-based evaluations of these patients (Fins, 2019c). In that light, the 2018 guidelines call for improved diagnostic accuracy and standards of care. This is an important affirmative statement for a population for whom diagnostic or therapeutic efforts have historically been viewed as invariably futile. Seeking to reverse this presumption of futility, the guidelines call for the identification, prevention, and amelioration of confounding conditions that interfere with diagnosis, such as unrecognized seizures. They also call for better diagnostic accuracy using the vetted Coma Recovery Scale-Revised (CRS-R) that has unique advantages over the Glasgow Coma and Outcome Scales as well as careful use of emerging neuroimaging methods. Perhaps more critically, the guidelines urge clinicians to avoid and mitigate complications that adversely affect morbidity and mortality like aspiration pneumonia, bedsores, and urinary tract infections. Finally, the guidelines recommend that clinicians engage in dialogue with families about care options including palliation (Fins and Pohl, 2015).

Case Analysis

Despite all of the advances in the field over the past two decades, patients with severe brain injury remain vulnerable to substandard care and precipitous decisions to withhold or withdraw care before their prognosis is clear. Outcome studies have shown that over 20% of patients with the most grievous injuries can regain functional independence (Fins, 2015).

Tragically, this collective knowledge deficit is compounded by the infusion of ideology into an already fraught situation. In this case, Dr. Longwood seeks to steer the patient's wife away from ongoing care and in the process conflates the brain states we have just carefully sought to distinguish. Even if we presume that Dr. Longwood's intentions were nonmaleficent, in seeking to prevent harm he may have also precluded benefit or avoided treatment decisions that might have been therapeutic. In short, his editorializing might have led to a self-fulfilling outcome.

Given these beliefs, how much more difficult would it be to hear that her husband's eye-opening emergence from coma into the vegetative state and possibly progression into MCS were favorable early signs? The point, then, is not to preordain the outcome but to provide guidance to families, follow the facts, using good evidence-based distinctions, and then make moral valuations about care.

The healthcare ethics committee (HEC), through the consult service, can help by convening the clinical team in order to reach a consensus on the facts and work with them to explain the patient's current situation and prospects for recovery and rehabilitation. It would also be useful to ask a specialist in brain rehabilitation to provide additional input. Some acute care and rehabilitation hospitals have even begun to communicate about patient outcomes after discharge to counter the bias that can arise in the acute care setting. This is an important organizational ethics reform that can improve perspectives across the care continuum and improve handoffs on discharge.

The fundamental challenge, then, is not one outcome or another but the pursuit of balance, compassion, and transparency when guiding families through this difficult terrain (Fins, 2019a).

Questions for Discussion

1. Conceptual: How do the differences in disorders make a moral difference for how the HEC should respond to these cases?
2. Pragmatic: What kinds of policies related to disorders of consciousness might be useful to your hospital? Who are the stakeholders who should be involved in the creation and/or revision of these policies?
3. Strategic: What are some strategies to educate hospital staff about how to best communicate the differences in states of consciousness to families?

References

Adams ZM, Fins JJ (2017) The historical origins of the vegetative state: Received wisdom and the utility of the text. *Journal of the History of the Neurosciences*, 26(2): 140–153.

Classen J, Doyle K, Matory A, et al. (2019). Detection of brain activation in unresponsive patients with acute brain injury. *New England Journal of Medicine*, 380(26): 2497–2505.

Edlow BL, Fins JJ (2018). Assessment of covert consciousness in the intensive care unit: Clinical and ethical considerations. *Journal of Head Trauma and Rehabilitation*, 33(6): 424–434.

Fins JJ (2015). *Rights Come to Mind: Brain Injury, Ethics and the Struggle for Consciousness*. New York: Cambridge University Press.

Fins JJ (2019a). Disorders of consciousness in clinical practice: Ethical, legal and policy considerations. In Posner JP, Saper CB, Claussen J, Schiff ND, eds., *Plum and Posner's Diagnosis of Stupor and Coma*, 5th ed. New York: Oxford University Press, 449–477.

Fins JJ (2019b). Disorders of consciousness, Past, present, and future. *Cambridge Quarterly of Healthcare Ethics*, 28(4): 603–615.

Fins JJ (2019c). When no one notices: Disorders of consciousness and the chronic vegetative state. *The Hastings Center Report*, 49(4): 14–17.

Fins JJ (2020). Cruzan and the other evidentiary standard: A reconsideration of a landmark case given advances in the classification of disorders of consciousness and the evolution of disability law. *Southern Methodist University Law Review*, 73(1): 91–118.

Fins JJ, Bernat JL (2018). Ethical, palliative, and policy considerations in disorders of consciousness. *Neurology*, 91(10): 471–475.

Fins JJ, Pohl BR (2015). Neuro-palliative care and disorders of consciousness. In Hanks G, Cherny NI, Christakis NA, Fallon M, Kassa S, Portenoy RK, eds., *Oxford Textbook of Palliative Medicine*, 5th ed. Oxford University Press, 285–291.

Giacino JT, Ashwal S, Childs N, et al. (2002). The minimally conscious state: Definition and diagnostic criteria. *Neurology*, 58(3): 349–353.

Giacino JT, Fins JJ, Laureys S, Schiff ND (2014). Disorders of consciousness after acquired brain injury: The state of the science. *Nature Reviews Neurology*, 10(2): 99–114.

Giacino JT, Katz DI, Schiff ND, et al. (2018). Practice guideline: Disorders of consciousness. *Neurology*, 91(10): 450–460.

Jennett B, Plum F (1972). Persistent vegetative state after brain damage: A syndrome in search of a name. *Lancet*, 1(7753): 734–737.

Multi-Society Task Force on PVS. (1994). Medical aspects of the persistent vegetative state (Parts 1 and 2). *New England Journal of Medicine*, 330(21): 1499–1508 and 330(22): 1572–1579.

Schiff ND (2015). Cognitive motor dissociation following severe brain injury. *JAMA Neurology*, 72(12): 1413–1415.

Schiff ND, Fins JJ (2016). Brain death and disorders of consciousness. *Current Biology*, 26(13): R572–R576.

17

Ethical Issues in Reproduction

Anne Drapkin Lyerly

Objectives

Upon reading and considering the content of this chapter, the reader should be able to:

1. Identify the major ethical positions specific to reproductive decision-making, including the moral status of the fetus, the status of the pregnant woman,[1] and the maternal-fetal relationship.
2. Describe the ethical challenges associated with contraception and pregnancy termination, including the legal and cultural context surrounding conscientious refusal.
3. Describe the ethical challenges associated with conception and loss, including management decisions in the context of significant fetal anomalies.
4. Describe the ethical challenges involved in the management of pregnancy, including potential conflicts between maternal health needs or behaviors and fetal well-being, and decisions about mode of delivery.

Case 1

T.D. is a 22-year-old woman who presented to the emergency room after being raped by a coworker. She underwent a full rape work-up; although standard procedure is to offer her emergency contraception, the emergency room physician felt that doing so would be a conflict of conscience for him, so he refused to write the order. The nursing staff raised concerns that the physician was putting his own interests before those of his patient and failing to provide standard care. The physician countered that it is his right – even his obligation – to act in accordance with his conscience.

Case 2

L.G. is a 28-year-old with a history of multiple miscarriages. In her last pregnancy, a cerclage (a stitch around the cervix) was placed; she carried the pregnancy to term and delivered a healthy child. Now pregnant at 14 weeks, she had planned cerclage placement

---

I am grateful to my colleague Arlene Davis for generously sharing her wisdom from many years serving as an ethics committee member and chair.

[1] While I use the term "woman" throughout this chapter, it is important to recognize that not all individuals who can become pregnant identify as women. The considerations in this chapter are meant to be exclusive to all who may become pregnant, regardless of gender identity.

again; however, an ultrasound revealed an anencephalic fetus. The patient declined abortion and requested the cerclage be placed, but her doctor refused, arguing the risks of cerclage placement (anesthesia, infection) were not justified absent the possibility of meaningful life for her child.

Case 3

S.B. was in her 25th week of pregnancy when she developed signs of preterm labor. She was also a smoker. Her doctor recommended admission to the hospital for bed rest and immediate smoking cessation. The patient declined, noting she had two small children at home to care for. Believing S.B.'s behavior would endanger the fetus, the doctor was considering legal action to force the patient to comply with medical recommendations.

Case 4

A.F. was pregnant with her second child. She delivered her first baby vaginally, which she found traumatic though she and her baby had excellent medical outcomes. After careful consideration, she requested a cesarean delivery for her second birth. Her doctor felt that performing a cesarean delivery absent medical indications would be unethical; he would be willing to refer her to another physician, but none of the available doctors was willing to perform the surgery.

Introduction

Few areas of medicine raise issues more contentious than those generated by the intersection of health care and reproduction. From decisions about disposal of reproductive tissue, to the provision of contraception and abortion, to delivery decisions at the threshold of fetal viability, to issues about intervention and care in pregnancies to be carried to term, the potential for disagreement – and deep disagreement – may lead to requests for input from healthcare ethics committees (HECs).

In this chapter, I discuss a variety of ethical issues that commonly arise in reproductive medicine, and introduce considerations often helpful in identifying ethical pathways forward for those involved. The first section provides a topography of such considerations: the moral status of the fetus, the status of the woman, and the moral implications of the maternal-fetal relationship. Drawing on the cases above, the subsequent three sections apply these considerations to three areas of reproductive medicine: contraception and abortion, conception and loss, and pregnancy and delivery.

Considerations Relevant to Reproductive Ethics: A Brief Topography

When questions of ethics arise in reproductive medicine, they often become difficult and divisive questions. Understanding the taxonomy of these concerns may better prepare an HEC to address them through consultation, education, and policy.

One of the first considerations often raised is the *moral status* of the fetus or embryo. Moral status is a term used to capture the extent to which the fetus or embryo should be given the respect or protections afforded to born human beings. Some hold the view that full moral status is conferred at fertilization or conception – that early embryos deserve the same respect and protection as born children. Others hold the view that gestating humans have no intrinsic moral status, even late in pregnancy, or that that moral status is achieved with certain capacities, such as consciousness (or "sentience"). Still others hold a *gradualist* view – that moral status is something that develops as the embryo does, until near term when the fetus is deserving of the same, or nearly the same, moral protection due to newborns (Little, 2008). These disparate views can be the genesis for conflicts that the ethics committee is asked to address.

However, resolving ethical dilemmas in reproductive medicine does not turn exclusively on the moral status of the fetus. At least two other considerations, often overlooked, may help to solve ethical conflicts, even in the face of polarized views about obligations to the unborn. Both relate to the "unique conditions" under which the fetus lives – namely within the body of a pregnant woman (Little, 2008).

The first of these other considerations is the status of the pregnant woman. Over the last several decades, a curious pattern has emerged in debates about reproductive ethics. Oftentimes, as clinicians and ethicists tussle over obligations to fetuses or embryos, the woman herself – and obligations of others to *her* – fade from view (Mahowald, 1995). In some cases, she is considered not at all – she is for practical purposes invisible. When debate arose about whether it was ethical to perform surgery on fetuses before birth, discussions revolved primarily around the severity of fetal disease and the risks of fetal harm from intervention and nonintervention, not on the impact of surgery on the woman herself. On point, a group of bioethicists critiqued the term "fetal surgery" and suggested that "maternal-fetal surgery" more accurately characterized the investigative practice, and might help orient attention to the pregnant woman, whose body and interests are also profoundly affected by prebirth intervention (Lyerly et al., 2001). The more inclusive term has since been adopted by leading organizations, such as the American College of Obstetricians and Gynecologists (ACOG) and National Institutes of Health (NIH). In other cases, the woman has been considered merely as a "vessel or vector." In the early days of the HIV epidemic, women were studied primarily in terms of their likelihood of infecting men or fetuses/children – indeed as *vectors*, but not as patients or subjects in their own right (Faden et al., 1996). Finally, women's views about what matters morally may not inform reproductive debates. In the 1990s stem cell debates included the perspectives of religious authorities, politicians, scientists, disease advocates; when IVF patients' views were finally included, their voices made clear that more than moral status was at stake when they made decisions about disposition of excess embryos.

But there is a second, if related (and similarly overlooked) consideration beyond moral status, namely the *relationship* between the pregnant woman and the entity she actually or potentially gestates. Physically, gestation involves use of a person's body by another, entailing profound physiologic shifts in the healthiest pregnancies, and in others, threats to health and life. Emotionally, reproduction is among the most private and personal matters that humans will face; decisions about whether and how to reproduce will invoke the ethics of relationships, of parenthood, of intimacy. Whatever the moral status of the embryo or fetus, its unique relationship with the pregnant woman should inform discussions about the provision of reproductive care.

Contraception and Abortion: The Debate over Conscientious Refusal

As reflected in Case 1, sometimes physicians and other healthcare workers will assert that providing legal or standard care would constitute a conflict of conscience for them. Though this occurs across medicine (e.g., in end-of-life care, pediatrics) the issue of conscientious refusal has gained particular attention in reproductive medicine, especially around the contested areas of contraception and abortion. The debate has been polarized, with one side claiming that physicians and other health workers who cannot provide such services should leave the profession, and the other that healthcare providers have a virtually absolute right to refuse.

Arguments against the latter view are several-fold. First, refusals may constitute a failure to respect a person's autonomy. In Case 1, the physician's refusal to dispense emergency contraception further (given the patient was raped) compromised the patient's ability to decide for herself whether and under what circumstances to become pregnant. Second, many refusals have the potential to harm patients. If the patient above did become pregnant, she would be faced with the choice – unpleasant for some, heart-wrenching for others – of whether to carry the pregnancy or obtain an abortion. And if she chose the latter, she would face the risks of a procedure that could have been avoided if emergency contraception had been made available to her in the emergency room. Third, sometimes judgments about the morality of an act are based on inaccurate understandings of science. For instance, many healthcare providers and pharmacists have based their objections to emergency contraception on a misunderstanding or mistrust of science. They believe that emergency contraception is an abortifacient, when the body of science points to prevention of fertilization as the primary mechanism of action. Finally, refusals have the potential to exacerbate discrimination, unjustly burdening socioeconomically or otherwise disadvantaged people. For example, "finding another doctor" may be particularly difficult for women whose access to care or resources is already limited. Moreover, where refusals are grounded in discriminatory views, they not only lack an ethical foundation but worsen existing disparities in gender and minority health.

While a full treatment of this issue is beyond the scope of this chapter, as Wicclair argues in Chapter 24, HECs may address these issues creating organizational structures that ensure access to professional services and minimize the need for individual practitioners to act in opposition to their conscience. Ethics committees may be in a position to help institutions to develop, for example, staffing and intradepartmental referral plans that ensure standard services like emergency contraception be available to victims of rape and other women for whom it is indicated.

Conception and Loss

Decisions about conception and loss raise complicated issues for providers and patients alike. Although up to one in three pregnancies end in miscarriage, little attention has been directed at understanding how best to care for patients who face it (Layne, 2003).

When prenatal imaging or diagnosis reveals an anomaly incompatible with life, requests to prolong pregnancy are often framed in terms of futility (see Chapter 15). If intervention will not improve the fetus's condition, the argument goes, physicians have no ethical obligation to provide requested care, and may in fact have an obligation to *refrain* from providing it. Such reflects the response of the obstetrician in Case 2 to the patient's request for cerclage placement.

Framed in this way, Case 2 raises several potential avenues for resolution. It is certainly possible, for example, that the patient's request stems from a lack of comprehension about the implications of the diagnosis, and highlights the importance of ensuring adequate disclosure and understanding. It is also possible that the patient and physician diverge in their understanding of what constitutes a meaningful life; for the patient, a short life without cerebral function may in fact be something she views as valuable, and may undergird her desires to bring her pregnancy to term.

But there is another way to frame the case, which brings to attention particular considerations in reproduction that are often overlooked. As noted in the *Topography* (above) moral status is but one consideration used to frame debates in reproductive ethics. Alternatively, placing the woman and her relationship to the fetus at the center of the discussion may lead to different questions – and answers. Indeed, the case discussion thus far uses the question of *life* as the language of contention: What is the status of an entity that does not have a brain? What does that tell us about the ethics of intervention? But when women make decisions about reproduction, they often attend not just to life, but to *relationships*: Regardless of the status of the fetus, what would it mean to responsibly proceed as a gestating woman, a mother-to-be?

By pulling away from questions of moral status we can begin to see how the patient's request – even if medically futile – might still be reasonable and beneficial. For one, carrying a pregnancy to term might allow the patient to go through the process of giving birth and mourning a loss. And in the cases such as the one described above, discussions with the ethics committee may prove enlightening. Further discussion with this patient may have revealed that all seven of her miscarriages happened unexpectedly and quickly (losses with an "incompetent cervix" are often physically painless and happen without the usual warnings of labor), throughout pregnancy, and laced her days with fear. Active pregnancy termination was not an option, but equally untenable was going through a pregnancy never knowing when she might deliver the child – on the floor of her kitchen, in the middle of the night, in the presence of her toddler, in the middle of a workday. The cerclage would allow her to exert some control over when she had the baby, and provide the opportunity to bid her child farewell in a space of peace and safety.

Pregnancy and Delivery: The Ethics of Intervention, Refused and Requested

Most of the time, pregnant women are the staunchest advocates for the health of the fetuses they carry. When they do not seem to be acting in the best interests of the fetus – as the physician in Case 3 posited of his patient – what is the appropriate response?

Over the past 30 years, doctors, lawyers and ethicists have discussed and disputed this question. Both legal precedent and ethical analysis have pointed to the same answer: Neither forced treatment nor intervention against the wishes of pregnant women is ever justified. ACOG affirmed this view in an Ethics Committee Opinion when it stated, "The

College opposes the use of coerced medical interventions for pregnant women, including the use of the courts to mandate medical interventions for unwilling patients" (ACOG Committee on Ethics, 2016/2019, 1190).

ACOG and others offer several reasons for this stance. The first is that pregnant women have legal and moral rights to informed consent and bodily integrity. Failure to attend to these rights – to access a fetus through the body of a pregnant woman without her consent – treats women as "vessels" or "nonpersons." The Supreme Court has long acknowledged the right of individuals to refuse intervention, including individuals who are pregnant. The landmark case was that of Angela Carder who, at 26 weeks pregnant and dying from cancer, was forced to undergo a cesarean delivery against her wishes and those of her family. She and the baby both died, and a District of Columbia appellate court subsequently vacated a lower court's decision to compel the delivery and stated that "in virtually all cases the question of what is to be done is to be decided by the patient – the pregnant woman, on behalf of herself and the fetus" (In re A.C., 573 A.2d. 1235 [DC 1990]).

But there are other strong reasons to oppose forced intervention. One is prognostic uncertainty: Medical knowledge and predictions of outcomes in obstetrics have stark limitations. Many have emphasized that conflicts such as those described above are more accurately described as being between patients and physicians, administrators or judges, *not* between women and fetuses. Women who refuse interventions will often do so because they believe (and correctly) that doing so is the best option – for the fetus, for the woman herself, and for her family, given what she values and the importance of risks and benefits in the context of her life. Further, outcomes in obstetrics are notoriously hard to predict, and the certainty with which doctors make recommendations is often linked with an uncertainty about the actual potential for harm.

In addition, many have argued that forced intervention does not make sense in terms of public policy or public health. Coercive approaches are disproportionately applied to disadvantaged populations, raising concerns of discrimination. Further, the use of coercive practices has the potential to discourage women from seeking prenatal care, and may create the potential for legal intervention to redress the breadth of health behaviors, common across the population. For instance, if a diabetic woman didn't adhere strictly enough to her insulin regimen (or a healthy diet, for that matter) when pregnant, would forced hospitalization be justified? Certainly not.

There are a number of strategies that can and should be used to attend to conflicts without involving the legal system, all of which an ethics committee can facilitate. These may include evidence-based strategies to enhance patient-centered communication, an interdisciplinary team approach, and robust risk-benefit analysis that attends to common distortions in risk reasoning around pregnancy (ACOG Committee on Ethics, 2016/2019).

While the right of competent pregnant patients to refuse medical interventions is clear, the appropriate response to a patient who requests an intervention other than what is usually recommended is less so. If some cases are easily dispensed with (a request for elective delivery remote from term), many cases, such as delivery decisions at term like the one described in Case 4, will be more complex. Patients may request that labor be induced for reasons that do not seem adequately pressing to a physician; they may request a trial of vaginal delivery in a setting where a physician believes such is unsafe; or they may request a cesarean for a first or later birth when attempted vaginal delivery would be standard and accepted care.

Debates over the ethics of providing cesareans in the absence of medical indications have garnered widespread attention, including consideration by a panel convened by the NIH. Those opposed have argued that it constitutes unnecessary surgery that has the potential to adversely affect the health of women and children, and that expanding choice might in fact constrict women's options in the long term. Others have countered that other riskier elective procedures are provided across medicine; that in today's obstetric climate, cesarean delivery is a likely outcome even with a trial of vaginal birth; and that the risks of either approach are not so different that they justify constraining women's choices in a circumstance where preferences around process will reasonably vary widely.

When determining how to sort through such requests around delivery, four considerations are relevant (Little et al., 2008). First are considerations of safety and efficacy, which include the extent to which a provider has the tools and expertise to manage the specific approach; further, notions of what is "safe" or "safest" will be shaped by how patients or providers value (or disvalue) possible outcomes. But choices in the clinic may have implications for other patients, which raises two other considerations. They include cost-effectiveness, which is especially important for options whose use would be prevalent (like cesarean), and externalities, or the broader clinical and social consequences of practices or policies that expand or restrict choice. Indeed, opponents of elective cesareans have worried that if the cesarean rate further increased and obstetrics became even more oriented to high-intervention approaches, access to vaginal delivery for the general population might be restricted. These later two considerations are important for policymakers, but should not be used to restrict choice in an individual clinical encounter. Ethics committee members can be helpful in emphasizing the importance of respecting the individual choice in clinical contexts, and also in helping institutions guard against general policies and practices that may narrow access to modes of delivery – including vaginal delivery – of value and benefit to childbearing women.

Perhaps of most pressing importance is the fourth consideration: what the patient prefers, including the extent to which she would trade off one set of possible outcomes for another, how important differences in such outcomes are to her, and which risks emerge for her as most pressing. Because birth, like death, is an arena in which personal values are often strongly held and varied, and where process matters in addition to outcome, priority should be given to maintaining a range of options within which a woman's values can be responsibly honored.

In the case of A.F. in Case 4, the *process* of vaginal birth may have been the issue. She had a prior vaginal birth in which outcomes were good – but it was the *process* that gave her pause about laboring again. Certainly, an in-depth discussion about what exactly concerned her and ways to avoid it would be critical to informed decision-making on her part and responsible action on that of the provider. However, blanket refusal to perform a procedure with risks comparable (though not equivalent) to a vaginal delivery would fail to adequately respect the patient's autonomy and incorporate her preferences into clinical decision-making.

Approaches for an Ethics Committee

The specific issues mentioned in this chapter may arise in consultations related to reproductive health care. Hopefully, the treatment of these issues will assist consultants in probing more deeply about the context and perspectives of all of the stakeholders involved as a way of reaching resolution. In addition, educating hospital stakeholders about the issues described in this chapter may serve as a proactive ethics mechanism to promote sensitivity and nuance in addressing patients as they present with needs in reproductive health care that may at first appear challenging to providers. Finally, engaging with institutional leaders to establish local policies about issues such as conscientious objection and consent requirements for labor and delivery may foster a compassionate and consistent approach to reproductive health care institution-wide, resulting in an ethical environment and culture where women feel respected and empowered.

Questions for Discussion

1. Conceptual: In what circumstances should a healthcare worker's refusal to provide a legal and medically-indicated reproductive service be protected? What are some alternatives to their directly providing care?
2. Pragmatic: What considerations should guide practitioners in evaluating women's preferences in the context of reproductive loss, particularly when they fall outside of standard care?
3. Strategic: When a pregnant woman refuses a medically-indicated intervention aimed at fetal health, how should providers/ethics committee members respond? What considerations should guide delivery decisions about whether to provide a requested service that falls outside usual recommendations for care?

References

American College of Obstetricians and Gynecologists Committee on Ethics. (2007; reaffirmed 2019). ACOG Committee Opinion #385: The limits of conscientious refusal in reproductive medicine. *Obstetrics and Gynecology*, 110(5): 1203–1208.

American College of Obstetricians and Gynecologists Committee on Ethics. (2016, reaffirmed 2019). ACOG Committee Opinion #664: Refusal of medically recommended treatment during pregnancy. *Obstetrics and Gynecology*, 127(6): 1189–1190.

Faden RR, Kass N, McGraw D (1996). Women as vessels and vectors: Lessons from the HIV epidemic. In Wolf SM, ed., *Feminism and Bioethics: Beyond Reproduction*. New York: Oxford University Press, 252–281.

Layne L (2003). *Motherhood Lost: A Feminist Account of Pregnancy Loss in America*. New York: Routledge.

Little MO (2008). Abortion and the margins of personhood. *Rutgers Law Journal*, 39: 331–348.

Little MO, Lyerly AD, Mitchell LM, et al. (2008). Mode of delivery: Toward responsible inclusion of patient preferences. *Obstetrics and Gynecology*, 112(4): 913–918.

Lyerly AD, Gates E, Cefalo RC, Sugarman J (2001). Toward the ethical evaluation and use of maternal-fetal surgery. *Obstetrics and Gynecology*, 98(4): 689–697.

Mahowald MB (1995). As if there were fetuses without women: A remedial essay. In Callahan J, ed., *Reproduction, Ethics and the Law: Feminist Perspectives*. Bloomington: Indiana University Press, 199–218.

Chapter 8

Ethical Issues in Neonatology

18

John D. Lantos

Objectives

Upon reading and considering the content of this chapter, the reader should be able to:

1. Understand what makes the neonatal ICU (NICU) ethically unique.
2. Recognize ways in which improved prenatal diagnosis may change neonatal care and may create additional ethical challenges.
3. Describe different clinical populations in the NICU and the implication for ethical decision-making.

Case 1

A healthy 25-year-old married woman who had good prenatal care goes into labor at 24 weeks and 3 days of gestation. The dates were established by two ultrasounds done at 8 and 16 weeks of gestation. She and her husband have a healthy 3-year-old at home. Both parents are informed that the doctors recommend antenatal steroids and, if there is any fetal distress, a C-section. They are also informed that, once the baby is born, it will likely require intubation and mechanical ventilation. After thoughtful discussion that included the woman, her husband, the neonatologists, and the obstetrician, the woman opts not to receive steroids and requests that, if her baby is born before 25 weeks, only comfort care be provided.

A baby girl is born by vaginal delivery. In the delivery room, the baby has a heart rate of 130 and a weak cry. The baby's birthweight is 750 grams. Should the doctors follow the parents' wishes for palliative care, or should they intubate the baby and provide mechanical ventilation and other NICU care?

Case 2

A baby is born at 39 weeks' gestation after a prenatal diagnosis of trisomy 18 diagnosed by amniocentesis. At birth, he was noted to have a heart murmur and was subsequently diagnosed with a large perimembranous ventricular septal defect (VSD). An EEG showed seizure activity. He was placed on phenobarbital. Head ultrasound showed prominent extra-axial fluid, but no evidence of a bleed. Genetics counseled the parents that most infants with trisomy 18 do not survive until their first birthday, although approximately 10% of affected children do survive longer. The doctors ask that the palliative care team meet with the parents, and recommend that the child receive only palliative care. The parents reject this recommendation and, instead, request that their baby have cardiac surgery to repair the VSD. Should the heart surgery be performed, or should the doctors only provide palliative care?

Introduction

These two cases illustrate a number of crucial features about the ethical dilemmas that arise in the NICU. They highlight the ways in which ethical dilemmas for newborns are similar in some ways and different in other ways from ethical dilemmas in other clinical settings. In discussing these cases, I will try to highlight the features that ought to be of concern to healthcare ethics committees (HECs).

First, as in other settings, an ethical "dilemma" only draws the attention of an ethics consultant when there is a disagreement between relevant stakeholders. One could argue that every birth of a baby at 23–24 weeks of gestation should be considered an ethical dilemma. In most cases, however, doctors and parents agree on an appropriate course of action. The decisions they reach might be different in different cases. Some hospitals have policies mandating or proscribing resuscitation at particular gestational ages. Obstetricians and neonatologists have differing attitudes about whether to insist on life-sustaining treatment or palliative care. But, when doctors and parents agree, it is generally not considered a dilemma. Certainly, when there is agreement, nobody would call an ethics consultant to ratify (or critique) the agreement. Ethics consultations are often requested when the key players cannot agree. Recognition of these precursors of ethics consultation influences the ways in which HECs may respond.

A second feature of these two cases is unique to neonatal bioethics. Many ethical controversies in the NICU begin with decisions that must be made – and are made – during pregnancy. In Case 1, the baby's prognosis was influenced by the decision of the parents to forgo antenatal steroids and C-section. Presumably, they also refused fetal monitoring. If they had accepted these, the baby's prognosis would have been better than it was without them. To the extent that the proper ethical resolution of the conflict turns on the baby's prognosis, it is impossible to separate those antenatal decisions from the postnatal situation. The ethical and legal considerations that inform discussions of whether to override treatment refusals by a pregnant woman for herself are quite different from those that go into discussions of whether to override treatment refusals for her baby. Her decisions should be respected in deference to her autonomy. Decisions for the baby should reflect considerations of what is in the baby's best interest. The effects of these prenatal decisions are even more striking in the second case. Most cases of trisomy 18 – and many other congenital syndromes and anomalies – can be diagnosed prenatally. Prenatal decisions about whether to pursue such diagnoses and, if the diagnoses are made, whether to terminate the pregnancy, are common, legally sanctioned, and well accepted by most doctors and citizens.

For the purposes of neonatal bioethics, it is important to recognize the ways that prenatal decisions, which adhere to a set of moral guidelines different from postnatal decisions, can shape those postnatal decisions. Pregnant women can refuse treatments that are clearly beneficial for the fetus and that will lead to better outcomes for the baby, even though they may not be legally permitted to refuse similar treatments for an already born baby if those treatments are thought to be clearly beneficial. The decision to refuse steroids in Case 1 changes the baby's prognosis. The parents' decisions to both permit prenatal diagnosis and then not to terminate the pregnancy in Case 2 are important factors in understanding the moral commitments that shape postnatal options in this case.

Another important feature of these two cases is one that is common to ethics consultations in other pediatric settings, but different from involving patients who are competent (or who were once-competent) adults. The focus in neonatal and pediatric cases is on whether or not the treatment is likely to be beneficial to the baby, rather than on the patient's or parents' values and preferences. Put another way, beneficence is the primary concern in pediatrics and autonomy in older patients.

This focus turns on the baby's prognosis for survival and for various forms of medical or neurocognitive impairment. If the likely outcome is deemed sufficiently good, then the treatment is considered legally and morally obligatory. If the likely outcome is sufficiently bad, treatment may be legally and morally optional. It may even be considered futile.

The classification of treatment as futile is complicated and controversial (see Chapter 15). There is debate, for example, about whether any congenital anomaly can be considered "lethal" or "incompatible with life" in the age of high-tech NICU and pediatric ICU care. But there is widespread agreement that treatment of babies born at less than 22 weeks of gestational age is futile. Most doctors will refuse to provide intensive care for babies born before 22 weeks. The law upholds these refusals. When such cases go to court, which is rare, the courts have upheld the doctors. In general, the ambiguity of futility determinations in the NICU is similar to ambiguities in other clinical settings.

The obligatory nature of treatment in situations where the prognosis is good is unique to pediatrics and reflects the prioritization of the baby's interests over the parents' legal authority to make medical decisions for their children. Competent adults can refuse medical treatment even when doctors think that treatment will be beneficial based upon the principle of respect for autonomy. Parents do not have the same right to refuse treatment for their children. The key question in the NICU (or other pediatric settings) then, is not whether the parents are reasonable and competent but, instead, whether the benefits of treatment are sufficiently clear as to make treatment morally obligatory regardless of the parents' capabilities, views, values, and preferences.

Case 1 and Case 2 illustrate the two most common types of cases that generate moral controversy in the NICU – decisions for babies at the borderline of viability and decisions for babies with congenital anomalies or syndromes that are associated with long-term morbidity and mortality. In either case, the process of resolving the cases is similar. Data must be gathered on the likely outcome for the baby with or without treatment. Then, a judgment must be made about whether the outcomes are sufficiently dichotomous and unambiguous as to leave no room for discretion or, alternatively, whether the cases fall into an ethical and regulatory "gray zone." For these two particular conditions, very good data exist to define the prognosis fairly precisely. They are, thus, good paradigm cases for determining what sorts of outcomes ought to be considered so good that treatment is obligatory, or so bad that treatment is considered futile.

With prematurity, interpretation dilemmas arise because the precise prognosis is a probabilistic assessment of likely outcomes. For babies like the baby in Case 1, there is a quantifiable probability of either an excellent outcome, a dismal one, or something in between. The key question is the likelihood of each. In the second case, by contrast, the key question is whether the outcomes are sufficiently good to deem treatment nonfutile – or sufficiently bad to argue that treatment is painful and harmful without any compensatory benefit. If the latter, then treatment should be considered futile and doctors should refuse to provide it even if the parents want it.

In theory – and in many professional guidelines – doctors ought to defer to parents when a case is thought to be one in the gray zone. However, doctors are the ones who determine the boundaries of the gray zone. It is fairly well established that doctors do not agree with one another about where those boundaries should be drawn.

Answers to these questions must be based upon the facts but, as I shall argue below, must go beyond mere consideration of facts.

Facts about Babies at the Borderline of Viability

Good ethical reasoning must start with good facts. But facts, in a situation like this, are not straightforward. As noted above, they depend, in part, upon the decisions that are made prenatally. Babies whose mothers were treated with steroids prenatally do better than babies whose mothers were not. Premature babies born by C-section do better than those born vaginally. Other factors also influence prognosis. Generally, girls do better than boys at any given birthweight and gestational age. In many studies, Black babies have better outcomes than white babies. Parental socioeconomic status and educational background exert influence on neurocognitive outcomes. Babies born in tertiary care centers do better than babies born in hospitals without similar technology and expertise. Even in tertiary care centers, the philosophy of the center might influence outcome. Those that generally treat babies at 23 weeks of gestation, for example, have better outcomes for such babies than those that don't. These factors create a certain tension when doctors, parents, or bioethicists talk about "the facts." The most statistically robust "facts" are those that come from large, multicenter studies. The most personally relevant facts in any particular case are those that are applicable to the particular baby, the particular institution, and the particular clinical situation. The former are easier to get. The latter ought to be determinative.

One of the studies that is most widely used to determine prognosis for babies at the borderline of viability is based on work from the Neonatal Research Network (NRN) of the National Institute of Child Health and Development (NICHD) (Tyson et al., 2008). Researchers used retrospective data on outcomes within the NRN to calculate outcomes for babies after consideration of five factors – birthweight, gestational age, gender, singleton versus multiple gestation, and the use of antenatal steroids. They have converted their analysis into a publicly available, internet-based application that can be used to give the prognosis for survival and for neurologic impairment, given those five variables (https://www.nichd.nih.gov/research/supported/EPBO). Using this tool, one could assess the prognosis for the baby in Case 1. That work has recently been updated by including outcomes from the hospitals that participated in the Vermont Oxford Network during the years 2006–2012. For a singleton female born at 24 weeks' gestation, with a birthweight of 750 g, and without antenatal steroids, the predicted survival rate is 68% if the baby is given mechanical ventilation. Of the babies born in these circumstances who are given mechanical ventilation, 60% of survivors will have good neurological outcomes (that is, no impairment or only mild impairment). Only 3%–5% of survivors will have severe impairment (www.nichd.nih.gov/research/supported/EPBO/use/ accessed July 21, 2021). If antenatal steroids had been given, the predicted survival rate would have been 80%. In that situation, 75% of babies would survive without severe neurodevelopmental impairment. It should be remembered that these numbers are based on outcomes in the years 2006–2012.

These general statistics mask variations among hospitals. Even within the NRN, which consists only of tertiary care hospitals in the United States, there is tremendous variability in which babies are treated and on outcomes. For babies born at any particular gestational age, survival rates differ between hospitals. At 22 weeks, survival rates range from zero at one hospital to 50% at another. At 23 weeks, the range is 24%–47%. At 24 weeks, it is 47%–69% (Rysavy et al., 2015). The differences reflect different philosophies of treatment. Hospitals with the lowest survival rates are those that do not offer active treatment and NICU admission to the tiniest babies.

Predictions of neurodevelopmental impairments among survivors also hide significant interhospital variation. The NRN has not published hospital-specific data on long-term outcomes, but it does analyze differences in some of the predictors of neurodevelopmental problems. The percentage of babies who had Grade IV intracranial hemorrhages ranged from 3% to 67% between centers. The percentage of babies with severe retinopathy ranged from 0% to 20%.

HEC members who are called to consult in such a case ought to be aware of tools like the NICHD neonatal calculator. They should also be aware of the limitations of these tools. The percentages ought to be the starting point for a judgment about whether or not treatment is morally obligatory. But only a starting point. Local data ought to be considered. There ought to be some deference given to parental motivations – that is, for the reasons that they give for what they do. HEC members ought to ascertain whether or not the parents understand their baby's prognosis. Importantly, the doctor's views ought to be interrogated with equal rigor and attention to detail. Are they making decisions that are consistent with the professional consensus about similar cases? Or does the doctor have idiosyncratic views that ought to be recognized as such?

Ultimately, HEC members must pull together the best facts and then seek to understand the motivations of doctors and parents for their views of what ought or ought not to be done in each case.

Facts about Babies with Trisomy 18 and other Life-Limiting Congenital Anomalies

Until recently, many doctors referred to trisomy 18 as a "lethal congenital anomaly." It was common for doctors to say that all babies with this anomaly died within the first year of life. McGraw and Perlman note, for example, that, until recently, "there was tacit consensus among those providing neonatal intensive care that these were lethal trisomies and therefore were classified as conditions for which resuscitation was not indicated" (McGraw and Perlman, 2008, 1109).

That is starting to change. A strict interpretation of lethality would mean that no baby with the anomaly could survive, even with intensive care treatment and life support. Few congenital anomalies meet those criteria. Medical technology has advanced to the point where even babies with anencephaly can sometimes be kept alive for months or years. Today, we know that the likelihood of prolonged survival for a baby with trisomy 18 may be influenced not just by the underlying condition but also by the treatment decisions that are made. That is similar to the situation with extremely premature babies.

In the age of the Internet, clinical studies by doctors are not the only source of data about outcomes. Families of babies with trisomies have formed their own research networks, and publish their own results on websites (see, for example, www.trisomy.org/ and www.hopefortrisomy13and18.org). There are differences between the "facts" found in the peer-reviewed scientific literature and the "facts" found on these "lay" websites that gather data from parents. Two commonly cited studies from the medical literature claim that the 1-year survival rate for babies with trisomy 18 is less than 10% (Rosa et al., 2011). In one study, over half the babies had do-not-attempt-resuscitation orders (Hsaio et al., 2009). By contrast, the website called TRIS (for tracking rare incidence syndromes), based at Southern Illinois University, reports that half of babies with trisomies live for years (http://web.coehs.siu.edu/Grants/TRIS/index.html). Furthermore, the categorizations between "academic" and "lay" literature are not so straightforwardly dichotomous. Some such websites are based in academic institutions and publish their results in peer-reviewed journals.

Although there is disagreement about life expectancy, there is no disagreement about the likelihood or degree of neurocognitive impairment. All babies with trisomy 18 have profound neurocognitive impairment. Decisions about whether or not to treat those medical and surgical problems depend upon an assessment of the baby's quality of life, given the profound neurocognitive deficits. Thus, unlike the situation for babies at the borderline of viability, the possible outcomes in cases of trisomy cover a much narrower spectrum. Life expectancy is shorter, and there is no possibility of future cognitive function in the normal range.

As in Case 1, the consultant has a delicate role to play in trying to determine whether the doctors and parents are making decisions based upon facts or upon misunderstandings. For both, values are important, but generally values should reflect a given fact pattern, which is not determined by values. HEC members can serve as a neutral sounding board for all parties.

Values and Disagreements in Neonatal Treatment Decisions

It is abundantly clear that different doctors, different doctor groups, and different professional societies make different recommendations for the treatment of babies born at the borderline of viability. This is true within countries and between countries. While most older policies assumed that survival was unlikely for babies born at 22 weeks of gestation, more recent data (Rysavy et al., 2015) show that, with active treatment, many such babies survive. Further, although there is general agreement that treatment is morally obligatory after 25 completed weeks of gestation, differences in practices persist. In Switzerland and the Netherlands, both C-sections and resuscitation are considered optional at 25 weeks and provided only when parents demand them. In most countries, 23–24 weeks are a sort of gray zone, where recommendations suggest resuscitation on an "individual basis" and "according to the parents' wishes." In Germany, every preterm neonate is a candidate for treatment, regardless of gestational age. In Sweden, neonatal intensive care is offered to all babies at 22 weeks and above. Of babies born at 22 weeks who receive intensive care, 58% survive. Most survivors do not have severe disabilities (Norman et al., 2019).

Similar practice variations can be seen within countries, too. In the United States, for example, some centers recommend palliative care only at 23 and 24 weeks (Kaempf et al., 2009), while other centers recommend routine resuscitation at these gestational ages (Batton et al., 2011). Even within centers, some doctors may be more willing to provide palliative care than others, or more insistent on providing intensive care (Rysavy et al., 2015).

There is similar disagreement among doctors, hospitals, and centers regarding the treatment of babies with trisomies. Some recommend palliative care. Some leave it up to the parents. These decisions reflect both the physicians' assessments of the medical facts in the case and also their own religious beliefs or other value commitments (Donohue et al., 2010).

Parents have similar differences in their views. Most parents who receive a prenatal diagnosis of trisomy 18 choose to terminate pregnancy. Others choose to carry the pregnancy to term. After birth, some choose palliative care while others want all available life support.

In both situations – babies born at the borderline of viability and babies born with life-limiting conditions – the potential exists for intractable value disagreements between parents and healthcare professionals (Janvier et al., 2011).

Implications for Ethics Consultation

So, what are HEC members to do when an intractable disagreement arises in a situation that is well recognized to be ethically controversial but that only rarely leads to an intractable disagreement? The first questions the HEC member must ask are, "Why this case? Why now? What is so different and so difficult in this case that the experienced practitioners felt the need of outside assistance to resolve an intractable disagreement?"

The HEC member in the NICU has a number of tasks. The first is to answer questions about the "standards of care." The consultant must determine if the particular features of the case make it different from the generic case of "a baby at the borderline of viability" or "a baby with trisomy 18." Those generic cases are ones in which the consultant can confidently say that, as of 2019, in the United States, reasonable people disagree in ways that place these cases squarely in the gray zone, also known as the "zone of parental discretion" (McDougall et al., 2018). If that is the case, then the consultant can confidently argue that parental preferences should prevail as long as the parents have been informed about and seem to understand the implications of their choices.

If the HEC member is going to say more than that, then they must shoulder the burden of proving why this particular case is atypical and thus does not belong in the zone of parental discretion.

Not all babies with trisomy 18 are the same. They can have a range of severe congenital anomalies that may make treatment particularly inappropriate. Not all 24-weekers are the same, for similar reasons. Some pregnancies may be complicated by significant maternal health problems. Babies may be at higher risk than average as a result.

If the HEC member confirms that the case is one that truly belongs in the zone of parental discretion, then they must support the parents' right to make the decision. To do this, it will be crucial to help doctors, nurses, and parents to clarify their own values and the role that those values should play. This can often lead to appropriate compromise and consensus.

Ethical dilemmas in neonatal intensive care engage people's deepest moral commitments, strongest emotions, brightest hopes, and darkest fears. The ethicist must work with those powerful forces, keeping an eye out always for the baby's interests. Each case should become part of an institutional pattern of decisions that reflect the collective moral wisdom of physicians, the community, and the ethics consultant.

Questions for Discussion

1. Conceptual: How should we understand neonatal "best interests"? Should we balance the interests of the parents/family and the neonate, and if so, how?
2. Pragmatic: What are the standard clinical practices at your institution for babies born at the threshold of viability? How might you discover this information?
3. Strategic: How would you elicit the underlying values of the parents and the healthcare providers when ethical issues arise in neonatal treatment decision-making?

References

Batton DG, DeWitte DB, Pryce CJ (2011). One hundred consecutive infants born at 23 weeks and resuscitated. *American Journal of Perinatology*, 28(4): 299–304.

Donohue P, Boss R, Aucott S, Keene E, Teague P (2010). The impact of neonatologists' religiosity and spirituality on health care delivery for high-risk neonates. *Journal of Palliative Medicine*, 13(10): 1219–1224.

Hsiao CC, Tsao LY, Chen HN, Chiu HY, Chang WC (2009). Changing clinical presentations and survival pattern in trisomy 18. *Pediatrics and Neonatology*, 50(4): 147–151.

Janvier A, Okah F, Farlow B, Lantos JD (2011). An infant with trisomy 18 and a ventricular septal defect. *Pediatrics*, 127(4): 754–759.

Kaempf JW, Tomlinson MW, Campbell B, Ferguson L, Stewart VT (2009). Counseling pregnant women who may deliver extremely premature infants: Medical care guidelines, family choices, and neonatal outcomes. *Pediatrics*, 123(6): 1509–1515.

McDougall R, Gillam L, Spriggs M, Delany C (2018). The zone of parental discretion and the complexity of paediatrics: A response to Alderson. *Clinical Ethics*, 13(4): 172–174.

McGraw MP, Perlman JM (2008). Attitudes of neonatologists toward delivery room management of confirmed trisomy 18: Potential factors influencing a changing dynamic. *Pediatrics*, 121(6): 1106–1110.

Norman M, Hallberg B, Abrahamsson T, et al. (2019). Association between year of birth and 1-year survival among extremely preterm infants in Sweden during 2004–2007 and 2014–2016. *JAMA*, 321(12): 1188–1199.

Rosa RF, Rosa RC, Lorenzen MB, et al. (2011). Trisomy 18: Experience of a reference hospital from the south of Brazil. *American Journal of Medical Genetics A*, 155A(7): 1529–1535.

Rysavy R, Li L, Bell EF, et al. (2015). Between-hospital variation in treatment and outcomes in extremely preterm infants. *New England Journal of Medicine*, 372(19): 1801–1811.

Tyson JE, Parikh NA, Langer J (2008). Intensive care for extreme prematurity – moving beyond gestational age. *New England Journal of Medicine*, 358: 1672–1681.

19

Ethical Issues in Pediatrics

Douglas S. Diekema and D. Micah Hester

Objectives

Upon reading and considering the content of this chapter, the reader should be able to:

1. Describe the ethical scope and limits of parental authority.
2. Navigate the challenge of using the "best interest standard" when authoritative parties disagree on what is best for the child.
3. Discuss the role of pediatric assent and implications of the mature minor doctrine.

Case 1

Tommy was 3 years old when he was hit by a car, resulting in severe traumatic brain injury (TBI). Two weeks into his ICU stay, Tommy's parents were presented with the option to forego life-sustaining treatments (FLST). After a few days of reflecting and discussing the issue, they had determined that stopping the ventilator was best, but by that time there was a new ICU physician who, after review of Tommy's condition, did not think that FLST was warranted. With more intensive therapy, Tommy was able to breathe without the ventilator, and he was moved to the rehabilitation unit. Because of his TBI, however, he maintained a requirement for tube feeding. Brain scans indicated problems with the basal ganglia, and Tommy's parents suggested that continued existence in his condition was not in his best interest and asked the palliative care physician about the possibility of stopping his tube feedings. At the same time, the physical and occupational therapists working with Tommy, as well as nurses and social workers from the pediatric ICU (PICU) who came to visit him in rehab, believed they saw slight but noticeable improvements in his cognitive status – possibly tracking, smiling, and reacting to some stimuli. The entire unit, as well as these PICU staff members, is concerned about the ethics of what the parents are requesting.

Case 2

Yasmine is a 2-month-old visiting her pediatrician, Dr. Jones, for the first time. Her parents have been told by their church pastor that some vaccines violate religious tenets and, after doing some research online, they have also decided that the medical risk is too high, especially since the chance of her getting any of the vaccine-preventable diseases is so low. Dr. Jones explains that the risks of vaccination have been misstated on the Internet, that there are few risks of any significance, and that there is a real risk to Yasmine should she not get vaccinated. Further, the "herd immunity" that protects both Yasmine and others in the community is compromised whenever a child does not get her shots. Yasmine's parents explain that they have read some very convincing articles, and that medicine can't promise she won't become autistic or come down with some immune deficiency. That, for them, is too great a risk to take with their child.

Case 3

A 14-year-old girl, Anna, has been living with acute lymphoblastic leukemia (ALL) for 3 years. She has recently been admitted to the Children's Hospital after complaining of fatigue and lethargy. In the hospital, she is found to have relapsed for the second time, and her prognosis for survival at this point is very unlikely, even with the most aggressive treatment available. Her parents decide not to begin any treatment for her ALL and ask the medical staff not to tell her that her ALL has returned nor about the dire prognosis.

Concerns about ethics in the care of children have been central to modern bioethics since its inception over 50 years ago. Key milestones in pediatric bioethics include the controversy over the Willowbrook hepatitis experiments in the 1960s, acknowledgment of the importance of "assent" for children participating in research by the National Commission in the 1970s, and the Baby Doe regulations regarding the treatment of neonates in the 1980s. Despite the prominence of pediatric cases and issues, development of bioethical reasoning during the first 30 years was heavily focused on issues surrounding adults with decisional capacity and the principle of respect for autonomy. In fact, most of the groundbreaking judicial opinions about end-of-life decisions prior to the year 2000 focused on protecting the rights of adults to make autonomous decisions about their own medical care (Menikoff, 2002).

Many healthcare ethics committees (HECs) operate in an environment primarily oriented toward the care of adult patients, and as a result, the ethics education of many HEC members is primarily adult-focused. Along with the chapter on neonatal issues (Chapter 18), this chapter focuses on unique considerations in pediatric ethics, considerations that can differ, subtly though importantly, from situations involving adult patients.

Children Are Not Simply "Little Adults": Highlighting Key Differences

It may sound trivial, but it is no small matter to recognize that children are not just adults-in-miniature. While some cases involving children have features that are analogous in the adult world, there are other cases where a traditional adult approach will simply not do justice to the unique aspects of caring for children.

The powerful hold of the principle of respect for autonomy on medical ethics is a testament to the adult-centered emphasis of medical ethics. Of course, there are other theories, models, and principles of ethics, but none completely escapes the fact that they were created with adults in mind and tend to be applied similarly.

Take the case of Tommy (Case 1, above) who lies in a hospital after a severe TBI, and is unable to speak for himself. Clearly, someone else must make his healthcare

Table 19.1 Adults versus pediatric – differing ethical presumptions

Adult Care Ethical Presumptions	Pediatric Care Ethical Presumptions
• Presumption of *patient autonomy* ▪ Presume maturity/ownership of values ▪ Presume full accountability • Ethically: presume obligation to respect	• Presumption of *patient incapacity* ▪ Presume patient immaturity/innocence/lack of medical decision-making ability ▪ Presume lack of values development ▪ Presume need to protect
• Presume *family insight* into the patient's values • Greater potential for conflict between *respecting autonomy* and "best interests"	• Presumption of *parental authority* over the child's values development • Greater potential for conflict between *parental authority* and "best interests"

decisions. Now, the same would be true if Tommy were 30 years old. But something morally substantive changes when we think about a 3-year-old Tommy versus a 30-year-old Tommy. At 30, he would still require another person to make decisions for him and we would seek an appropriate "surrogate" (aka "proxy"). Our expectation of the surrogate would be to attempt to bring Tommy's voice into a conversation where he, in fact, cannot speak. We ask of this surrogate that they try to respond the way Tommy would respond if he could do so himself – to make decisions based on his values and interests, extending his autonomy as far as it can be stretched. If Tommy is 3, however, his decision maker is not tasked with the same responsibility. Both 3-year-old and 30-year-old Tommy require others to make decisions for them, but honoring the patient's autonomy in that process makes little sense for 3-year-old Tommy. Whereas Tommy the 30-year-old (all other things being equal) presumably would have had decisional capacity before his TBI and, as such, would be presumed to own the values that he believed in and acted upon at that time in his life, for Tommy the 3-year-old, no such presumption of capacity or values-ownership exists. Even a 30-year-old Tommy who had never possessed decision-making capacity because of injury or disability would have a history and a lifetime of basic preferences on which a surrogate could base decisions. Thus, in the younger Tommy's case we turn to someone with "authority" to make decisions for him – typically parents. Parents are not expected to speak in Tommy's voice but to address his "best interests." The prevailing principle for providers, then, becomes beneficence, not respect for autonomy. These facts about the basic presumptions regarding minors and the responsibilities that follow from them create a different moral space when making pediatric decisions. Table 19.1 illustrates some of these differences.

The Role of Parents

The decision-making process for children typically contains an element not seen as frequently in adult-care situations – namely, the need to look toward someone other than the patient for consent. Legally, this default assumption of parental decision-making is often phrased as a parental *right* to make decisions, but ethically, it might be better characterized as a parental *responsibility*.[1] While rights can be exercised as desired, responsibilities place a moral claim on those who possess them, in this case to seek the good of the child.

The basic presumption in favor of parental decision-making has legal, social, and ethical grounding. It is generally accepted that parents should serve as the default decision makers for their children because the role of parenting requires protecting and raising children. Parents have more invested in their own children than other people do; they typically know their own children better than others; and they almost always want what is best for them. Moreover, parental values are often imparted to children, and thus, most children ultimately share some common values with their families (Nelson and Nelson, 1995).

Traditionally, parents are expected to make decisions for their child based on what they discern to be the child's "best interest" (Salter, 2012). The "best interest standard" is a *guidance* principle – that is, a principle designed to aid parents (and surrogates for adult patients) as they make decisions and provide consent on behalf of someone for whom they exercise decision-making authority (Buchanan and Brock, 1990). The term "best interest" is ubiquitous in medical care, and yet it is not without vagueness and controversy. On the one hand, it is often interpreted as maximizing the welfare of a child, an ideal that cannot always be met in a world of constrained resources and in families where optimizing the interest of the whole may occasionally mean doing less than what is "best" for some members. However "best" interest is interpreted, most would agree that it requires making medical decisions with the welfare of the child as a primary consideration. This raises another problem with the application of the best interest standard. In fact, many cases that come before ethics consultants and committees involving parents who refuse to provide consent on behalf of a child are situations where the medical team and the parents *disagree* about which course of action is best for the child. In Case 2 above, the physician believes strongly that vaccination will benefit Yasmine and the community. The parents, however, disagree, and have concluded that not allowing Yasmine to be vaccinated serves her interests. Which path, in fact, leads to Yasmine's best interest? Similarly, a parent who is a Jehovah's Witness truly has the best interest of their child in mind in refusing to consent to a life-saving transfusion. They have simply weighed the harms and benefits (factoring the impact on the child's spiritual welfare) differently than most medical teams would. Parents are tasked with pursuing the best interest of their child, and healthcare professionals are obligated to seek the good of the patient. When these parties differ in their conceptions of what will benefit the child, the best interest standard is not so much the solution as a source of disagreement.

There will be times where a parental refusal of consent should be challenged. On rare occasions, a parent may not be capable of understanding the medical issues or adequately weighing risks and benefits. In other cases, parents may find themselves in situations where they must balance the welfare of their child against other interests. And perhaps

---

[1] NB: the parental right (or authority) to make decisions should not be confused with the oft-used concept of "parental autonomy" (Ross, 1998, 2019). Given that "autonomy" is the concept of "*self*-determination," the only sense that a phrase "parental autonomy" can make is if we are talking about parents making decisions about *themselves as parents*. Parents making decisions about their children are making "other-regarding" decisions and, thus, are not exercising "autonomy" but "authority."

most commonly, parents may believe they are acting in the best interest of a child, but members of the medical team strongly disagree with that assessment. Because of that, there remains a need for *intervention* principles as well (Buchanan and Brock, 1990).

The Limits of Provider and Parental Authority

Unless it has been revoked through state action, parents have the legal authority to authorize medical evaluation and treatment for their children. While this is usually described as parental permission, rather than consent, it nonetheless falls under the legal doctrine of informed consent. This is important, because except in emergency situations where a delay would result in significant suffering or harm to the child, the physician cannot do anything to a child without the permission of the child's parent (or legal guardian). Unconsented touching (whether for medical evaluation or treatment) without consent is generally considered a legal battery. Thus, in situations where a parent has refused to consent, a clinician or institution must either tolerate the parent's decision (while continuing to work with the family and perhaps gain their approval) or follow legal avenues to overturn the parental refusal of consent. Only the state can *order* a parent to comply with medical recommendations.

On the other hand, parental authority is not unlimited, and when a parent or guardian fails to provide adequate care for a child, the state may intervene. All states have child abuse and neglect laws that represent the boundary of parental decision-making authority. If a parent refuses to authorize necessary medical care for a child, the state can authorize medical care over their objection under a claim of medical neglect. This can occur in different ways, but most frequently either includes involvement of child protective agencies or a judicial order.

Intervention Principles

In cases where parents have refused to consent to evaluation or treatment, the most important decision faced by the clinician, institution, or ethics consultant is whether the parents' refusal of the recommended management strategy falls below a minimally acceptable threshold of medical care, for example may constitute medical neglect. The important question is not, "what is best for this child?" but "how can we identify when decisions exceed parental authority?"

In Case 2, for example, Dr. Jones clearly disagrees with Yasmine's parents about their decision to refuse vaccinations. Even though Dr. Jones believes in the benefit of vaccinations for Yasmine, absent parental consent, Dr. Jones is not empowered to overturn the parents' decision. Instead, Dr. Jones is left with two acceptable options: (1) attempt persuasion, based on evidence and other considerations, or (2) seek the intervention of state agencies to require the vaccination. However, courts and state agencies generally grant parents significant discretion. They generally place a high burden to prove that the medical treatment is necessary before compelling treatment over parental objections, and they rarely override parents unless imminent action is necessary to prevent a potentially serious harm.

The key decision facing ethics consultants and clinicians is under what circumstances they should seek to engage the state to force treatment on a child. This requires an *intervention principle*. The proper role of an intervention principle is to identify the boundaries around the decisions a parent is permitted to make. There are a number of suggested thresholds for intervention. For example, Ross (1998, 2019) argues that state intervention should be limited to cases in which children are deprived of basic needs or when parental decisions to refuse a treatment place the child at high risk for serious and significant morbidity and the treatment is of proven efficacy with a high likelihood of success. Still, others have suggested loss of health or some other major interest, deprivation of basic needs, and deprivation of future opportunities or freedoms.

One suggested intervention principle has become known as the "harm principle." According to the harm principle, parental decisions should be tolerated except in those cases where the decision of a parent places the child at significant risk of a serious harm as compared to other options (like the one suggested by the medical team). How should one define a significant risk of serious harm? Feinberg (1984) suggests that serious harm includes intervention with interests necessary for more ultimate goals like physical health and vigor, integrity and normal functioning of one's body, absence of absorbing pain and suffering or grotesque disfigurement, minimal intellectual acuity, and emotional stability.

In addition to demonstrating that a parent's refusal to consent would place the child at significant risk of serious harm, institutions or individuals challenging a parental decision should provide evidence of efficacy for the preferred intervention and demonstrate that the proposed course of action is required imminently and is likely to prevent harm. Finally, all alternatives short of state action must have been exhausted and every effort made to seek a mutually acceptable solution to the child's medical problem (Diekema, 2004). State involvement represents a serious challenge to parental authority and family integrity. Such actions will generally be perceived as disrespectful and adversarial by parents, and may adversely affect the family's future interactions with medical professionals. Such action should be undertaken only after careful and thoughtful deliberation.

We must acknowledge that parental authority has fairly broad scope, and given that none of us has the hold on "truth," and that the story of their medical care is not the sum total of any patient's life story, it may be necessary to allow parental decision-making to hold sway even when doubts remain about whether those decisions are, in fact, best for the child. Here, then, is the place of the harm principle, setting a threshold for harm below which we cannot allow parents to go. Above that threshold, however, the most we can do ethically is attempt to persuade parents, giving reasons why we believe some other viable path is best.

Parental Requests for Nonstandard Interventions

Parents who make requests of healthcare professionals that the professional may be uncomfortable carrying out pose a slightly different issue. Because these are situations where a parent is requesting something of a provider, professionals have a good deal more freedom to exercise their own judgment and need not engage state agencies to exercise coercive power. These generally represent "hands off" situations rather than "hands on" situations. These situations may require ethical justification, but rarely require legal permission.

In general, professionals can reasonably refuse a parent's request for a specific test or treatment regimen if, in the provider's professional judgment, the request falls outside of the realm of accepted professional practice (Buchanan and Brock, 1990, 143), the likelihood of harm to the patient greatly exceeds the likelihood of benefit to the patient (Beauchamp and Childress, 2012, 169–171), the request falls outside of the realm of the provider's expertise of training (in such cases, a referral should be provided), the intervention would not work (based on the best available data), or cooperating with the request would harm someone else (public health threat, poor use of available resources) while failing to benefit the child-patient. In addition, providers may also refuse to participate in management requests to which they ethically object (see further, Chapter 24, herein).

That being said, providers should consider accommodating parents when the parents request a test or intervention that is not likely to harm the child, does not significantly harm others, and where some potential for benefit is possible that has not yet been demonstrated through medical studies. Even in these situations, it is always appropriate to limit interventions to those within the scope of the provider's practice or the established standard of care.

Older Children and Teens: Issues Related to Developing Capacity

As children enter the teen years, their desire and ability to be involved in their own medical care increases. At a minimum, they deserve to be respected. As such, groups like the American Academy of Pediatrics have suggested that we consider developmental maturity when working with pediatric patients (Katz et al., 2016). One recommendation is that, roughly speaking, young children into their early school-aged years should be informed about what is happening to them to the extent they can understand. Under certain conditions, older adolescents should also be offered some level of involvement in decision-making. In Case 3, Anna's parents attempt to protect her from the harm that might follow from the news of relapse. However, at 14, with multiple admissions, her personal knowledge and experience with her disease is possibly quite robust. Excluding her from this information and the decisions that follow from it ignores or devalues her own experience and maturity with this disease, and could be quite harmful if she feels isolated.

In most states, there are some statutory categories that exist to allow some minors to make decisions in all or some defined medical situations. Most states have laws that set out certain conditions (like emancipation, marriage, military service, or even incarceration) that allow a minor to provide medical consent for themselves without the involvement of a parent. All states also have statutes that allow minors (in some states with a lower age limit) to consent for care in specific medical situations. These include consent for evaluation and treatment of sexually transmitted diseases, evaluation and management of pregnancy and pregnancy-related conditions, and evaluation and management of substance abuse and psychiatric conditions. These latter exceptions to the requirement for parental consent are not based on presumed maturity or capacity of the minor, but rather the public health implications of having adolescents unable to receive care for these conditions in situations where they wish not to involve their parents.

Barring these exceptions, the majority of medical encounters with minors require parental consent, and parental choices will generally prevail. However, the distinction noted above between parental refusals and parental requests remains an important one. It would be ill-advised (barring state intervention or a statutory or judicial exception) to treat a child or adolescent without parental consent. However, a provider has more freedom to consider the child's voice in situations where a parent requests a medical intervention on behalf of their child, particularly one that is not essential to the child's health. A 6-year-old who refuses a shot for tetanus after stepping on a dirty nail will most likely receive the shot regardless, not only on grounds of their inability to understand risks and benefits and potential consequences of refusing but also on the basis of the strong medical indications for the tetanus vaccination in these circumstances. But the same is not the case for the 16-year-old who refuses to get a medroxyprogesterone acetate (aka Depo-Provera) shot because her mother wants to protect her from getting pregnant. In that case, the provider should strongly consider withholding the treatment unless the daughter and mother can come to an agreement. In this case, the adolescent may be capable of making the decision, forcing her to undergo the treatment against her wishes would be inherently disrespectful and potentially traumatic, and the treatment itself is generally considered a choice, not a necessity.

To accommodate the developing capacity of select adolescents to make at least some medical decisions, some states have also adopted, either in statute or common law, some form of a "mature minor doctrine" (where other authority-granting conditions for minors do not already apply). The doctrine can be summarized as follows:

> Any minor who is capable of understanding their treatment options, is experienced enough to weigh the consequences to them of those options, and is mature enough to cope with the information, deliberation, and outcomes should have authority to make the decision at hand.

Since the doctrine is not recognized in every state, it is important for ethics consultants to be aware of the existence and nature of a mature minor doctrine within their jurisdiction.

So, what if Anna's case was a bit different? Instead of ALL, let's assume Anna has Hodgkin's and has been given one round of chemotherapy. Even though remission occurs 80% of the time after several rounds of chemotherapy, Anna, together with her parents, has decided that she does not want to undergo further chemotherapy. Given how ill she felt receiving the first round of chemotherapy, she has concluded that it is not good for her. She prefers to try some alternative, homeopathic treatment options instead. Anna is an intelligent girl, seems capable of making careful decisions, and states clearly that she understands the possible consequences of her decision; she is unconvinced that chemotherapy will benefit her, and the websites of other Hodgkin's patients have convinced her (and her parents) to try another method.

Whether adolescents should be allowed to refuse lifesaving treatments for any reason, including religious belief, remains controversial. Most would agree that adolescents should be involved in discussions about their health care and should be offered the opportunity to voice their feelings, opinions, and concerns and they should be provided reasonable opportunities to make choices and have those choices respected. On the other hand, there is reason to question whether any adolescent is truly mature enough to refuse lifesaving treatment in situations where there is likely to be a good prognosis with a proven intervention (Diekema, 2020) .

Many factors would be relevant in determining whether an adolescent possesses sufficient maturity to make a life-altering medical decision. Minimally, healthcare providers should require a high level of psychosocial maturity and consider the adolescent's ability to understand and reason, project meaningfully into the future, express a relatively settled set of values and beliefs, and demonstrate that their decision is driven more by long-term interests than short-term concerns. The chances of a good outcome with treatment and the burden of the proposed interventions are also relevant considerations. In general, healthcare professionals should be reluctant to allow an adolescent to refuse interventions in a situation where they would challenge the same decision being made by their parents (Diekema, 2020). That being said, the use of physical force is rarely justified in adolescents, particularly if it is required repeatedly to ensure treatment. In these situations, a healthcare provider may decide to forgo lifesaving interventions simply because the harm done by using force may not be justified by the potential benefit, particularly in a setting of long-term therapy that requires the cooperation and investment of the adolescent over time.

In Anna's case, vigorous debate might ensue with regard to whether child protective services should be notified. If Anna were younger, that would be the likely outcome based upon an application of the harm principle. But in this case, Anna also has a strong opinion, and given her apparent level of maturity, she is at least owed a careful hearing and respectful conversation. However, when it comes to whether state intervention should be sought, reasonable people may disagree (see Ross et al., 2009). Such decisions are challenging, and they demand reflection, discussion, and principled determinations. A full ethics committee hearing might be best in a case like this, with Anna and her parents invited to bring their arguments. In the end, however, it is far from clear that we should allow Anna's opinion to alter our course in a situation where we would not allow the same decision made by her parents to go unchallenged.

Conclusion

It is important to recognize not only the physiological but ethical differences between adult and pediatric care. Pediatrics creates a unique moral space in which patients, families, and practitioners operate, and this space is characterized by an ethic of protection, the importance of limited parental authority, and (over time) the developing maturity and participation of the patients themselves. HECs in hospitals that provide care to pediatric patients should regularly offer targeted education in the arena of pediatric ethics in order to maintain a sensitivity to the subtle but important moral differences that exist when caring for pediatric patients, and crafting or reviewing policies that impact the care of those children.

Questions for Discussion

1. Conceptual: In what ways can your HEC better prepare for pediatric cases and policies in your institution? What are the appropriate roles of "best interest" and "harm" in pediatric cases?
2. Pragmatic: In what ways is parental authority respected within your institution and HEC? Is too much deference paid to parental decisions?
3. Strategic: In what ways is teenage decision-making respected in your institution and by your HEC? What kinds of situations challenge how we care for teenagers?

References

Beauchamp TL, Childress JF (2012). *Principles of Biomedical Ethics*, 7th ed. New York: Oxford University Press.

Buchanan A, Brock D (1990). *Deciding for Others: The Ethics of Surrogate Decision Making*. New York: Oxford University Press.

Diekema DS (2004). Parental refusals of medical treatments: The harm principle as threshold for state intervention. *Theoretical Medicine and Bioethics*, 25(4): 243–264.

Diekema DS (2020). Adolescent brain development and medical decision-making. *Pediatrics*, 146(2, Suppl. 1): S18–S24.

Feinberg J (1984). *Harm to Others: The Moral Limits of the Criminal Law*. New York: Oxford University Press.

Katz AL, Webb SA, The American Academy of Pediatrics Committee on Bioethics. (2016). Technical report: Informed consent in decision-making in pediatric practice. *Pediatrics*, 138(2): e20161485.

Menikoff J (2002). *Law & Bioethics: An Introduction*. Washington, DC: Georgetown University Press.

Nelson HL, Nelson JL (1995). *The Patient in the Family*. New York: Routledge.

Ross LF (1998). *Children, Families, and Health Care Decision Making*. New York: Oxford University Press.

Ross LF (2019). Better than best (interest standard) in pediatric decision making. *Journal of Clinical Ethics*, 30(3): 183–195.

Ross LF, Blustein J, Clayton EW (2009). Adolescent decision making. *Cambridge Quarterly of Healthcare Ethics*, 18(3): 302–322, 18(4): 432–442.

Salter E (2012). Deciding for a child: A comprehensive analysis of the best interest standard. *Theoretical Medicine and Bioethics*, 33(3): 179–198.

Neuroethics

20

Paul J. Ford

Objectives

Upon reading and considering the content of this chapter, the reader should be able to:

1. Identify the ethical challenges in the increasing complexity of brain injury and the complexity in restoring patients to full functioning.
2. Apply the concept of neurodiversity to the ethical analysis of prognosis and continuing care needs for patients with brain injury and other neuropsychological illnesses.

Case 1   Futile Surgery and Self-Fulfilling Prophecy?

Sarah is a 50-year-old who was found unconscious in her garden by her adult daughters, who rush her to the emergency department. After a clinical evaluation, including brain imaging, it is determined that Sarah has a moderate, dominant-sided, intracerebral hemorrhage (ICH) with increasing intracranial pressures. If a surgical intervention is not undertaken to alleviate the intracranial pressure, Sarah's brain will be damaged in a life-threatening way (herniation). With the surgery, Sarah's outcome is uncertain; because of brain complexity and plasticity, the ICU team believes there is no way of knowing the real functional outcome for Sarah unless they intervene and assess her over time. Yet the family has consulted the Internet and found reports that say patients with this type of ICH have extremely high mortality rates. Since Sarah has always stated that she is against medical intervention that would be futile to survival, the family decline the surgery despite a plea by the ICU team to proceed. The ICU team asks the ethics committee to permit the surgical decompression against family objections.

Case 2   Neurodiversity: Energetic Kid or Attention Deficit?

Antoine was brought in after a significant leg injury suffered while he and his parents were on vacation. He had run off ahead of his parents on a hike and fell off a short ledge, resulting in a compound fracture. Antoine was diagnosed with autism when he was 3 years old; at 12, he now attends a school for children with special needs. While in the hospital, Antoine can be pretty loud on occasions, and if he could he would hit the nurse call button as often as possible. He also loves to do logic puzzles that a child life specialist brought him and he plays chess with the social worker. His mother tells the physician on the hospital ward that he is prone to act out, and so at home they have been prescribed a medication

---

The author is grateful to the editors for helping craft the primary case in this chapter.

Case 2 (*cont.*)

to "level out" his behaviors, but this also means he rarely reads much or plays many games. She does ask if they can give him that medication in the hospital because she is embarrassed by his loud behavior and is concerned it is too disruptive to the staff and other patients. The staff does not think it is too bothersome and like the interactions they have with Antoine. However, Mom begins to insist on giving the medications. The healthcare ethics committee (HEC) is called by the child life specialist who is concerned that the mother's request is not what is best for Antoine.

Introduction

As defined by Judy Illes and Stephanie Bird (2006, 511), "neuroethics is concerned with ethical, legal and social implications of neuroscience research findings, and with the nature of the research itself." Subsequent to this definition, it has become clear that some of the implications of neuroscience have a direct effect on clinical care. This is especially true when focused on neuropsychiatric illnesses, which cover a broad range of conditions that are treated by psychiatry, neurology, psychology, neurosurgery, neurooncology, neuroendocrinology, and rehabilitation medicine. These areas treat chronic, acute, and congenital health conditions across the lifespan. For instance, brain malformation or perinatal strokes can occur in the youngest of patients and have sequela throughout a lifetime. Late in life, neurodegenerative diseases such as Parkinson's or Alzheimer's commonly arise and create many challenges for patients and families. Between these bookends we have pain disorders, epilepsies, traumatic injuries, vascular insults, and schizophrenia as further examples of the varieties of illnesses that fall under this broad rubric. These conditions all involve the brain in some way as a central processing unit and as an organizer of experiences for the individual. They also involve elements of control and experience that become altered or at risk of loss for the individual.

For the purposes of this chapter, neuropsychiatric illness encompasses the broad spectrum of health issues that include those things that have been traditionally thought of as primarily neurological or primarily psychiatric. These are complex disorders that have often been stigmatized; in fact, some would argue that mere differences of cognitive ability, mental health, and mental states have been pathologized or feared. Regardless, there is a complicated bidirectional interplay of physiology and complex behavior in these conditions. As such, HECs increasingly encounter complex clinical neuroscience cases that involve value assumptions and prognostic uncertainty. Therefore, an HEC should be attentive to all the potentially related neuropsychiatric disciplines when approaching the most complex cases.

Ethical issues that involve the brain and its processes are further complicated by the rapidly evolving scientific and clinical findings that challenge prognosis. This is coupled with the fact that brains tend to be quite plastic – that is, able to adapt in ways not otherwise anticipated. In addition, sometimes brain injuries are not reliably demonstrable through technological imaging, so the "pictures" of what is going on can be misleading. All of this uncertainty can be complicated by value judgments or assumptions about what makes a life valuable or worth living. It is these considerations that makes the area of neuroethics particularly rich and is why HEC members should pay special attention to conditions that involve the nervous system. In what follows, we will use the cases from the beginning of the chapter to explore how these ethical issues often come into play in clinical practice.

Neuroexceptionalism

The privacy and intimacy of a person's mind is typically taken as foundational to a person and to their self-determination. Because of their contribution to the very foundation of identity, some argue that nervous systems are fundamentally different from other bodily systems in ways that require us to value them differently from other systems. This suggests that we should develop or insist upon special protections and considerations because of the central and direct role the nervous system plays in our experiences and understanding of our identity (Tovino, 2007). This has come to be known as "neuroexceptionalism," and this exceptionalism is further justified because of the incredible complexity of interactions and outcomes that can occur from even small nervous system alterations.

One risk of such exceptionalism, however, is that it can lead to valuing cognitive and experiential abilities in ways that can unwittingly devalue those persons whose brain and nervous system are compromised in some way. That is, when placing so much import-ance on the "exceptional" abilities of the brain, people may demonstrate biases that are blind to neurodiversity because they lean toward what have come to be called "neuro-typical" traits and against neurodisabilities. This happens precisely because of the high value placed on the brain's ability for creation of deep understandings through process-ing of facts and emotive content, which can result in the belief that lacking such ability for deep understanding (whether through genetic/congenital conditions, trauma, or mental illnesses) means that such persons have lesser qualities of life or may, themselves, may not be full "persons" at all.

Given that emergency and critical care departments are often the location of a wide variety of acute neuroethics cases that arise from strokes, trauma, seizures, and cardiopul-monary arrests – resulting in compromises of cognition and leading to end-of-life decision-making – Sarah's case (Case 1) has similarities to the discussions in other chapters. For the purpose of this chapter, however, Sarah's case should be evaluated by inspecting our intuitive biases about the brain and surrounding technology, as well as reevaluating the facts through the lens of neurodiversity, plasticity, and clinical uncertainty.

Uncertainty of Knowledge and Outcome: Biases

Left unchecked, brain herniation will lead to Sarah meeting neurological criteria for death. She is on a ventilator, and while surgery seems to be an option, the family's concerns about reported outcomes invoke a concern for physiological futility regarding the surgery. Even with all their research, what the family may not understand or appreciate is the validity of the literature they have researched and, thus, the uncertainty of how the brain could recover. Most studies in the 1980s–2000s did not account for the high rate of early withdrawal of life-sustaining therapy, which has been described as a self-fulfilling prophecy that can inappropriately drive decision-making if the underlying value assumptions are opaque (Jacobs et al., 2017). Some of those value assumptions presume that diminished cognitive and experiential capacities are unacceptable states of existence for humans to inhabit. It is only within the last decade, however, that research-ers and clinicians have come to recognize that the natural history and outcomes of ICH are, in fact, unknown. Thus, reading outdated, poorly grounded literature can perpetuate the pernicious side of neuroexceptionalism, where any significant diminishment would be seen as resulting in an unacceptable quality of life. If this kind of value assumption drives the research, the data and their interpretations will, even if only unconsciously, tend to support dire outcomes.

HECs, then, should remain acutely aware of the possibility of underlying value assumptions that can result from unexplored neuroexceptionalism of providers, families, and HEC members themselves as they navigate difficult decisions with, about, and for patients. Transparently identifying interests and values in published literature as well as practice will help to mitigate biases during HEC discussions. In Sarah's case the HEC should help the family and healthcare team carefully evaluate the underlying assumptions. These assumptions might be about a life worth living with a difference in neurological function rather than simply judging if Sarah will return to the same functional self as she was before the ICH. On an institutional level, the committee needs to consider the boundary between protecting those with cognitive disability from dying because of biases against their cognitive state and preserving both patients' rights for self-determination and stewardship of best medical practices and resources.

Imaging: Damages and Plasticity

Once Sarah's family was educated on the reasonably high probability of survival with aggressive intervention, the family still worried that Sarah might lose language ability, which they believed would be unacceptable to her. The family asked to see the pictures of the brain damage in hopes of better understanding her condition.

Although neuroimaging can be helpful in some cases – for example, using brain images may be a useful indicator of loss of large amounts of structure or identifier of herniation of the brain stem – very small differences in size and location of neurological injury can have dramatically different effects. For anatomic location correlating to specific human function, there are broad variations between brains. Save for acting as a broad educational tool, a generic brain "atlas" purporting to show a map of specific areas of the brain that control specific functions is far too general to aid in understanding an individual patient's condition. Further, brains do not work in discrete parts but as circuits. As such, a specific location of damage must also be considered in conjunction with connectivity to other areas. One clear example of the circuitry of the brain is the expression of language where Broca's area plays a central role – substantial damage at that location results in expressive aphasia (inability to express language). However, Broca's area alone, while necessary for language, is not itself sufficient: it is but one node in the circuitry. Thus, it is possible to have Broca's area completely undamaged yet not be able to speak because a different part of the pathway no longer functions.

To further complicate matters, a variety of circuits may run through a single area that can be affected. For instance, the thalamus is the intersection of several pathways for circuits, and as such a stroke near, or in, the thalamus may affect a wide variety of functions in unpredictable ways. So, even if damage is seen in the thalamus or Broca's area, it often needs to be paired with a physical examination of function in order to evaluate the type and degree of impairment. In such cases, imaging alone may be ineffective in explaining the challenges of the current neurological condition of the patient.

One more complication is that brains retain some plasticity for new learning, which means that if one circuit is disrupted the brain may eventually partially recover function through developing alternate circuits. This is particularly pronounced in young children with brain injury where there can be very dramatic reprogramming of functions, including language dominance transferring between hemispheres. As the brain ages the degree of plasticity decreases, but even in a case like that of Sarah, who is 50 years old, there is no good ability to predict whether some recovery is possible in the context of her ICH. There are some known limitations to plasticity. In this case it would be important to know if Sarah had previous conditions, particularly when she was a child, that might have prompted a reconfiguration of the brain circuits. This information might be important as clinicians interpret the imaging and may affect the reasonable speculations regarding the outcomes of the damage.

Unfortunately, while the above shows why images of damage to the brain may not be easy to decipher, the flip side of imaging results is that it can be easy to confuse the lack of clear visual damage as proof that a brain is healthy. Because brain imaging only gives a limited view, when imaging shows no clear damage, certain types of damage may not show up on a brain image or may only show up later. Clinicians should, thus, say only that the imaging shows no evidence that would preclude the patient from recovery, avoiding categorical statements about lack of damage to the brain.

Finally, with new data being generated about the brain's basic electrical functioning through initiatives such as the National Institutes of Health (NIH) Human Connectome Project (see Connectome Programs | Blueprint [NIH], n.d.), any interpretation of and communication about imaging of the brain will continue to become increasingly confusing. And while promising, these initiatives generate maps of pathways whose functional utility is currently unclear – which speaks to caution in clinical application.

The HEC has a role in ensuring that families fully appreciate the subtlety of what knowledge images provide and the limitations of that knowledge. Further, the HEC has an opportunity to help clinicians be careful with their communication to avoid expressing their own biases while conveying neuroimaging information. This is especially important given that all this uncertainty and complexity means that patients and families have a higher than usual dependence on the integrity of the specialist to act as interpreter. HECs can help practitioners, patients, and families bring out into the open the insights and limits of current knowledge and practice surrounding imaging and interpretation. In this way, Sarah's family may come to see how best to put the imaging studies into the context of current medical progress and limitations as well as Sarah's own values and interests.

Neurodiversity

It is not novel to say that human variation goes beyond differences of physical features. People differ in cognitive abilities, behavioral/social responses, and emotive reactions; such variation is known as neurodiversity. And while the variations among us are obvious, the pressure, even requirement, to conform to neurotypical norms is significant. This pressure results in the kinds of biases in individuals and society discussed above, but the pressure is all the more troubling for those who are behaviorally and neurologically altered, at times leading to choices that result in significant loss of aspects of their personalities and experiences that they value. In his blog post, "An Experimental Autism Treatment Cost Me My Marriage," John Robison, who has been diagnosed on the autism spectrum, challenges the pressure to "normalize" emotions, which in turn raises the issue of acceptance of neurodiversity (Robison, 2016). In his post, Robison explains that he participated in a research study of noninvasive transcranial magnetic stimulation (TMS) of the brain. During his time in the study he gained the ability to experience emotional cues for the first time (though no scientific evidence currently exists that would explain TMS having this effect), an experience previously unavailable to him. He reports that these newfound emotional cues interfered with the relationship he had with his wife and in the end resulted in his divorce. Robison's narrative highlights that for a person who has structured a life in the absence of neurotypical abilities, and thereby created habits and patterns of actions and emotions in absence of those abilities, the new and sudden acquisition of a neuroability can prove harmful rather than beneficial. In Robison's case, interfering with a particular social neurofunctioning upset a kind of accommodating balance he had developed over his life. Clearly, such changes effect specific outcomes for individuals, but they do not stop there. As a concern about devaluing neurodiversity, these kinds of social/neuro differences should be carefully considered before medicine and its interventions are initiated, and there should be greater promotion of the acknowledgment and acceptance of neurodiversity by society.

Robinson's account shows how developing a new or enhancing an existing ability can have unexpected and troubling results, but eliminating certain behaviors or symptoms can be equally problematic. So, while in some cases symptoms or behaviors may be viewed as pathological by medicine or certain social groups, any particular individual or group may highly value them as part of their experiences. Such can be the case of a patient with temporal lobe epilepsy that produces ecstatic religious experiences. Seizures and the resulting "ecstasies" from this condition can be challenging for the individual and disturbing to observers. Such patients can be candidates to have a portion of the temporal lobe surgically removed to control seizures. Many patients celebrate the loss of these experiences as a benefit because they find the experiences as intrusive. Occasionally, however, even if surgery eliminates the seizures, some patients may view it as a failure because it eliminates the valued ecstatic religious experiences as well. Like so many other medical interventions, then, good informed-consent processes are necessary, and must be sensitive enough to the patient's interests and values so as to help the patient determine whether the surgical outcome is best understood as a risk or a benefit.

These examples all continue to push the biases that may be embedded in what is considered the "better" life worth experiencing. Antoine (Case 2) faces an intervention that would have him better conform to societal expectations, but that might alter how he experiences the world, and that alteration can be frustrating, even disturbing, to kids (Singh, 2006). From the case description, no one has asked Antoine about his experiences or his goals, and that's a suggestion the HEC might make. As stated, the dilemma presents a dichotomy: provide the medication Antoine's mother wants to reduce his behavioral problems or follow the medical team's inclinations not to medicate a normally functioning 12-year-old boy. The HEC may be able to identify a third option that is responsive to systemic biases and accepts a broader range of normal behavior, even if that option is beyond the purview of the HEC to enact.

In general, when faced with a neurobehavioral ethical dilemma the HECs should evaluate the degree to which a patient should be changed and to what degree the actual societal structure needs to change to accommodate diversity. Robison's blog and the epilepsy example push committee members to be open to how neuropsychiatric side effects could be either a harm or a benefit depending on the patient's own perspective and way of living in the world. These considerations hinge on being cognizant of the incredible variation of neurodiversity that exists and accepting variation as an acceptable part of the social order – and then providing necessary resources to support Antoine and his mother as part of this process.

Coda: Functional Diseases

There are illnesses that have psychological roots but that are experienced and expressed physiologically. These disorders are often termed "functional" and can have symptoms that present very similarly to diseases like epilepsy, stroke, pain, movement disorders, multiple sclerosis, postural tachycardia syndrome (POTS), fibromyalgia, etc. These illnesses do not fit into either of the traditional neurological or psychiatric practices and therefore these patients are sometimes "orphaned" by not having a central clinical home for their condition and, while rare, HEC members should be prepared to address topics related to these mental illnesses that carry a strong social stigma and medical misunderstanding, in part because they have substantial somatic manifestations.

One example that brings these issues into stark relief is psychogenic nonepileptic seizures (PNES). PNES can occur in conjunction with epilepsy seizures or without the presence of epilepsy. Individuals with PNES experience loss of control that can present exactly like epilepsy seizures. However, these seizure events occur without an EEG correlate (the electrical "storm" that is measured through EEG in epilepsy) and hence are not caused by epileptic brain activity. The patient is not "faking" a seizure or "malingering." Instead, in PNES the source of seizure is a psychological/emotional state that manifests as seizure movements. The only proven therapy for PNES involves cognitive behavioral interventions rather than pharmaceuticals. Individuals with PNES suffer greater rates of disability than those with epilepsy and they create a high burden on emergency departments. The patient with a functional disorder can be at risk for poor continuity of care and excessive testing, as well as being stigmatized when seeking medical care.

Collaboration between mental health professionals and neurologists is important, even necessary, in order to avoid the injustices that occur when patients with functional disorders get bounced back and forth between services. The HEC can provide support for clinicians as they attempt to avoid overtesting, which can be a defensive medicine approach, as well as assure flexibility for exceptions to be made in creating multi-disciplinary approaches that will be consistent.

Conclusion

Variations in humans present as illnesses as well as mere differences. HECs need to recognize the ways in which society views some emotional and behavioral differences as pathological and some as acceptable. When faced with complex neuroethics cases with high levels of uncertainty, the biases as well as the roots of uncertainty should be carefully analyzed in terms of the underlying neuroethical biases. This includes reminding stake-holders of the limits of knowledge of emerging technologies and humility on the ability to predict neurological outcomes. HECs have a responsibility to help resolve ethical dilemmas, identify system biases, and guide more respectful practices that will embrace the spectrum of human thriving that is possible.

Questions for Discussion

1. Conceptual: How do we know the difference between a person living their own true existence and one who has an illness for which we must intervene? In particular, what are the limits to self-determination when a patient's neuropsychiatric illness may influence a decision?

2. Pragmatic: How can your hospital best fulfill the obligations to provide the right level of testing and treatment (not too little or too much) for patients with functional neurological disorders without a stable primary medical service as a home?

3. Strategic: How should a committee prepare to address the complex real-time neuroethics issues that arise in the clinic? What procedures, expertise, practice are needed to fully account for the inherent uncertainty?

References

Connectome Programs | Blueprint (NIH). (n.d.) https://neuroscienceblueprint.nih .gov/human-connectome/connectome-programs (accessed November 23, 2020).

Illes J, Bird SJ (2006). Neuroethics: A modern context for ethics in neuroscience. *Trends in Neurosciences*, 29(9): 511–517.

Jacobs BS, Poggesi A, Terry JB (2017). Max-ICH score: Can it prevent self-fulfilling prophecy in ICH? *Neurology*, 89(5): 417–418.

Robison JE (2016, March 18). An experimental autism treatment cost me my marriage. https://well.blogs.nytimes.com/2016/03/18/ an-experimental-autism-treatment-cost-me-my-marriage/

Singh I (2006). Will the "real boy" please behave: Dosing dilemmas for parents of boys with ADHD. *American Journal of Bioethics and Humanities*, 5(3): 34–47.

Tovino SA (2007). Functional neuroimaging information: A case for neuro exceptionalism? *Scholarly Works*, 76. https://scholars.law.unlv.edu/facpub/76

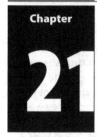

Chapter

Ethical Issues in Clinical Genetics

Thomas May, Kelly East, Whitley Kelley, and Jana Craig

Objectives

Upon reading and considering the content of this chapter, the reader should be able to:

1. Identify the ethical issues raised by genetic testing.
2. Discuss the use and consequences of genetic information for patients and their relatives.
3. Mitigate risk of discrimination toward persons who test positive for variants associated with genetic conditions.

Case 1

Carmen is a healthy 25-year-old woman with a family history of early-onset breast cancer. Her mother, maternal grandmother, two maternal aunts, and a maternal cousin each developed breast cancer before the age of 45, with two of these relatives receiving diagnoses in their 30s. Extensive genetic testing in these relatives has been unable to determine whether there is an identifiable genetic variant contributing to the development of breast cancer in this family. Carmen's gynecologist, realizing Carmen's significantly increased risk, would like to begin an aggressive screening regimen for her to include annual mammograms and breast MRIs. Carmen, however, has felt reassured by her family members' negative genetic test results and would like to be managed based on the general population guidelines, including waiting until age 40 to begin receiving mammograms. Carmen's gynecologist is concerned that this approach may cause a potential future breast cancer to be identified at a later stage, when it is more difficult to treat.

Case 2

Kiana was 37 years old when she suddenly passed out while in an exercise class. She was unresponsive and had no pulse. Fortunately, another person in the exercise class was able to perform CPR until emergency personnel could arrive. Kiana was resuscitated and determined to have suffered a sudden cardiac arrest. Given her young age and lack of known risk factors for a cardiac arrest, genetic testing was performed to look for a possible underlying genetic cause. Genetic testing finds that Kiana harbors a disease-causing variant in the *KCNQ1* gene associated with Long QT Syndrome, that causes an abnormal

---

Thomas May's work was supported by grant 5G13LM012445–02 from the National Library of Medicine and National Human Genome Research Institute.

heart rhythm. Kiana has no known family history of heart problems or sudden death; however, very little is known about relatives on her father's side of the family. Based on this diagnosis, Kiana's sister and brother, as well as other family members, are at risk of having the same condition. When the physician discloses the genetic test result to Kiana, she says that she does not plan on discussing the result and risk with her brother or sister. The physician expresses concern that her sister and brother are unknowingly at significant risk of severe heart complications including sudden death, and could be monitored if they were aware of their risk. Kiana is adamant she does not want to them to know. The physician also personally knows Kiana's family and talks with her brother on a regular basis, and feels a professional and personal obligation to warn these family members about their health risk.

Case 3

Finn was recently born prematurely at 30 weeks and is being cared for in the neonatal ICU (NICU). Two weeks into Finn's NICU stay, his father, Derek, asked the neonatology team whether any genetic testing would be ordered on Finn. Derek explained that he has a family history of Huntington's Disease (HD). Derek's mom passed away from the disease and Derek recently had genetic testing himself that found he also has the HD-causing genetic variant and will develop the disease during his lifetime. Derek is worried that he has passed the condition on to Finn, and would like for Finn to be tested to find out for sure, though he understands that the results of this test would not impact Finn's care in the NICU. The neonatologist is concerned about the ethics of testing an infant for HD, despite the significant risk.

Ethical issues in genetics are studied and addressed under the rubric of what is commonly referred to as "ELSI": the Ethical, Legal, and Social Implications of genetics. In this chapter, we will focus on a subset of ELSI issues in genetic medicine that surround common applications of genetics in general clinical settings. Common ethical issues arising for healthcare ethics committee (HEC) members from genetic technology gravitate toward concerns to assure that genetic testing results are utilized in ethically appropriate ways to identify risk, and develop treatment or health maintenance plans consistent with patient values. This will most commonly take the general form of: (1) protecting against harms that are motivated by unreliable results; (2) promoting informed consent by addressing misunderstanding, misapplication, or unwarranted reaction to genetic testing results on the part of either patients, their families, or members of the healthcare team; or (3) assuring that patient privacy is maintained and applied in appropriate circumstances.

We will examine these three general areas of concern in the context of the above-described scenarios, each of which contains elements relevant in different ways to all three of the general issues described in the preceding paragraph. Ethics committees and consultants should readily recognize the moral dilemmas presented in each of the scenarios. They are familiar to us as conflicts or tensions between important moral values, most notably protecting privacy, confidentiality, and personal autonomy on the one hand and potentially preventing or limiting significant harms on the other.

Each of the scenarios above could be brought to the attention of an ethics committee via their ethics consultation service. For those committees that are also involved in policy development and review, one could take a proactive step in helping their organization think through some of these anticipated difficulties before they become everyday occurrences.

Protecting against Harms

The first ethical issue facing the use of genetic testing in a clinical setting concerns the issue of reliability, which in clinical genetics most commonly centers on the potential for false positive and false negative results. Such results raise ethical issues because they undermine the translation of test results to desired health outcomes, which is at the heart of ethical concerns to protect patient rights to informed consent. Simply put, "steering the direction of one's life" requires a reasonably accurate grasp of the context within which one exists. Inaccurate results undermine this, and thus are a threat to patient autonomy/informed consent (May and Fullerton, 2021).

To illustrate the relation of reliability to desired outcomes, consider a slight modification to Case 1 where an increased risk of breast cancer is indeed identified based on a positive BRCA result, motivating a prophylactic double mastectomy and/or salpingo-oophorectomy to prevent ovarian cancer. The first issue of concern is whether this positive result was confirmed. The genetics literature has found that 40% of variants reported in direct-to-consumer raw data reflected false positive results, emphasizing the importance of confirmation (Tandy-Connor et al., 2018). In some of these cases, acceptance of test results by surgeons that were not fully educated about the limitations of different testing platforms, false positive rates, or the role of clinical confirmation resulted in unwarranted prophylactic surgeries of the types just described; prophylactic surgeries that have profound ramifications for both reproduction and self-image (May and Fullerton, 2021). In these cases, it is recommended to seek input from a genetic specialist, such as a genetic counselor where available, to assess the interpretation of results, especially if these reflect nonclinical reports such as "raw data" or results from a laboratory that is not CLIA certified.

We should take this opportunity to comment on ethics committee education and composition. It is well established that ethics committees should be multidisciplinary groups, bringing together different perspectives, expertise, ideas, and focus. They are also responsible for self-education as this discussion makes clear: Novel situations may require moral knowledge and moral reasoning applied in new ways. Ethics committees may acquire familiarity and expertise in a myriad of ways. One method is by regularly revisiting the multidisciplinary composition of the committee. It is worth noting that genetic counselors and others involved in genetic medicine may be valuable outright additions to committees. It may also serve to utilize consultants both to educate the committees and also to help address specific policy challenges or difficult ethics-related cases as demonstrated above.

Case 2 raises similar issues due to different levels of confidence about different types of gene–disease associations. The American College of Medical Genetics and Genomics has issued guidelines that are commonly used by genetic testing laboratories to make a final determination of the likelihood that a genetic variant contributes to a disease or disease risk (Richards et al., 2015). This framework utilizes a series of evidence lines to determine whether a variant falls into one of five categories: benign (not thought to contribute to disease risk), likely benign, pathogenic (thought to contribute to disease risk), likely pathogenic, and variant of uncertain significance (contribution to disease risk is unknown or unclear). Categories are based on level and types of evidence identified for each gene–disease association. Because of this, a variant's classification is subject to change in this rapidly evolving field. Given that laboratories commonly will report variants that fall into any of the last three categories on this list, one can imagine confusion about which action(s), if any, should be taken based on a variant's classification.

For example, consider Case 2. For an individual who has experienced symptoms of a likely inherited disease and received a test result, the knowledge of whether their result is "pathogenic/likely pathogenic" (typically managed the same way) versus "a variant of uncertain significance" has profound implications for protection from harm. A variant of uncertain significance that is acted upon without the evidence to support its definitive association with disease can essentially render it as a false positive in a symptomatic individual (i.e., the genetic contribution to disease is still unknown, and more testing may still be necessary), or might increase the risk of falsely reassuring other (pre-symptomatic) family members who receive negative results for this particular variant, when risk might be associated with some other variant not yet identified (that is, the negative test result is only for a specific familial variant of uncertain significance, while the actual genetic contribution "running in this family" may as yet be unknown or unidentified).

Case 3 raises the potential of harm both through threat to a child's "right to an open future," and through potential ramifications for insurability and employment (May and Fullerton, 2021). As discussed in greater detail below, each of these potential harms are consequences of threats to patient informed consent and privacy. In terms of harm, control over access to (privacy) and utilization of (informed consent) a person's genetic information is essential to fair opportunity, violation of either potentially resulting in discriminatory treatment that limits access to insurance and employment opportunities, or potential for stigmatization with its accompanying social challenges.

Promoting Informed Consent

Perhaps the most important ethical issue for clinical genetics is the issue of context for test results. Context underlies informed consent in clinical genetics as it establishes the framework for understanding benefit and the translation of test results to desired health outcomes. For example, the absolute versus relative risk associated with genetic variants identified is of paramount importance in many preventive contexts. Most gene–disease associations are complex and subtle, conferring slight additional risk that itself varies depending on lifestyle, environment, and the presence and/or absence of other gene variants. In a *Los Angeles Times* op-ed, H. Gilbert Welch and Wylie Burke describe an example of a 50% increase in risk associated with a particular genetic variant, but then go on to specify that this increase is from a 4% to a 6% chance of manifesting the disease (Welch and Burke, 2015). While an increase in risk of 50% might seem very significant and worthy of action, an absolute increase from a 4% to a 6% chance of manifesting a condition does not warrant drastic prophylactic intervention (the side effects or adverse events from which may well be greater than the risk of manifesting the condition). Because *how* information is presented can frame how its significance is interpreted and acted upon, it is important to be mindful of such framing, such as the absolute versus relative risk context just described.

Additionally, unwarranted reassurance from genetic test results can undermine compliance with screening that could be lifesaving through early detection. Consider for example, the choice made by the patient in Case 1, to forego increased screening and surveillance on the basis of BRCA-negative results. Although we can identify some disease–gene associations, not all such associations have been identified. This limitation makes recognition of testing limitations of paramount importance in a situation like that reflected by Case 1.

While a positive BRCA result identifies definite increased risk (estimated 65%+ lifetime chance of manifesting breast cancer), BRCA-associated breast cancer represents only a small fraction of breast cancer cases (the Centers for Disease Control and Prevention [CDC] estimates only 3% of breast cancer cases are related to BRCA muta-tions) (CDC, n.d.). A negative BRCA result, then, means that you are, at best, still at "population risk" of breast cancer, including inherited breast cancer (and may even be at increased risk due to other inherited conditions, that have not yet been identified or are not yet detectable). In this circumstance, the patient's extensive family history of breast cancer remains indicative of increased risk. The BRCA test results are only useful for identifying risk related to this limited form of breast cancer. Only if it were known that the patient's family history of breast cancer was specifically tied to BRCA would these results constitute a legitimate reason not to undergo increased screening/surveillance. Many HECs may see this situation as analogous to those involving end-of-life discus-sions wherein for true informed consent patients and their families need to know not only the clinical facts of their circumstances, but should also try to see these facts in the context of their values, experiences, and ideals.

For Cases 2 and 3, the most important issues surround individual preferences to know or not know their genetic predispositions. Myriad studies have documented wide variation between individuals in terms of desire to know about different types of genetic predisposition and risk (Roberts et al., 2018). This is especially true where the risk or predisposition is "not actionable," as is the case in Case 3 (Huntington's Disease), meaning that there is no known effective treatment or cure, or other behavioral steps to mitigate risk stemming from the condition. Here, it should be noted that the exercise of informed consent may at times involve the use of decision strategies that exclude or emphasize certain reasons for action (e.g., second-order reasoning – see Raz, 1990). Such exercise of informed consent is familiar to HECs in other contexts, such as advance directives (May, 2009).

Another important consideration stems from the extended pertinence of test results to individuals and populations beyond the individual tested (May, 2012). Even when actionable (as in Case 2), the desire to know about pathological predisposition varies between individuals. The importance of this variation can be seen in controversies surrounding American College of Medical Genetics and Genomics (ACMG) recommen-dations for reporting of secondary and incidental findings. In 2013, the ACMG pub-lished guidelines for reporting of secondary and incidental findings from clinical exome and genome sequencing, that recommended mandatory (automatic) evaluation and reporting of 56 gene variants (later revised to 59) that are highly associated with pathological conditions for which effective treatments exist, and which are often not recognized at early stages through symptomology (Kalia et al., 2017). Justification of these recommendations centered on the idea of medical benefit and a fiduciary duty to report relevant deleterious health information. However, even though limited to highly "penetrant" pathological conditions, these recommendations were vehemently criticized as paternalistic because they ran counter to the idea of patient autonomy and informed consent, resulting in modification of the recommendations to include the right of patients to "opt out" of these secondary or incidental results (Wolf et al., 2013; May, 2015). Here, it is important to note that, for example, a child's right to an open future, or other second-order decisions strategies (as discussed above) may emphasize rights to genetic ignorance (May and Spellecy, 2006). Thus, in regard to Case 2, it is important to ascertain the sibling's desire to know about their potential genetic predisposition to the condition in question even where the tested individual has agreed to share their genetic testing results.

In regard to Case 3, it is important to consider the ability of the patient to form and express preferences for knowing about nonactionable genetic predispositions. While "nonactionable" in terms of mitigating deleterious effects of the condition, many people find predispositional information "actionable" in other contexts: adopting life plans that are plausibly realizable, for example, or motivating estate planning, etc. Other individuals, however, find such information to be burdensome, tainting their ability to enjoy life as it happens and placing a dark cloud over even short-term rewards. For this reason, absent utility for diagnosis of present conditions or childhood-onset debilitating disease, a joint Working Group formed by the American College of Pediatrics (AAP) and the ACMG recommended against predispositional genetic testing of children in order to maintain the child's "right to an open future" (AAP Committee on Bioethics et al., 2013; Ross et al., 2013).

Assuring Patient Privacy

Cases 1 and 2 have the most direct and obvious implications for privacy, as each involves issues related to the implications of one person's genetic test for other (biologically related) individuals. Here, clinical genetics faces challenges that are less common in other areas of clinical medicine. Unlike most traditional tests, genetic tests often have direct implications for others. Consider, for example, a chest x-ray done to diagnose potential pneumonia. Imagine that the x-ray identifies a spot on the lung likely to be lung cancer. The results of this imaging test might have indirect implications for the welfare of the patient's family members (they are likely to be sad and experience anxiety, etc. due to a potential lung cancer diagnosis), but the imaging results are not suggestive that others have this condition (although the fact that patient was a heavy smoker who subjected family members to second-hand smoke, for example, might be relevant – again, indirectly). In contrast, a genetic test that identifies, for example, a BRCA variant associated with breast cancer, has (because it is inherited) direct implications for the likelihood that the same variant might be present in biological siblings, offspring, or parents. This raises questions about the duty to warn, and how this duty might be influenced by patient preferences.

Case 3 raises issues of potential consequence to insurability, and employability. There are many conditions that, like Huntington's Disease, represent the likelihood of substantially increased health-related problems that will be costly for insurers, and problematic for employers (due to likely increased absenteeism and/or potential decreased productivity related to health problems). Recognizing these threats, the USA passed into law the Genetic Information Nondiscrimination Act of 2008 (GINA), which protects individuals from having their genetic information used against them by health insurance companies or potential employers. However, GINA does not apply to long-term, life, or disability insurance, or to employers with fewer than 15 employees, limiting its protection. In addition, the enforceability of GINA is questionable, as the burden lies upon the person wronged to establish that the information has been misused, something that is easy to deny and difficult to prove. For these reasons, concerns about insurance companies or employers learning about genetic test results are commonly identified as significant reasons for refusing genetic testing, particularly in the context of screening and prevention. HECs should seek ways to educate themselves about these issues – indeed, all of the specialized issues discussed in this chapter – in addition to seeking out colleagues with greater expertise (if they do not already exist on the committee), in order to ensure that their respective healthcare organizations are prepared to address these complex issues in a thoughtful, ethical and informed manner.

As medical applications of genetics rapidly move from the research realm to the clinical, the prominence of ELSI issues for clinical ethicists will inevitably increase. As seen throughout this chapter, these issues will at times pose novel challenges, but many will pose familiar challenges that require thoughtful attention to how our "toolbox" of moral concepts is applied in novel contexts. We hope to have illuminated in this chapter the key issues pertinent to addressing issues arising in this emerging area of clinical practice. HECs would do well to identify potential expert resources to assist in the development of institutional policies and practice standards, as well as articulation of professional expectations in these emerging areas. See Chapter 26 for advice concerning how to identify such expert resources.

Questions for Discussion

1. Conceptual: What are the different potential "harms" that should be protected against when genetic testing is undertaken?
2. Pragmatic: How might ethics committees help raise awareness of the uncertainties and complexities of interpreting genetic test results?
3. Strategic: Given the limitations of the Genetic Information Nondiscrimination Act (GINA), what additional steps might help to mitigate "risk" of one's genetic information being used in deleterious ways?

References

AAP Committee on Bioethics, Committee on Genetics, and the ACMG Social, Ethical and Legal Issues Committee. (2013). Ethical and policy issues in genetic testing and screening of children. *Pediatrics*, 131(3): 620–622.

Centers for Disease Control and Prevention. (n.d.). Hereditary breast and ovarian cancer: BRCA 1 and BRCA 2. www.cdc .gov/genomics/disease/breast_ovarian_ cancer/genes_hboc.htm (accessed September 1, 2020).

Kalia SS, Adelman K, Bale SJ, et al. (2017). Recommendations for reporting of secondary findings in clinical exome and genome sequencing, 2016 update (ACMG SF v2.0): A policy statement of the American College of Medical Genetics and Genomics. *Genetics in Medicine*, 19(2): 249–255.

May T (2009). *Bioethics in a Liberal Society*. Baltimore: Johns Hopkins University Press.

May T (2012). Re-thinking clinical risk for DNA sequencing. *American Journal of Bioethics*, 12(10): 24–26.

May T (2015). On the justifiability of ACMG recommendations for reporting of incidental findings in clinical exome and genome sequencing. *Journal of Law, Medicine and Ethics*, 43(1): 134–142.

May T, Fullerton SM (2021). Ethical considerations in the use of direct-to-consumer genetic testing for adopted persons. *Adoption Quarterly*, 24(1): 89–100.

May T, Spellecy R (2006). Autonomy, full information, and genetic ignorance in reproductive medicine. *Monist*, 6(1): 466–481.

Raz J (1990). *Practical Reason and Norms*. Princeton University Press.

Richards S, Aziz N, Bale S, et al. (2015). Standards and guidelines for the interpretation of sequence variants: A joint consensus recommendation of the American College of Medical Genetics and Genomics and the Association for Molecular Pathology. *Genetics in Medicine*, 17(5): 405–424.

Ross LF, Saal HM, Davis KL, et al. (2013). Technical report: Ethical and policy issues in genetic testing and screening of children. *Genetics in Medicine*, 15(3): 234–245.

Roberts JS, Robinson JO, Diamond PM, et al. (2018). Patient understanding of, satisfaction with, and perceived utility of whole-genome sequencing: Findings from the MedSeq Project. *Genetics in Medicine*, 20(9): 1069–1076.

Tandy-Connor S, Guiltinan J, Krempeley K, et al. (2018). False-positive results released by direct-to-consumer genetic tests highlight the importance of clinical confirmation testing for appropriate patient care. *Genetics in Medicine*, 20(12): 1515–1521.

Welch HG, Burke W (2015, April 27). Op-ed: Why whole-genome testing hurts more than it helps. *Los Angeles Times*. www.latimes.com/opinion/op-ed/la-oe-welch-problems-predictive-medicine-20150428-story.html

Wolf SM, Annas GJ, Elias S (2013). Respecting patient autonomy in clinical genomics: New recommendations on incidental findings go astray. *Science*, 340(6136): 1049–1050.

Chapter

22

Challenging Issues in Surgical Ethics
Intraoperative Decision-Making, Innovative Surgery, and High-Risk Operations near the End of Life

Darryl Schuitevoerder and Peter Angelos

Objectives

Upon reading and considering the content of this chapter, the reader should be able to:

1. Analyze the complexities of intraoperative decision-making when faced with unexpected findings.
2. Describe the importance of shared decision-making, disclosure, and informed consent when surgeons perform novel techniques or use innovative technologies during operative care.
3. Assess the challenges for deciding whether or not to pursue operative interventions in both high-risk patients and patients nearing the end of life.

Case

A 44-year-old patient is seen for persistent right upper quadrant pain that is associated with food. After several visits to her primary care provider, she is referred to a gastrointestinal specialist, where it is confirmed that her clinical history and work-up are consistent with symptomatic cholelithiasis. A laparoscopic cholecystectomy is recommended. She is referred for surgery, and during the consultation the surgeon describes the procedure, its risks, benefits, and alternatives, and obtains her informed consent to proceed with the operation. During surgery, on laparoscopic exploration of the abdominal cavity, she is noted to have a dilated and fluid-filled appendix concerning for an appendiceal tumor. There was no prior discussion with the patient surrounding anything except performing the cholecystectomy. How should the surgeon proceed?

Introduction

For centuries, surgery and medicine existed in overlapping but different professional spheres, but of course, in modern medicine, this is no longer the case. Thus, surgery and surgical interventions are generally governed by the same ethical norms that govern most medical practice. However, how those norms are applied and balanced often differ between standard medical and surgical care.

For example, as in internal medicine or family practice, so too in surgery the process of disclosure and information sharing is firmly grounded in the moral obligation to respect patient autonomy. Through the process patients are educated by their physician about the diagnosis, necessary intervention, risks associated with intervention, and alternative treatments. After obtaining this information, the patient weighs the options and then, with the aid of recommendations provided by the physician, decides for or against available interventions, such as surgery.

However, what is often absent in practice is a broader conversation about what is important to that particular patient and what quality of life means to them. This last aspect of informed decision-making is of paramount importance when deciding whether or not to pursue operative interventions, because (as can be seen by the case at the beginning of this chapter) surgery often presents unique challenges: information not available perioperatively becomes clear during a procedure, and only by understanding the patient's overall goals, values, and priorities will the surgeon be able to proceed in a manner consistent with the patient's desires. Once the patient is under anesthesia, they no longer have capacity to change their mind or make further decisions. This vulnerability is unique to procedure- and surgical-based medical practices. The patient is putting trust in the surgeon and expects that the surgeon will, in good faith, perform the stated procedure as described at a time when the patient no longer has capacity. This relationship and trust are stressed in the setting of unforeseen circumstances encountered in the operating room when the patient is unable to voice desires, and the surgeon, while relying on prior discussion as well as the core bioethical principles, must do what they believe is in the patient's best interest given the situation.

Another aspect that differs when the intervention is surgical compared to medical management of disease is the responsibility for adverse outcomes. For example, consider the following two clinical scenarios. A patient presents to the emergency department having suffered a myocardial infarction. Despite appropriate medical management the patient develops congestive heart failure, requires placement of a left ventricular assist device, and experiences a significant decrease in quality of life. While this outcome is clearly undesirable, it is a known risk with cardiovascular health issues. Thus, unless there was some element of malpractice or neglect, the physician would not be considered responsible for this poor outcome.

In contrast to this, however, consider a patient who presents to the emergency department with acute cholecystitis. She undergoes a laparoscopic cholecystectomy during which the common bile duct is transected. This complication results in a prolonged hospitalization, a subsequent major operation, and potential long-term effects on her quality of life. This outcome is similarly undesirable, and is also a known risk of the procedure; however, despite the surgeon not causing the cholecystitis, one would place direct responsibility of this poor outcome on the shoulders of the surgeon. Perhaps this is what Bosk noted when he wrote in *Forgive and Remember*, "When the patient of an internist dies, the natural question his colleagues ask is, 'what happened?' When the patient of a surgeon dies his colleagues ask, 'what did you do?'" (Bosk, 1979, 30). This question becomes all the more striking when a surgeon uses a novel technique or relatively new device with which they have little experience.

This chapter will explore three areas of surgical practice that require a nuanced attention to how we work with ethical norms in medicine, in order to come to good medical and ethical outcomes: decision-making about surgical interventions; handling unexpected findings during surgery; and the use of innovative surgical techniques.

Ethical Aspects Surrounding Operative Interventions – Especially in High-Risk Patients or Patients Nearing the End of Life

Once again, an ethical cornerstone of surgery is the importance of respecting patient autonomy, informed consent, and shared decision-making. As such, considering benefits and risks relative to an individual patient's values and their concept of a reasonable quality of life allows for a more complete understanding of the possible outcomes and how a proposed operation may affect the patient's life moving forward. Such a nuanced approach goes beyond saying, "Your risk for serious complication is 20%, which includes heart attack, stroke, pneumonia, need for reoperation," and instead includes translating this cold data into tangible outcomes. If these complications should arise it could mean a prolonged hospital course, require an extended ICU stay, a period of mechanical ventilation, several weeks to months of physical rehabilitation, and likely discharge to an inpatient nursing home for further recovery. This approach paints a more descriptive picture and is likely to be more useful to the patient than binary outcomes.

Dr. Gretchen Schwarze has described a "Best Case/Worst Case" framework for providing this information in high-risk surgical situations. In this approach two parallel paths are graphically depicted, one representing the surgical option and one if the decision is made for nonoperative management. For each option, a best-case, most likely case, and worst-case scenario is described as a series of events or a plausible story that includes the outcome of treatment and the events experienced in order to get to that outcome. Through this structured framework for approaching difficult discussions and clinical scenarios, the Best Case/Worst Case improves objective measures of shared decision-making, and was found by a majority of surgeons to be superior than their prior approach to these discussions (Kruser et al., 2017; Taylor et al., 2017).

Consider the clinical scenario in which a 75-year-old patient with coronary artery disease, COPD, diabetes, and hypertension is diagnosed with lung cancer for which an operation could remove the tumor. From a medical point of view, the patient's best option for long-term survival is to have surgery, and this is explained to them. However, it is very likely that the patient will require lifelong oxygen supplementation and will need to be in assisted living after the initial recovery. This particular patient may highly value complete independence and decide to forego surgery and focus on other management strategies that may better preserve their anticipated quality of life even though this may impact their longevity. Another patient in a similar situation may value the option that gives them the greatest chance for long-term survival over challenges with being in assisted living and on supplemental oxygen.

Similar situations may occur in a patient who is felt to be nearing the end of life. Indeed, it has been shown that up to 20% of patients older than 65 who undergo an abdominal operation for an urgent or emergent indication die within 30 days (Cooper et al., 2015). End-of-life care is often associated with significant financial expense and can potentially be burdensome to the patient. End-of-life care commonly includes operations or procedures; data demonstrate that over 30% of Medicare beneficiaries undergo surgery during the last year of life and 8% undergo a procedure in the final week of life. These interventions are almost certainly undertaken in order to provide medical care deemed to be in the patient's best interest. However, given the overarching societal sentiment that death must be avoided at all costs rather than accepted as part of life, it may be the case that patients choose high-risk surgery because they believe that this is what is expected. It may, in fact, be the case that, after holding detailed discussions with patients, providing the opportunity to explore what meaningful life is to them and covering the various potential outcomes, many of these hospitalizations, interventions, and operations might be able to be avoided. In such cases, beneficence may mean pursuing treatments that prioritize quality of life over length of life. In order to help quantify perioperative risk, clinical risk calculators can be helpful adjuncts to clinical conversation with patients and are frequently used to provide objective and tangible estimates of perioperative risk (ACS NSQIP Surgical Risk Calculator, 2020).

Especially in end-of-life settings or when faced with high-risk operations, physicians should take the time to evaluate what meaningful life is to that particular patient and clearly explain possible outcomes so that decisions will be reflective of the patient's values. Such an approach will assist in making appropriate care decisions when faced with difficult scenarios in frail elderly patients, those with significant comorbidities, or those at the end of life.

Intraoperative Decision-Making When Faced with Unexpected Findings

As noted, when discussing surgical options with patients, the discussion generally includes detailing the diagnosis, both surgical and nonsurgical options for management, and the risks and benefits inherent with the various options. As part of this process, physicians deliver information related to the procedure, including details a reasonable patient would find to be important as well as any specifics relevant to that individual patient. Subsequently the risks versus the benefits of the operation are discussed in detail.

While it is possible for unexpected yet potential complications of an agreed-upon operation to arise, sometimes these issues can be anticipated, and a broad preoperative conversation might provide the surgeon license to deal with such complications. A different situation may arise in which the surgeon is performing an operation on an unrelated organ system and sees a concerning finding in another organ or area of the body that is not part of or included in the agreed-upon procedure. Consider the case above, in which a patient is undergoing a laparoscopic cholecystectomy and during the case the patient is noted to have a mucus-filled and enlarged appendix concerning for tumor. In this situation, the surgeon has several options in addition to performing the planned cholecystectomy: (1) proceed with the appendectomy and explain the situation to the patient and the patient's family/surrogate after the case; (2) call the patient's surrogate, describe the findings, make a recommendation to perform appendectomy, and request permission to do so; (3) do not perform the appendectomy and allow the patient to wake up from the procedure, discuss the findings seen in the appendix, and recommend an additional operation at a later date to perform the appendectomy.

Though one could argue that an appendectomy was not part of the preoperative discussion and, as such, consent should be obtained prior to proceeding, to put the patient through subsequent general anesthesia and procedure instead of performing a relatively straightforward operation seems inconsistent with the principle of beneficence. Thus, most surgeons would opt for option 1 or 2. Such a move does seem problematic in the face of the requirement to respect patient autonomy, but is justified because the surgery is generally low risk with high reward.

Of course, even when a simple and low-risk procedure like an appendectomy is performed, a complication related directly to that portion of the procedure can occur, and the surgeon may have difficulty explaining how beneficence took precedence over respecting the patient's autonomy and seeking informed consent from a surrogate decision maker prior to proceeding. In this light, it is important to note that there are several situations in which the surgeon should *not* proceed without obtaining consent from the patient themself, such as when additional procedures would lead to loss of reproductive ability or cause significant patient disability (Langerman et al., 2016). In addition, when the impact on the patient's life is expected to be great, the importance of the patient actually making the decision becomes greater than the importance of avoiding a second operation. When the morbidity of the additional procedure is expected to be significant, the best course of action is to finish the current operation, stop, and wake the patient from anesthesia. Even though such an approach may necessitate greater risks to the patient, the patient is afforded the opportunity to participate in the decision, ask pertinent questions, and exercise autonomy in making the decision for or against a subsequent operation.

Novel Techniques and the Use of Innovative Technologies in Operative Care

From the outset we describe the importance of informed consent and respect for patient autonomy, leading to shared decision-making in surgical care. When discussing the use of novel techniques or innovative technologies in operative care, the importance of this process becomes even more evident. However, when considering innovative surgical approaches, there is often a lack of knowledge of what the true risks of the procedure are. As a result, the informed consent process required to respect the patient's autonomy must be altered given the lack of knowledge about what the actual risks and benefits of the novel surgical technique are.

The ethical basis for this desire to push boundaries for the sake of patients' welfare is beneficence. In modern surgery, however, it is sometimes not clear what the actual benefits to an individual patient will be of adopting a new surgical technique. Consider, for example, the transition from performing open cholecystectomy to laparoscopic cholecystectomy as the standard approach for management of patients with sequelae of gallstones. The laparoscopic approach was presented to patients as affording the benefit of less pain, shorter hospital length of stay, smaller incisions, and shorter period of time with physical limitations and time away from work. Given these benefits, it is easy to see why patients readily consented to this innovative procedure even when surgeons had very little experience with the operations. However, early in the learning process the procedure resulted in an initial increased rate of common bile duct injuries (Bernard and Hartman, 1993). Even though surgeons demonstrated respect for their patients' autonomous choices by obtaining informed consent, patients were actually being put at greater risk of this complication by virtue of their surgeons' lack of experience with what was then a novel technique. From the perspective of a patient needing their gallbladder taken out, having it done laparoscopically during the initial learning phase of the new operation actually meant that, even though many patients did not suffer complications, every patient was taking on more risk than the traditional method.

Any new operation raises the question of whether the risks to patients today will be higher than known and whether more patients will be harmed during the early phases of adopting a new technique. Balancing risk to individual patients and the rewards of long-term outcomes is a significant challenge in innovative surgical techniques. A learning curve is unavoidable with new operations; however, how much increased risk is acceptable in the short term to improve patient care in the long term and what measures can be implemented to improve safety and shorten the learning curve as much as possible during this initial learning phase? A current example is robotic surgery, which, when compared to the laparoscopic approach, offers a three-dimensional view, enhanced image magnification, wristed instruments with a greater degree of freedom of motion, and instrument stabilization. However, there is a documented learning curve that varies significantly depending on the experience of the surgeon and the complexity of the procedure performed. There is also a dearth of quality data comparing and documenting the robotic approach to the current standard of care, the open or laparoscopic approach, and indeed much of the rationale for robotic safety is derived from the data supporting laparoscopy, which has a different learning curve. Recent data have shown inferior outcomes after radical hysterectomy for early cervical cancer using the robotic platform (Ramirez et al., 2018), prompting the US Food & Drug Administration (US FDA) to issue a warning statement about the utility of robotic assistance for cancer operations (US FDA, 2019). Accordingly, surgeons who were employing robotic assistance to perform these procedures are now forced to adopt a new technique until more data confirm or refute these early findings.

There are a number of articles and arguments relating to the ethics of innovation as it implies to research and systemic implementation of innovation (Karpowicz et al., 2016; Reijers et al., 2018); however, little is written regarding the ethics surrounding the process of devising and developing innovative technology or techniques on a more granular or individual level. The message as it relates to providers, patients, and healthcare ethics committees (HECs) is that when considering using the assistance of developing or new technology during surgical procedures, a detailed discussion about the safety, efficacy, and surgeon's experience needs to be held with the patient preoperatively. Without this step, the patient is unable to make a truly informed decision about whether they should opt for the standard approach or undergo the procedure with the assistance of novel technology. While surgeons may be reluctant to disclose their amount of prior experience and where they are on the learning curve, this information is vital in allowing the patient to make an informed decision, as these factors are highly likely to impact the success of the procedure and the patient outcome. Thus, respect for patient autonomy requires full disclosure without patient prompting and should be strongly encouraged when surgeons discuss the use of new techniques and technologies with their patients.

Ethical issues surrounding innovative techniques and novel technology should involve discussion with the HEC. It is important for the HEC to acquire information regarding several important questions:

1. Is the technology being utilized the current standard of care, widely performed although not yet standard of care, or truly experimental? And what is the current standard of care for treating the patient's problem?
2. What was discussed and disclosed during the preoperative discussion?
3. If there was an adverse outcome, did the fact that new technology was utilized cause or lead to the adverse outcome?

Answers to these questions and consideration of essential ethical norms ground the guidance that HECs can give regarding the performance of innovative surgical procedures. Further, the HEC may want to consider policies for the use of innovative practices so that there are checks and balances in the system, providing valuable oversight that does not exist now, since such practices fall outside of research oversight.

Conclusion

In the above clinical settings several core principles are emphasized and are of great importance. The concept of shared decision-making and respect for patient autonomy has been emphasized throughout this chapter and is of paramount importance. It reflects a fundamental respect for the patient's autonomy and their innate ability to determine what is in their own best interest aided by clinical information and support from the physician or surgeon. Whether for regular surgical interventions, high-risk situations, or end-of-life conditions, shared decision-making is the right norm of practice. But not all situations in surgery can be anticipated ahead of the operation itself. When confronted with unexpected findings during surgery, the surgeon must balance respect for autonomy with beneficence and nonmaleficence in light of the new findings. This balancing can lead to surgeons performing interventions not otherwise directly authorized by the patient but supported by good moral reasoning. Further, full disclosure when discussing the use of surgical innovation or novel approaches to existing procedures is also critically important, especially when the risks may not be fully known. In our experience, patients are frequently excited by novel techniques and are often eager participants even if the surgeon has limited experience. Appreciation of this fact requires surgeons to be very circumspect in how they discuss the unknown risks of new techniques and technologies with their patients. Further beyond respect for autonomy, there will be situations in which the principle of nonmaleficence demands that surgeons are not to offer surgical interventions to a patient even if the patient wants the operation. This is an important part of the surgeon's expert authority – namely, to determine the limits of the craft in relation to the patient's own conditions – and, as such, demands careful moral consideration to exercise that authority responsibly.

Questions for Discussion

1. Conceptual: What does shared decision-making (SDM) mean in relation to surgery? Do all surgeries necessitate robust SDM? How does SDM apply in cases of innovative surgeries?
2. Pragmatic: When faced with unexpected findings in the operating room, how should respect for autonomy be weighed relative to beneficence and nonmaleficence in determining how to proceed?
3. Strategic: How would the HEC go about developing policies for the use of innovative techniques and novel technologies? Who should be part of the discussion, and what features would a policy contain?

References

ACS NSQIP Surgical Risk Calculator. (2020). https://riskcalculator.facs.org/RiskCalculator/PatientInfo.jsp (accessed March 2020).

Bernard HR, Hartman TW. (1993). Complications after laparoscopic cholecystectomy. *American Journal of Surgery*, 165(4): 533–535.

Bosk C. (1979). *Forgive and Remember.* University of Chicago Press.

Cooper Z, Mitchell SL, Gorges RJ, Rosenthal RA, Lipsitz SR, Kelley AS (2015). Predictors of mortality up to 1 year after emergency major abdominal surgery in older adults. *Journal of the American Geriatrics Society,* 63(12): 2572–2579.

Karpowicz L, Bell E, Racine E (2016). Ethics oversight mechanisms for surgical innovation: A systematic and comparative review of arguments. *Journal of Empirical Research on Human Research Ethics,* 11(2): 135–164.

Kruser JM, Taylor LJ, Campbell TC, et al. (2017). "Best case/worst case": Training surgeons to use a novel communication tool for high-risk acute surgical problems. *Journal of Pain and Symptom Management,* 53(4): 711–719 e715.

Langerman A, Siegler M, Angelos P (2016). Intraoperative decision making: The decision to perform additional, unplanned procedures on anesthetized patients. *Journal of the American College of Surgeons,* 222(5): 956–960.

Ramirez PT, Frumovitz M, Pareja R, et al. (2018). Minimally invasive versus abdominal radical hysterectomy for cervical cancer. *New England Journal of Medicine,* 379(20): 1895–1904.

Reijers W, Wright D, Brey P, et al. (2018). Methods for practising ethics in research and innovation: A literature review, critical analysis and recommendations. *Science and Engineering Ethics,* 24(5): 1437–1481.

Taylor LJ, Nabozny MJ, Steffens NM, et al. (2017). A framework to improve surgeon communication in high-stakes surgical decisions: Best case/worst case. *JAMA Surgery,* 152(6): 531–538.

US Food & Drug Administration. (2019). Caution when using robotically-asssisted surgical devices in women's health including mastectomy and other cancer-related surgeries: FDA safety communication. www.fda.gov/medical-devices/safety-communications/caution-when-using-robotically-assisted-surgical-devices-womens-health-including-mastectomy-and (accessed March 15, 2020).

Chapter

23 Psychiatric Ethics

Cynthia M. A. Geppert

Objectives

Upon reading and considering the content of this chapter, the reader should be able to:

1. Distinguish the ethical issues of patients with mental illness from those presented by patients with other medical and neurological conditions.
2. Recognize the primary ethical obstacles to providing health care for patients with mental illness and potential strategies to overcome them.
3. Formulate approaches to address the ethical challenges of patients with mental illness as a comorbidity to other healthcare issues.

Case 1

Mr. J is a 56-year-old man with chronic paranoid schizophrenia who presents to the emergency department of a community hospital because he is having difficulty walking. Mr. J has been walking up to 25 miles a day around the Texas city where he lives. Mr. J's foot is so swollen that his cowboy boot has to be cut off revealing wet gangrene of the lower extremity. Infectious disease and orthopedics services are called to consult and recommend below the knee amputation. They think there is almost no chance antibiotics could treat the massive infection and that without emergent amputation the infection will rapidly spread to other parts of the body resulting in life-threatening sepsis. Mr. J is adamant that he will not consent to amputation because "all I need is to walk more, that will heal my foot." He repeatedly says, "I don't want to die, but the walking will cure me." The on-call psychiatrist evaluates Mr. J and finds he lacks decision-making capacity to refuse a life-saving amputation as he is displaying inconsistent reasoning and does not appreciate that without amputation he will die. The emergency room physician contacts the patient's mother who is listed in the medical record as his surrogate decision maker. She clearly understands the gravity of the predicament and is willing to come to the hospital immediately to provide informed consent for the surgery. The orthopedic surgeon still refuses to amputate: "The man told me no, and I am not holding a patient down and cutting off his leg no matter what his mother or a psychiatrist says." The emergency department physician calls the healthcare ethics committee (HEC) for an ethics consultation.

Case 2

Mr. C is a 49-year-old intermittently homeless man with a long history of intravenous methamphetamine and heroin use who is hospitalized for the third time in 5 years for infective endocarditis. He underwent a tricuspid valve replacement 2 years before, but the new valve is now infected and must be replaced. Mr. C has always declined substance use treatment and inconsistently frequents needle-exchange facilities. The senior cardiologist believes a second valve replacement is clinically indicated but recommends against it on the grounds this valve will also become infected. The cardiologist writes in the medical chart that "such an expensive intervention should not be offered to drug addicts who refuse treatment; it is an unethical waste of valuable resources." The nurse caring for Mr. C, Jane, is appalled when she reads the cardiology note. The unit social worker suggests making a contract with the patient to enter substance use treatment as a condition for valve replacement; Jane is not sure that is ethical either as it seems coercive to her. She contacts the HEC to ask for help in thinking through this difficult situation.

Case 3

Ms. S is a 27-year-old woman who is in the hospital after attempting suicide. Ms. S has bipolar I disorder severe with psychotic features as well as alcohol use disorder, and she took all of her psychiatric medications along with alcohol. Initially stabilized for acute kidney failure due to lithium toxicity on the ICU, she has been cared for on the medical floor for several days and is approaching discharge. The psychiatric consultant, Dr. P, who has been following the patient, believes she is still suicidal and is at high risk for harming herself if she is not transferred to the psychiatric unit for further stabilization. The patient tearfully refuses transfer, saying she "cannot stand to be locked up." Dr. P evaluates Ms. S and determines she does not have decision-making capacity to refuse psychiatric hospitalization. After multiple failed attempts to persuade Ms. S to agree to voluntary admission to the psychiatric unit, Dr. P decides he must then admit her involuntarily for her own safety and files the required commitment paperwork. The senior medicine resident, Dr. J, is the same age as Ms. S and has gotten to know her over the time she has been on the ward. She tells the psychiatrist that if Ms. S had refused a medical admission, her choice would be respected; as such, a person with mental illness should have the same right. Further, if she wants to kill herself that is her choice. Frustrated when Dr. P tells her "the admission is for her own good," Dr. J calls the HEC asking for an ethics review of psychiatric paternalism.

Introduction: Why HECs Need to Know about Psychiatric Ethics

There are three important reasons that HEC members, especially those who do ethics consultation, need to know about psychiatric ethics. The first is that psychiatric or mental health ethics is a neglected topic in bioethics education, healthcare ethics textbooks, and the training of HECs. When it is taught it is usually peripheral to other issues like confidentiality or a contributing factor to case presentations focused on concerns such as difficult discharges. The second reason this gap in knowledge needs to be addressed is that patients with psychiatric and addictive disorders are commonly encountered in every healthcare environment from outpatient clinics to ICUs. As of 2016 almost 10 million patients on inpatient medical and surgical units suffered from a principal or secondary mental or substance use disorder. Depression, alcohol use disorder, and schizophrenia were the three most frequent diagnoses and often were co-occurring with other chronic medical conditions like diabetes and cardiac disease (Owens et al., 2019).

A similar representation of patients with substance use and mental health disorders can be found in residential programs, nursing homes, rehabilitation hospitals, and primary care practices, among other medical settings. It is nearly impossible for members of an HEC not to be called into ethics consults or have to address policy questions related to psychiatric ethics. This chapter provides an introduction to issues in clinical psychiatric ethics for HEC members.

Why Psychiatric Ethics Is Different

Of the three important reasons to understand psychiatric ethics, the third and most ethically salient reason to learn about psychiatric ethics is that psychiatry presents important clinical, social, and legal challenges not found in typical medical care, and these challenges make the psychiatric ethics different from other medical specialties. Chronic conditions like heart failure, obstructive pulmonary diseases, or even cancer rarely result in a diminishment and/or impairment of fundamental aspects of human functioning and cognitive capacity or when they do it is much later in the disease process. However, in patients with substance use disorders and serious mental illnesses thinking, willing, perceiving, judging, and feeling can all be severely impacted, interfering with the ability of psychiatric patients to care for themselves, to relate to family and friends, to act safely and appropriately, to interact in the larger community, to hold a job, and to keep stable housing or avoid incarceration. And while this level of fundamental neuropsychiatric dysfunction does occur in some patients with neurological illnesses, patients whose major neurocognitive disorder presents with behavioral disturbances, delusions, or other psychiatric symptomology tend to be treated as psychiatric patients, while those patients without these symptoms are more likely managed on medical or neurological services or in nursing home units (Treloar et al., 2010). Ultimately, patients identified as having a mental health disorder simply pose different challenges to practitioners and society than patients whose initial presentation may have features that are similar but are seen as primarily medical patients. These substantive challenges require a particular standard of professional conduct in order to protect the rights and interests of patients (Radden and Sadler, 2010).

Using the introductory cases to illustrate the unique challenges the bulk of this chapter will explore four significant challenges in psychiatry that raise issues in psychiatric ethics. They are:

1. The evaluation of decision-making capacity in patients with mental and substance use disorders is often more complex and nuanced than are assessments of patients with medical and neurological conditions.
2. Patients with addiction and mental illness tend to be more socially stigmatized than patients with medical and neurological conditions.
3. The nature of the psychiatric therapeutic relationship is more easily exploitable due to the vulnerability of patients and the power the psychiatrist wields.
4. The law plays a more prominent and determinative role in psychiatry than in almost any other type of medical practice.

Complexities in Evaluating Decision-Making Capacity

A fundamental ethical obligation in healthcare ethics is that healthcare practitioners respect the informed decisions of patients with decisional capacity. To uphold this duty on behalf of patients with varying levels of neuropsychiatric dysfunction from mental health and addictive disorders requires careful evaluation of the potential for these disorders to decrease the ability of patients to make informed and authentic choices about their health care. HEC members play a crucial role for these patients in assuring that those with meaningful deficits in decision-making have an authorized surrogate decision maker or a sound and authoritative policy and legal process to make decisions in accordance with their values and interests (Geppert et al., 2016).

Although studies have found that many patients with serious mental illness often experience more difficulty making decisions than patients with medical illnesses, many practitioners assume that patients with specific diagnoses such as schizophrenia or dementia automatically lack the ability to make any decisions. However, research suggests that there is no clear correlation between having a particular psychiatric or substance use diagnosis and the lack of capacity. Further, with decision aids – such as family support, repeated discussions, and audiovisuals – many psychiatric patients can make a wide variety of medical decisions. It is imperative that HEC members recognize that mental health patients fall across a spectrum of capacity, and that ethics consults can help remove obstacles that prevent psychiatric patients from exercising self-determination to their fullest ability. HEC members can educate practitioners that lack of capacity must be assessed – not assumed – especially in patients with addictive and psychiatric disorders. Cognitive domains are those most adversely affected in most medical patients whose capacity is questioned or questionable. Patients with psychiatric and addictive disorders may perform well on standard cognitive testing and yet have profoundly impaired volitional and emotional abilities. For example, the depth of depression that drove Ms. S to a suicide attempt may have so depleted her usual coping skills that she is overwhelmed with anxiety even considering being on the psychiatric unit. Members of the HEC assist the practitioners in the difficult ethical task of not only promoting the ability of patients with psychiatric and addictive disorders to make their own decisions when they have capacity to do so, but also with maximizing their potential for sound decision-making. For example, the ethics consultants could recommend that medicine keep Ms. S on the ward a few days longer while psychiatry adjusts her medications and provides supportive therapy with the goal that she agrees to a voluntary admission and/or her risk of suicide decreases.

Assessments of decision-making capacity are based on the criteria noted in Chapter 11 on capacity, but in patients with neuropsychiatric conditions, there are often complexities and nuances requiring a higher level of experience and expertise precisely because these disorders impair and diminish the very components of executive function that are involved in complex medical decision-making. Taking Mr. J's case as our example, it would likely be easier for all the clinicians to recognize a lack of decision-making capacity if Mr. J's refusal was based on a paranoid delusion that aliens had invaded his leg or in response to a command hallucination that said the world would explode if he allowed amputation. As presented, however, Mr. J's situation is more challenging. He understands what amputation means and that it is being recommended, and he clearly can communicate his choice against the procedure. As such, the surgeon, who is probably not well versed in the literature on capacity evaluations and the full range of ethical concerns that surround this issue, is satisfied with these lower-order capacities and refuses to provide the surgery against the patient's wishes. However, the psychiatric evaluation reveals that Mr. J lacks the higher-order capacities of reasoning and appreciation required to make an informed refusal of a life-saving intervention. This is illustrated by his inability to explain rationally how walking will cure an infection or to grasp that surgery is the only medical option to stop the spread of infection and remain alive. A type of soft paternalism that would never be normative for a patient suffering from uncontrolled diabetes or heart disease may be ethically warranted in some patients with psychiatric and addictive disorders. When a patient makes what from a medical perspective is a poor decision or an irrational choice we generally presume they are exercising their self-determination as they see fit. This is frequently true of patients with psychiatric and addictive disorders as well – the patient with chronic substance use and post-traumatic stress disorder who while capable feels safer and freer on the street than in shelters. Yet there are also cases like that of Mr. J and perhaps Ms. S in which as a result of the disorder the individual is not able to make choices and decisions that reflect their most fundamental values and interests. Mr. J lives to walk and yet his paranoia and disorganization are cardinal symptoms of schizophrenia that preclude him from making a decision that has the greatest long-term likelihood of allowing him to return to his former lifestyle.

Stigmatization

The American public, including those in the healthcare professions, stigmatize persons with psychiatric and addictive disorders. While there are signs of change in these attitudes, prevailing beliefs, such as that persons with serious mental illness are violent or the inability to stop using substances is a moral failing or a crime, become root causes of the healthcare inequalities these populations continue to experience (Committee on the Science of Changing Behavioral Health Social Norms et al., 2016). Mr. C's case is a clear example of a form of healthcare discrimination spurred on by social bias toward people suffering from addictions. A healthcare practitioner who blamed a patient for developing ALS or brain cancer would be considered not just unethical but inhumane. It is thought acceptable in many healthcare settings to assert that when serious health problems like endocarditis occur in and are associated with addiction that the individual is responsible for their plight and thus withholding even life-sustaining treatment is ethically justifiable. These are value judgments about what sorts of persons and lives are worthy of receiving health care that are often masked and rationalized as resource allocation decisions.

Of course, stewardship of scarce and expensive healthcare resources is an important ethical priority for any healthcare institution. Ideally, organizational ethics discussions would address these macro-concerns and include HEC members, institutional administration, and community stakeholders. However, micro-decisions – bedside decisions – are different. These decisions are prone to implicit, unconscious biases, and the ethics consultants in Mr. C's case would do well to point out that allowing a single clinician to make a micro-allocation decision at the bedside of a critically ill patient requires ethical justification and reflection, not mere individual authority. The HEC should emphasize the need for the decision to offer a valve replacement to be made on clinical grounds, and not on nonmaterial factors such as a hypothetical reinfection that a person who injects drugs will reinfect the valve. And should the surgeon still determine that a valve replacement is unwarranted, the HEC should support the right of the patient to appeal such a decision so that there is some oversight that corrects for potential bias of the surgeon (Buchman and Lynch, 2018). From a policy perspective, HECs may want to proactively develop protocols that ensure a fair, evidence based, consistent, and transparent process for allocating scarce resources.

In some states patients with life-threatening substance use can be involuntarily committed. Mr C. is simply too ill to participate in substance use treatment and, outside a court order, it is difficult to see how, once the valve is replaced, the patient can be compelled to participate in addiction therapy. The question then is: Should the state get involved? Many ethicists would say that state involvement is probably not warranted in these cases. However, it is tempting, even necessary, with patients like Mr. C to try a number of different strategies. The social worker's suggestion that the valve replacement be conditioned on the patient's agreeing to enter substance use treatment comes from the desire to find a way to get him the treatment his body needs while trying to maximize positive outcomes. However, even though research shows that coerced addiction treatment is at least as successful as care that is voluntary, it is ethically problematic precisely because for patients like Mr. C, the "bargain" can be coercive. Thus, renewed attempts to engage the patient in treatment and reliably utilize harm reduction techniques are preferable.

Power and Vulnerability

The state and society grant psychiatrists enormous legal powers that go beyond the scope of other medical specialties. Conversely, most people who are ill and in pain are more vulnerable than they would be when healthy and happy; mental suffering is among the most intense and anguishing afflictions of the human condition. In hope of relief from this anguish psychiatric patients often share with their psychiatrists and other mental health professionals the most intimate, disturbing, and sensitive secrets including histories of sexual abuse and parental neglect, family discord and shame, and their most private hopes and fears. Deep, often buried, waves of emotion may surface in transference and countertransference that characterize the dynamic of the psychotherapeutic alliance. The relationship between a patient and a psychiatrist or other mental health professional is perforce closer, more intense, and more personal, than that of a patient with their surgeon or primary care provider. Such intimacy, trust, and openness on the part of the patient is necessary if the psychiatrist is to diagnose accurately the patient's illness and develop a biopsychosocial treatment plan that is empathic, efficacious, patient-centered, and clinically appropriate. At the same time, it places the patient in a significant position of dependency and vulnerability that is easy to exploit. As such, a psychiatrist, especially in psychotherapy, must adhere to the highest principles of ethical conduct and professional boundaries (Gabbard et al., 2012).

Given this heightened vulnerability of patients with psychiatric and mental disorders, how can the exercise of psychiatric power to hospitalize and/or administer medication against the wishes and will of a patient ever be justified? Practitioners unfamiliar with psychiatric practice may. like Dr. J (the chief resident in Ms S's case), be morally troubled at the prospect.

States, following *parens patriae* (the state should protect those who cannot protect themselves) as well as an exercise of *police powers* (exercise of state control over liberty) (Testa and West, 2010), have developed involuntary commitment laws to protect those who are of danger to self or others and have a diagnosed mental illness. Ms. S's psychiatrist, Dr. P, is acting in accordance with this legal principle, but is motivated by the clinical ethics principle of beneficence ("this is for her good"). It is important, though, to separate involuntary commitment from involuntary treatment, as most states and most ethicists agree that persons who are involuntarily committed may still retain the ability, and therefore the right, to determine whether or not they want treatment.

In Ms. S's case, the resident, Dr. J, is articulating a position grounded in civil rights, while Dr. P is concerned about protecting the patient from harm. HEC members who understand the legal principles and ethical reasoning that support involuntary commitment can help assure staff that Ms. S will receive due process. For example, should Dr. P press forward with a petition for involuntary commitment, there will be a court hearing within a reasonable time frame in which Ms. S will have legal representation and a judge will decide whether or not she must remain on the psychiatric unit. In the case of Ms. S, it appears that Dr. P and Dr. J prioritize different fundamental ethical values: Dr. J wants to respect his patient's autonomy while Dr. P wants to prevent her from harming herself. A deeper analysis will show that Dr. P believes Ms. S is so psychologically vulnerable due to her severe depression that she is not able to act autonomously or protect herself. The only real ethical warrant for involuntary hospitalization is therapeutic to restore the patient's psychological resources to the point that they can truly make their own choices. HEC members, through their consultations, can emphasize and help bridge the gap between medical and psychiatric ethics: translating the essential values that healthcare professional share into the unique nuance of the psychiatric context.

Law and Ethics in Psychiatry

Civil commitment dramatically illustrates how prominent and even prescriptive a function the law serves in psychiatric practice; the law frames what a psychiatrist can and even must do differently than in other medical specialties. In many jurisdictions, even if it is against their medical judgment, psychiatrists and other mental health professionals are not only permitted but mandated to breach patient confidentiality under warn and protect laws (aka "Tarasoff" laws). Legal and economic forces are increasingly pressuring psychiatrists to take steps that may not always be in the best interest of the patients. Utilization reviewers may demand that patients be discharged who are no longer an acute danger to themselves or others but who are still psychiatrically unstable or, in the case of persons with addiction, who have been detoxified only without even beginning the real treatment of their disorder. While these pressures are not unique to psychiatric practice the nature of the disorders amplifies the uncertainty of practitioner's judgment. Forensic experts have shown that outside of imminent threat, there is not a solid scientific basis to make reliable predictions about which patients will harm themselves or others. Yet increasingly, professional peer review bodies, medical licensing boards, and courts are holding psychiatrists accountable for these acts. In most other branches of medicine, it is accepted and expected that a practitioner can exercise all their knowledge and skill and a patient will still succumb to their disease. The same standard often does not apply in psychiatry.

Further, legal statutes delimit who and how informed consent can be obtained differently in psychiatric patients than other patient groups. For instance, in some states a healthcare proxy named in an advance directive may consent for medical but not psychiatric treatments. Some states have restrictive requirements on the administration of electroconvulsive therapy despite its long track record of life-saving safety (Livingston et al., 2018). Similarly, psychiatric advance directives in which a patient with a recurrent mental illness can when stable express their treatment preferences and appoint a proxy decision maker in many jurisdictions are not afforded the same legal standing as would an advance directive for medical care, which has limited their utility (Swanson et al., 2006).

A significant problem is that these kinds of laws often reflect not science but a cultural suspicion of psychiatry that not infrequently results in patients not receiving the most effective treatment for their illness. The pervasiveness of the law that affects the ethics of psychiatric care makes it prudent for HECs to have a rudimentary understanding of the legal landscape and ready access to legal counsel and mental health experts knowledgeable about the applicable mental health laws in their states and the policies of their respective institutions (Appelbaum and Gutheil, 1992). HECs may want to develop policies and programs that assist patients with psychiatric and addictive disorders to engage in advance care planning, for both medical and psychiatric care, so that in the all too common crises situations like the cases presented here there is a process in place to follow. One way in which HECs can try to level the ethical playing field for patients with addiction and mental illness is to develop good working relationships with hospital attorneys, adult protective services, and other community organizations such as local chapters of the National Alliance for the Mentally Ill that can collaborate in offering education of practitioners and the HEC itself as well as advocating for patients within the healthcare system.

Conclusion

The chapter has reviewed four salient areas in which psychiatric ethics is distinctive: capacity, stigma, power and vulnerability, and law. HEC members who learn about these unique aspects will be better prepared to provide consultation and education and to develop organizational ethics policies that advance the competent and compassionate care of patients with psychiatric and addictive disorders.

Questions for Discussion

1. Conceptual: Provide counterarguments to the chapter's claim that psychiatric ethics is different than the ethics of other medical specialties.
2. Pragmatic: Identify the primary psychiatric ethical concerns currently facing your institution and how your HEC might proactively address them.
3. Strategic: How could you explain to the surgeon in Case 1 and Dr. J in Case 3 that a decision to amputate and to involuntarily hospitalize respectively actually honor many of the core ethical values they too are trying to defend?

References

Appelbaum P, Gutheil T (1992). *Clinical Handbook of Psychiatry and the Law*, 2nd ed. Baltimore: Williams & Wilkins.

Buchman DZ, Lynch MJ. (2018). An ethical bone to PICC: Considering a harm reduction approach for a second valve replacement for a person who uses drugs. *American Journal of Bioethics*, 18(1): 79–81.

Committee on the Science of Changing Behavioral Health Social Norms; Board on Behavioral, Cognitive, and Sensory Sciences; Division of Behavioral and Social Sciences and Education; National Academies of Science, Engineering, and Medicine. (2016). *Ending Discrimination against People with Mental and Substance Use Disorders: The Evidence for Stigma Change*. Washington, DC: National Academies Press.

Gabbard G, Roberts LW, Crisp-Han H, Ball V, Hobday G, Rachal F (2012). *Professionalism in Psychiatry*. Washington, DC: American Psychiatric Press.

Geppert C, Cohen M, Bourgeois J, Peterson M (2016). Bioethical challenges for psychiatrists: Determination of decisional capacity. *Psychiatric Times*, 33(7).

Livingston R, Wu C, Mu K, Coffey MJ (2018). Regulation of electroconvulsive therapy: A systematic review of US state laws. *Journal of ECT*, 34(1): 60–68.

Owens PL, Fingar KR, McDermott KW, Muhuri PK, Heslin KC (2019). Inpatient stays involving mental and substance use disorders, 2016: Statistical brief #249. In *Health Care Cost and Utilization Project*. Rockville, MD: Agency for Healthcare Research and Quality.

Radden J, Sadler J (2010). *The Virtuous Psychiatrist: Character Ethics in Psychiatric Practice*. New York: Oxford University Press.

Swanson JW, McCrary SV, Swartz MS, Elbogen EB, Van Dorn RA (2006). Superseding psychiatric advance directives: Ethical and legal considerations. *Journal of the American Academy of Psychiatry and Law*, 34(3): 385–394.

Testa M, West SG (2010). Civil commitment in the United States. *Psychiatry (Edgmont)*, 7(10): 30–40.

Treloar A, Crugel M, Prasanna A, et al. (2010). Ethical dilemmas: Should antipsychotics ever be prescribed for people with dementia? *British Journal of Psychiatry*, 197(2): 88–90.

24

Conscientious Objection

Mark R. Wicclair

Objectives

Upon reading and considering the content of this chapter, the reader should be able to:

1. Differentiate conscience-based refusals from other objections care providers use to justify an unwillingness to provide care.
2. Defend the conditions according to which conscientious refusals to provide care should be permitted in a healthcare setting.
3. Propose institutional policy addressing the appropriate exercise and limits of conscientious objection by healthcare providers.

Case 1

Dr. Gregory Phillips is a physician in the Fairview Hospital emergency department (ED). It is standard of care in the Fairview ED to offer emergency contraception (EC) to rape victims who present at the ED. However, Dr. Phillips has a moral objection to offering EC. He objects to providing EC to women who request it, and to informing women that there is medication to prevent pregnancy after rape. He requests an accommodation that will enable him to practice in the ED without violating his moral convictions.

Case 2

Carla Bronson is a Pinehurst Hospital ICU nurse. She is morally opposed to palliative sedation to unconsciousness (the administration of sedative medication to the point of unconsciousness in terminally ill patients). The hospital's end-of-life care policy requires offering palliative sedation to unconsciousness as an option for the relief of intractable symptoms when patients are in the final stages of a terminal illness and when symptoms cannot be alleviated by other means. Ms. Bronson requests an accommodation that will enable her to care for ICU patients without violating her moral convictions.

Introduction

Healthcare ethics committee (HEC) members frequently are called upon to provide guidance pertaining to conscientious objection. This guidance can include case consultation, policy creation, and education. For HEC members to effectively perform these functions, they will need to understand when an objection to providing a medical service is a conscientious objection, reasons for accommodating conscientious objectors, the need for ethical constraints on accommodation, and the basics of institutional manage-ment of conscientious objection. These issues are addressed in this chapter.

What Makes a Refusal to Provide a Medical Service a Conscientious Objection?

In health care, conscientious objection generally occurs when practitioners object to providing a legal, professionally accepted, and clinically appropriate medical service within the scope of their clinical competence – and their objection is based on their moral convictions. What makes Dr. Phillips' objection to offering EC and Ms. Bronson's objection to participating in palliative sedation to unconsciousness *conscientious objections* is that both objections are based on the practitioners' *moral convictions*. It does not matter whether their moral convictions are secular in nature or based on their religious beliefs. However, HEC members should consider an objection to providing a medical service a conscientious objection only if it is based on the practitioner's moral convictions. Healthcare professionals can object to providing a medical service for a variety of other reasons. Objections that are not conscientious objections include the following:

1. An objection to providing a medical service because it is not clinically indicated: Suppose a pediatrician refuses to provide a growth hormone when parents request it for their son who is well within the normal height range for his age. The parents request a growth hormone to increase their son's chances of becoming a basketball star. Or suppose a surgeon refuses to perform surgery on a brain tumor because they conclude that it is "inoperable." Insofar as both refusals are supported by accepted clinical norms and standard of care, they are not conscientious objections.

2. An objection to providing a medical service to avoid a substantial health risk to the practitioner: For example, if a physician or nurse refuses to treat patients with life-threatening infectious diseases such as Ebola and SARS because they do not want to put themselves at risk of dying, the refusal is not a conscientious objection. Although refusing to provide or assist in providing abortions commonly is based on moral objections, there are other reasons. For example, in view of the violence that has been directed against abortion providers in the USA, practitioners who are not morally opposed to abortion might refuse to provide or assist in providing abortions out of a concern for their safety. Insofar as a refusal is based on a concern for the practitioner's health or safety, it is not a conscientious objection.

3. An objection to providing a medical service for financial reasons: For example, if a practitioner refuses to treat Medicaid patients due to low reimbursement rates, the refusal is not a conscientious objection.

4. An objection to providing a medical service because it is illegal or contrary to the profession's code of ethics: If practitioners have no moral objection to physician-assisted death but refuse to provide it because it is illegal and/or violates the profession's code of ethics, the refusal is not conscience-based.

5. An objection to providing a service because it is beyond the scope of the practitioner's clinical competence: For example, if a general practitioner refuses to provide palliative services to patients in intractable pain because they lack the necessary training and expertise, the refusal is not a conscientious objection.

In sum, the physician's objection in Case 1 and the nurse's objection in Case 2 are paradigm instances of conscientious objections because their objections are based on their moral beliefs and the medical services to which they object are legal, professionally accepted, and clinically appropriate medical services within the scope of their clinical competence.

Why Accommodate Conscientious Objectors?

In the above cases, Dr. Phillips and Ms. Bronson are refusing to provide legal, professionally accepted, and clinically appropriate medical services within the scope of their clinical competence; and both services at issue are standard of care in their respective healthcare facilities. As such, one might well ask, why should they be accommodated?

The primary reason for accommodating Dr. Phillips and Ms. Bronson and other health professionals who conscientiously object to providing medical services is to enable them to practice without acting contrary to their conscience or core moral beliefs, thereby enabling them to maintain their moral integrity (Wicclair, 2011). Core moral beliefs are a person's fundamental moral beliefs. They comprise the subset of a person's moral beliefs that matter most to them, and they are integral to a person's understanding of who they are. As Jeffrey Blustein observes, when one acts against one's core moral beliefs or conscience, "one violates one's own fundamental moral or religious convictions, personal standards that one sees as an important part of oneself and by which one is prepared to judge oneself" (Blustein, 1993, 295). The loss of moral integrity associated with a violation of a person's core moral beliefs can be devastating. It can result in strong feelings of guilt, remorse, and shame, as well as loss of self-respect. It also can be experienced as an assault on one's self-conception or identity.

Suppose Dr. Phillips understands that the primary mechanism of EC is to prevent ovulation. Nevertheless, he believes that offering EC would make him complicit in a serious moral wrong because doing anything to prevent pregnancy after sexual intercourse – even after rape – is contrary to his core moral beliefs. Insofar as offering EC is contrary to Dr. Phillips' core moral beliefs, it would undermine his moral integrity. Next, suppose that Ms. Bronson believes that palliative sedation to unconsciousness is morally equivalent to unjustified killing and contrary to her conception of the goals of nursing. Insofar as participating in palliative sedation to unconsciousness is contrary to Ms. Bronson's core moral beliefs about unjustified killing and the goals of nursing, it would undermine her moral integrity.

However, actions that practitioners perceive to be morally wrong are not necessarily contrary to their core moral beliefs and do not necessarily undermine their moral integrity. The following case illustrates this point. Herbert Higgins is an 82-year-old patient in the ICU. He has advanced lung cancer and is in multi-organ failure. His adult children insist that the doctors do "everything," including providing hemodialysis, to keep their father alive. Dr. Stern, Mr. Higgins' attending physician, objects to providing hemodialysis. He believes that it would be morally wrong to provide hemodialysis because it would be wasteful and pointless in view of the patient's extremely poor prognosis. Providing dialysis, he believes, would not reflect wise stewardship of medical resources. Although Dr. Stern believes that it would be morally wrong, it would be a wrong of a type that he routinely tolerates, rather than a perceived grave injustice such as discrimination based on race or sexual orientation. Insofar as providing hemodialysis would not compromise Dr. Stern's deepest self-identifying moral convictions, providing it might result in moral distress, but it would not undermine his moral integrity. To be sure, healthcare facilities should adopt measures to alleviate or reduce moral distress. However, accommodation may not be the most appropriate measure to accomplish this important objective (Lewis-Newby et al., 2015).

Ethical Constraints on Accommodation

Although enabling clinicians to practice medicine without undermining their moral integrity provides a sound reason to accommodate health professionals such as Dr. Phillips and Ms. Bronson, there are also important reasons to limit or deny accommodation. First, a health professional's conscience-based refusal can have an unacceptable impact on patients. Depending on the circumstances, refusing to offer, provide, or participate in providing a legal, professionally accepted, and clinically appropriate medical service, or information about it, can undermine patient autonomy, health, and well-being. These are three core values of the health professions, which are advocated in major professional codes, such as the American Medical Association (AMA) *Code of Medical Ethics* (2017), the American Nurses Association (ANA) *Code of Ethics for Nurses with Interpretive Statements* (2015), and the *Ethical Guidance* of the General Medical Council (GMC) in the UK (2020). Accordingly, these three values set general constraints on accommodation.

Second, refusing to provide a medical service or information about it can be burdensome to colleagues, administrators (e.g., department heads or supervisors), and institutions. Health professionals who practice within institutions generally are members of teams and they all are members of the institution. Accordingly, burdens to others who practice and work within the institution can set justified limits to accommodation.

Depending on the specific circumstances, accommodation can impose substantial burdens on the health professionals who are called on to provide the information or service that an objector refuses to offer. For example, since offering EC to rape victims is standard of care in Fairview Hospital, accommodating Dr. Phillips will require other ED physicians to substitute for him. Other physicians may be required to be on call more frequently, and their workloads may increase significantly. Such changes can be a substantial hardship. The magnitude of the burden also can vary with the personal situations of the other physicians. For example, it might be more of a burden to physicians who have other substantial responsibilities (e.g., family, research, teaching, and/or community service) than to physicians with fewer other responsibilities. Similarly, to accommodate Ms. Bronson, it might be necessary to switch assignments with other nurses, which, depending on their life circumstances, might be a substantial hardship.

Depending on the specific circumstances, accommodation can also impose substantial burdens on supervisors, department heads, other administrators, and institutions. For example, to accommodate Ms. Bronson, the nursing supervisor will have to make the necessary work assignments, which may require significant modifications and rescheduling. It might even require hiring an additional (part-time) nurse, a potential burden to the institution. For similar reasons, accommodating Dr. Phillips also can be burdensome to department heads and other administrators. Moreover, as the frequency of requests for accommodation increases, the burden of making the necessary staffing and schedule changes can also increase.

Institutional Management of Requests for Accommodation

It is incumbent upon healthcare institutions to be prepared to respond to requests for accommodation from health professionals with conscientious objections. Fair, consistent, and transparent management of conscience-based refusals requires an institutional policy rather than ad hoc decision-making on a case-by-case basis. HECs can provide a valuable service by drafting conscientious objection policies that explain conscientious objection, clearly state the institution's objectives in relation to conscientious objection, provide guidelines for deciding when to grant requests for accommodation, and specify responsibilities and procedures. Another important HEC function with respect to conscientious objection is education. Hospital staff should be familiar with the institution's conscientious objection policy and should know what conscientious objection is, the institution's goals in relation to conscientious objections, reasons for accommodation, and when it should and should not be accommodated. The HEC can provide and facilitate staff education on these matters.

Institutional Policy Guidelines

Generally, institutional policies should be designed to protect the moral integrity of clinicians without placing excessive burdens on patients, surrogates, other clinicians, supervisors, department heads, and the institution (Wicclair, 2011, 2014). Another important aim is to prevent invidious discrimination. Institutional policies can promote these objectives by including five general requirements:

The *first requirement* states that conscience-based refusals will be accommodated only if a requested accommodation will not impede a patient's/surrogate's timely access to clinically appropriate information, counseling, and referral. It requires only that patients/surrogates must receive clinically appropriate information, counseling, and referral in a timely manner. It does not require that the objecting practitioner provide it. This can be a significant difference for health professionals with a moral objection to a medical service who believe that informing or counseling patients/surrogates about it or offering referrals makes them morally complicit in serious wrongdoing and thereby undermines their moral integrity.

The first requirement can be satisfied if there are alternative means for patients to receive information, counseling, and referral in a timely manner. For example, to accommodate Dr. Phillips and satisfy the first requirement, ED triage nurses could be instructed to assign rape victims to physicians who have no moral objection to informing patients about EC. However, implementing measures to satisfy the first requirement must also satisfy the third requirement, which considers burdens on other clinicians, supervisors, department heads, and the institution.

The *second requirement* states that conscience-based refusals will be accommodated only if a requested accommodation will not impede a patient's timely access to clinically appropriate healthcare services offered within the institution. The aim of this requirement is to protect patients and assure that accommodation does not significantly affect timely access to healthcare services. In the case of Dr. Phillips, the second requirement can be satisfied by implementing an arrangement that assures that whenever Dr. Phillips is on service, ED physicians who do not object to EC are on service and can offer EC in a timely manner to rape victims who present at the ED. In the case of Ms. Bronson, the second requirement can be satisfied by an arrangement that assures that whenever she is working in the ICU, a sufficient number of ICU nurses are on duty who have the relevant expertise and experience and who are willing and able to care for patients who are receiving palliative sedation to unconsciousness. However, arrangements designed to accommodate Dr. Phillips and Ms. Bronson must also satisfy the third requirement, which considers burdens on other clinicians, supervisors, department heads, and the institution.

What if a Pineview Hospital *intensivist* has a moral objection to palliative sedation to unconsciousness and believes that even if other intensivists offer and provide the procedure, informing them that a patient meets the criteria would make them complicit in a serious moral wrong? In that case, both the first and second requirements can be satisfied by an arrangement that assigns to nonobjecting members of the healthcare team the responsibility of reviewing the charts of the objecting intensivist's patients to identify those who meet the criteria for offering palliative sedation to unconsciousness. When patients who meet the criteria are identified, their care will be provided by intensivists who are willing and able to offer and provide the procedure. Once again, however, such an arrangement must also satisfy the third requirement, which considers burdens on other clinicians, supervisors, department heads, and the institution.

The *third requirement* states that conscience-based refusals will be accommodated only if they will not impose excessive burdens on other clinicians, supervisors, department heads, or the institution. This requirement sets context-dependent practical limits to accommodation. Whether an accommodation will impose excessive burdens depends on a variety of contextual factors, including the number of staff members whose clinical competencies overlap with those of the objector; the willingness of other practitioners to provide the medical service at issue; the number of health professionals within a service, a unit, and the institution who request accommodation; the frequency of such requests; the existing responsibilities and workloads of health professionals, administrators, and staff; and the availability of funds to pay overtime or hire additional staff.

For example, whether it is feasible to implement arrangements that can accommodate Dr. Phillips and Ms. Bronson is dependent on the hospitals' financial and staffing resources. It would be an excessive burden on other ED physicians if accommodating Dr. Phillips would require them to substantially increase the number of days that they are on-service. It would be an excessive burden on other ICU nurses if accommodating Ms. Bronson would require them to substantially increase their workload or the number of hours they work a week. Depending on the financial situation of Fairview Hospital, accommodating Dr. Phillips could impose an excessive burden on the hospital if it were to require hiring or contracting with an additional ED physician. Depending on the financial situation of Pinehurst Hospital, accommodating Ms. Bronson could impose an excessive burden on the hospital if it were to require offering overtime to nurses who are willing to care for patients who are receiving palliative sedation to unconsciousness. Similarly, depending on the financial and staffing resources of the hospital and its ICU, accommodating the intensivist who objects to palliative sedation to unconscious could impose excessive burdens on the hospital and ICU physicians. If Fairview and Pinehurst are large metropolitan university medical centers, it is more likely that accommodation will be possible without imposing excessive burdens on health professionals or the institution than if they are small rural community hospitals.

The *fourth requirement* states that whenever feasible, health professionals should provide advance notification to department heads or supervisors. This requirement enables department heads and supervisors to accommodate conscience-based objections with a minimum of inconvenience and disruption to the healthcare team and the institution. By facilitating continuity of services within the institution, advance notification also can minimize the burdens that patients will experience as a result of conscience-based refusals. Since advance notification can give practitioners who are asked to substitute more time to make necessary professional and personal adjustments, such notification also can minimize burdens to them. Advance notification also can increase the likelihood that staffing assignments and schedule changes can be made to facilitate accommodation. For example, Dr. Phillips should not wait to communicate his objection to EC until he is faced with caring for a rape victim. Notifying the department head in advance will decrease the risk that patients will not receive timely access to EC. It will also give the department head an opportunity to determine whether it is feasible to put arrangements into place that will accommodate Dr. Phillips. If Dr. Phillips were to announce his objection only when he is tasked with caring for a rape victim, accommodation might justifiably be denied because it would adversely affect the patient.

When health professionals do not object in principle to a medical intervention, such as abortion, donation after cardiac determination of death, palliative sedation to unconsciousness, or forgoing medically provided nutrition and hydration, advance notification can be more challenging but still not infeasible. For example, suppose a neonatal ICU (NICU) physician and an NICU nurse are not ethically opposed in principle to providing aggressive treatment to preterm neonates. Indeed, they both routinely provide such care. However, they both have conscience-based objections to continuing aggressive life support for one NICU patient, a preterm infant with very poor prognosis. Continued aggressive treatment is contrary to the physician's conception of "good medicine" and the nurse's conception of "good nursing practice." However, suppose aggressive life support does not violate established professional norms and is not clearly outside the boundaries of acceptable medical/nursing care. To facilitate advance notification of NICU administrators, the physician and the nurse should attempt to identify their respective general criteria for deciding when providing aggressive treatment to preterm newborns is contrary to their conceptions of "good medicine" and "good nursing practice," respectively, and they should attempt to determine whether their criteria correspond with established professional norms and the "culture" of the NICU. Generally, to facilitate advance notification, health professionals should attempt to anticipate the types of situations in which they are likely to request exemptions.

The *fifth requirement* states that conscience-based refusals will not be accommodated if accommodation would enable invidious discrimination. It is one thing for health professionals to object to providing a specific medical service (e.g., abortion or EC) and quite another thing to object to providing a medical service to African American or Muslim patients and yet be willing to provide the same medical service to white or Christian patients. Ethical codes of major health professions prohibit discrimination, and it is a settled view – one based on defensible and widely shared conceptions of justice, equality, dignity, and respect – that racial, ethnic, religious, and gender-based prejudice or bias are ethically wrong. Even if they are conscience-based (i.e., rooted in fundamental moral beliefs), accommodation for objections based on such discriminatory beliefs is unwarranted.

There is considerable agreement that it is wrong to discriminate against members of these "protected classes." However, currently, there is no similar agreement about whether antidiscrimination rules apply to members of other vulnerable and historically marginalized groups. It is beyond the scope of this chapter to resolve this issue or to specify the scope of "invidious discrimination." Suffice it to say that however it is specified, invidious discrimination should not be accommodated.

Some commentators claim that conscientious objection is incompatible with the obligations of health professionals. For example, Julian Savulescu claims: "If people are not prepared to offer legally permitted, efficient, and beneficial care to a patient because it conflicts with their values, they should not be doctors" (Savulescu, 2006, 294). However, this absolutist view is unwarranted if conscientious objectors can be accommodated without violating any of the five requirements (Wicclair, 2019).

Some commentators endorse an additional requirement: Health professionals must be able to explain their reasons and justify their moral objections. For example, Robert Card claims that an accommodation should be granted "only if the practitioner makes the objection and its reasoned basis public, and the justification offered for the exemption is subjected to assessment" (Card, 2017, 82). To be sure, a review of objectors' reasons can serve a useful function by giving objectors an opportunity to reflect on their reasons and determine whether they object for moral or other reasons. If their reasons are moral, a review can help objectors distinguish between core and peripheral moral convictions. However, it is one thing to require objectors to make their reasons public or to go on record, and quite another thing to require them to provide a justification that will satisfy someone else (e.g., a department head or members of an HEC). Insofar as other persons might not share an objector's moral and/or religious beliefs, the latter requirement risks introducing unwarranted arbitrariness and subjectivity and failing to respect the moral integrity of objectors.

A word of caution: The five requirements are offered as *ethical* guidelines. In the USA, several state and federal laws and regulations offer *legal* protections of conscientious objection that may or may not correspond to these ethical guidelines.

Procedures for Reviewing Requests for Accommodation

In some situations, there may be no need for a formal procedure to review and approve or deny requests for accommodation. For example, when an intensivist objects to continuing life support for a patient, it is common practice for the physician to arrange a transfer of care to an intensivist who is willing to continue life support, and if a physician is willing and able to accept the patient and continue life support, prior review and approval generally is not required. A similar practice is common when physicians object to discontinuing life support.

However, when health professionals are unwilling or unable to find willing substitutes or when accommodation requires more pervasive reallocations of responsibilities within a service, unit, or institution, it may be appropriate to require a formal review of requests for accommodation. Criteria for triggering a formal review process may differ from institution to institution, but each institution's conscientious objection policy should specify when formal approval is required.

The assignment of responsibility for an initial review of accommodation requests may vary depending on the size and culture of the institution and frequency of requests. Options include department heads and supervisors, a designated administrator or ombudsperson, or the institutional ethics committee. However, considerations of efficiency may favor limiting the role of the ethics committee to providing assistance with hard cases, hearing appeals, conducting periodic reviews of past decisions, and fine-tuning the policy. Whatever mechanism is chosen for initial review, it should be specified in the institution's conscientious objection policy.

If requests for accommodation are denied, health professionals should have an opportunity to appeal the decision. An opportunity for appeal can help to reduce the perception of arbitrariness as well as actual arbitrariness. It also can contribute to achieving the aim of properly determining when it is, and is not, justified to deny requests to accommodate. Institutional mechanisms for hearing appeals may differ from institution to institution, but each institution's conscientious objection policy should specify responsibilities and procedures. The institutional ethics committee is an appropriate body to hear appeals because its members should have relevant ethical expertise and familiarity with the institution's ethics policies. Moreover, review by a committee with a diverse membership may minimize the risk of bias and arbitrariness. Review by a committee with a diverse membership is especially appropriate insofar as requirements for accommodation are likely to include unspecified context-dependent terms such as "timely" and "excessive."

Conclusion

HEC members frequently are called upon to provide guidance pertaining to conscientious objection. This guidance can include case consultation, policy creation, and education. For HEC members to effectively perform these functions, they will need to understand when an objection to providing a medical service is a conscientious objection, reasons for accommodating conscientious objectors, the need for ethical constraints on accommodation, and the basics of institutional management of conscientious objection.

Healthcare professionals can refuse to provide a medical service for a variety of reasons. What makes a refusal a conscientious objection is that it is based on the practitioner's moral convictions. Conscientious objection in health care generally occurs when practitioners refuse to provide a legal, professionally accepted, and clinically appropriate medical service within the scope of their clinical competence because it violates their moral beliefs.

The primary reason for accommodating health professionals who have a conscientious objection is to give them moral space in which they can practice medicine without undermining their moral integrity. However, there are justified reasons to limit or deny accommodation. To protect patients and prevent excessive burdens to other members of the healthcare team, supervisors, department heads, and institutions, conscience-based refusals should be accommodated only if a requested accommodation will not: (1) impede a patient's/surrogate's timely access to clinically appropriate information, counseling, and referral; (2) impede a patient's timely access to clinically appropriate healthcare services offered within the institution; or (3) impose excessive burdens on other clinicians, supervisors, department heads, or the institution. In addition, whenever feasible, health professionals should provide advance notification to department heads or supervisors. Finally, accommodation should be denied if granting it would enable invidious discrimination.

Fair, consistent, and transparent management of conscience-based refusals requires an institutional policy. In some situations, there may be no need for a formal procedure to review and approve or deny requests for accommodation. Criteria for triggering a formal review process may differ from institution to institution, but each institution's conscientious objection policy should specify when formal approval is required. The assignment of responsibility for an initial review of accommodation requests may vary depending on the size and culture of the institution and frequency of requests. If requests for accommodation are denied, health professionals should have an opportunity to appeal the decision. The mechanisms for initial review and appeals should be specified in the institution's conscientious objection policy. Institutional ethics committees can play an important role by drafting conscientious objection policies, reviewing requests for accommodation and/or appeals, and facilitating staff education.

Questions for Discussion

1. Conceptual: If conscientious objection is about personal moral integrity, would it be ethically permissible for clinicians who have a moral objection to a medical service to communicate their objection to patients? To try to convince patients that the requested medical service is immoral?
2. Practical: Should clinicians who request accommodation be required to explain and justify their reasons, and if so, what should happen if they are unable to supply reasons?
3. Strategic: Given the varied missions of different hospital and health systems, what is the best way for institutions to express their mission-based values while still respecting the moral integrity of practitioners and meeting the healthcare needs of the communities they serve?

References

American Medical Association. (2017). *Code of Medical Ethics*. Chicago: American Medical Association.

American Nurses Association. (2015). *Code of Ethics for Nurses with Interpretive Statements*. Silver Spring, MD: American Nurses Association.

Blustein J (1993). Doing what the patient orders: Maintaining integrity in the doctor-patient relationship. *Bioethics*, 7(4): 290–314.

Card RF (2017). The inevitability of assessing reasons in debates about conscientious objection in medicine. *Cambridge Quarterly of Healthcare Ethics*, 26(1): 82–96.

General Medical Council. (2020). *Ethical Guidance*. www.gmc-uk.org/ethical-guidance (accessed September 26, 2019).

Lewis-Newby M, Wicclair M, Pope T, et al. (2015). An official American Thoracic Society policy statement: Managing conscientious objections in intensive care medicine. *American Journal of Respiratory and Critical Care Medicine*, 191(2): 219–227.

Savulescu J (2006). Conscientious objection in medicine. *British Medical Journal*, 332 (7536): 294–297.

Wicclair MR (2011). *Conscientious Objection in Health Care: An Ethical Analysis.* Cambridge University Press.

Wicclair M (2014). Managing conscientious objection in health care institutions. *HEC Forum,* 26(3): 267–283.

Wicclair M (2019). Preventing conscientious objection in medicine from running amok: A defense of reasonable accommodation. *Theoretical Medicine and Bioethics,* 40(6): 539–564.

Chapter

25

Ethics Committees and Distributive Justice

Nancy S. Jecker

Objectives

Upon reading and considering the content of this chapter, the reader should be able to:

1. Distinguish distributive justice questions from other types of ethical questions that healthcare ethics committees (HECs) face.
2. Identify competing conceptions of the health professional's ethical role in making cost containment and rationing decisions at the bedside.
3. Explain the importance of developing institutional policies to guide the distribution of scarce healthcare resources, and the response to uninsured and underserved patient groups.
4. Appeal to justice principles to formulate and defend a hospital policy for responding to uninsured and underserved patients.

A physician brings the following case to the ethics committee.[1]

Case

Mr. Nguyen, 54, presented to clinic with a devastating surgical complication: His abdominal incision had split open 1 week after emergency surgery. He was taken back to the operating room, and the deepest layer of his abdominal wall was sewn closed. Doctors treated the infection that had caused his wound to fall apart. Yet he still had a 3-inch crevice along the middle of his belly. Until the edges contracted and the gaping expanse filled in on its own, he and his wife were instructed to pack damp gauze into the wound daily to keep it clean and help it heal. A few weeks after discharge, Mr. Nguyen was seen in clinic by the treating physician, Dr. Morris, who noticed that the gauze was packed more loosely and changed less frequently than the patient had been instructed. What should have been white and fluffy looked dried and yellowed, and his wound was no longer clean and healthy, but covered with crusty patches. As the physician began to discuss with the patient the importance of dressing changes, the patient leaned over to interrupt. "Hey, Doc," Mr. Nguyen said, pointing to the pile of unopened gauzes the physician had brought into the room, "Could I have the extra? This stuff isn't cheap."

Dr. Morris subsequently learned that Mr. Nguyen had been cutting back on the gauze and changing the dressing less often because he couldn't afford the supplies. And while the physician had dutifully educated the patient about the science behind the treatments, the physician had been completely oblivious to how much Mr. Nguyen had to pay or if he could afford the expense.

---

[1] Adapted from Chen (2010).

Dr. Morris brought this case to the ethics committee. The patient continues to be seen in clinic, and the physician is wondering how to handle the case going forward. She tells the ethics committee that Mr. Nguyen's situation is probably representative of many uninsured and underserved patients the hospital serves. She felt that she, and perhaps other health professionals, had completely lost touch with the economic realities of their patients' lives. The physician wanted to know what her responsibility was in this situation and others like it. She had always believed that being a good doctor meant knowing the clinical facts down cold, and that worrying about other details would diminish her ability to do so. Now she was not so sure.

Introduction

This case raises a number of complex ethical questions for the HEC. When patients are unable to comply with best medical advice because they simply cannot afford the treatments prescribed, what should physicians do? To what extent are health professionals responsible for knowing about their patients' social and economic circumstances before prescribing a treatment plan? Does the patient have a responsibility to share such information? Is a hospital, which may be inundated with requests for financial assistance from the community it serves, obligated to help care for uninsured and underserved individuals? In the case of Mr. Nguyen, although the cost of providing needed wound dressing may seem minimal, what if many surgical patients served by the hospital need this kind of help? Are we, as a society, responsible for helping Mr. Nguyen and other patients who are uninsured and underserved to obtain needed health care?

These are clearly challenging questions, and it is far from clear how the ethics committee should respond. Mr. Nguyen's case may force the ethics committee to tread on unfamiliar ground by raising the broader question of what the HEC role should be in helping disadvantaged groups and by establishing a right to health care within the institution (Jecker, 2008). While it is easy to say that HECs should serve as advocates for patients and promote their best interests, it is more difficult to determine what the HEC's responsibility is in addressing larger justice issues.

In this chapter, I propose that much is to be gained by expanding, rather than restricting, the scope of the ethics committee's response. More expansive thinking not only enables us to map this case in a larger moral domain, it also enhances our understanding of the specific values and principles at stake. Cases like that of Mr. Nguyen force the committee to consider the just distribution of healthcare services, as well as the scope and limits of the hospital's and providers' responsibility to Mr. Nguyen. It can assist providers by educating and discussing economically challenging cases and can improve justice by ensuring a more transparent and consistent response to cases.

Understanding Justice: The Role of Providers

Dr. Morris was mistaken when she initially thought that attention to the economic and social dimensions of health care would interfere with being a "good doctor." Not only is it possible to learn about the economic and social aspects of patients' lives while immersed in the details of biology, physiology, and pharmacology, but in fact it is necessary to do so in order to be a good doctor. To see that this is so, it is helpful to begin by considering the scope and limits of the physician's role as patient advocate.

It is well established that a paramount responsibility of health professionals is to advocate on behalf of patients' best interests and to respect and support patients' preferences (Jecker, 1990). Clearly, it is in Mr. Nguyen's best interests to have the wound dressing he needs, and his noncompliance with instructions for wound dressing is based on socioeconomic barriers, not on patient preference. Mr. Nguyen is actively seeking to obtain the wound dressings that he cannot afford by asking the physician to give him the extra dressing. Suppose Dr. Morris responds to Mr. Nguyen by handing over the hospital supplies, perhaps opening the cabinet to pull out some additional boxes of sterile bandages, tape, and other materials, in an effort to do whatever it takes to get Mr. Nguyen the care he needs. This kind of response we shall call *unrestricted patient advocacy.*

1. **Unrestricted Advocacy:** This holds that the provider's primary responsibility is to advocate on behalf of the individual patient's best interests. Cost containment and rationing are simply incompatible with this role.

According to this understanding, patient advocacy imposes upon health professionals an obligation of fidelity. Fidelity requires faithfulness, loyalty, and unswerving allegiance to another person or to a bond between persons. The loyal health professional does everything possible to promote the welfare of their patient. It is not Dr. Morris's responsibility to control hospital costs, nor can she be expected to ration care effectively by saying no when Mr. Nguyen asks for medical supplies. According to this first view, the fact that a patient is uninsured or underinsured should have no effect on how a provider responds to meet the needs of the patient.

In defense of such a position, it can be said that as a physician, Dr. Morris is responsible to do whatever it takes to help her patient. One of the earliest formulations of the role and duties of physicians, the Hippocratic Oath, requires physicians to swear allegiance to the welfare of their patients: "I swear by Apollo . . . to follow that method of treatment which, according to my ability and judgment, I consider for the benefit of my patients, and abstain from whatever is deleterious and mischievous." To use the language of contemporary bioethics, ethical principles of beneficence and nonmaleficence support a recommendation that Dr. Morris's primary responsibility is to advocate on behalf of Mr. Nguyen's best interests.

Moreover, the alternative of placing providers in the role of society's gatekeepers, charged with containing costs and rationing care, has adverse effects, such as undermining trust in the provider–patient relationship. If Dr. Morris denies Mr. Nguyen the supplies he needs to take proper care of his incision, this may erode the patient's trust. Mr. Nguyen may begin to doubt that his doctor is putting his interests first. He may conclude that saving money for the hospital matters more to the doctor.

Finally, it is society at large, not healthcare workers, who have the ethical and political mandate to make allocation decisions. Moreover, health professionals do not have the training, knowledge, or expertise to ration care at the bedside of individual patients. Such decisions are best left to policy-makers at other levels within the healthcare institution and ultimately to the broader society.

A second and very different approach holds that restrictions on patient advocacy are ethically justified. Let us call this position restricted advocacy.

2. Restricted Advocacy: This holds that duties to patients are limited, and must be placed in a broader ethical context. Patient advocacy is qualified and restricted in light of other significant duties, including the duty to promote the welfare of society as a whole, or at a minimum to promote the welfare of other patients served by the institution.

In support of this position, it can be noted that a commitment to serve the public has always gone hand in hand with a commitment to advocate on behalf of individual patients. Thus, in its very first code of medical ethics, the American Medical Association held: "As good citizens, it is the duty of health professionals to be ever vigilant for the welfare of the community" (American Medical Association, Council on Ethical and Judicial Affairs, 2017). The American Nursing Association's Code for Nurses (2001, Provision 8) affirms a similar commitment: "The nurse collaborates with other health professionals and the public in promoting community, national, and international efforts to meet health needs."

In addition, it can be argued that health professionals, and physicians in particular, are recipients of numerous benefits from society. Massive amounts of money are regularly spent to fund medical education, the research on which medical practice rests, the institutions in which most medical activity occurs, and the demand for medical services. Accepting such benefits places health professionals under an obligation to benefit the society granting them. This stance allows for restrictions on individual patient care that are necessary to promote the good of the entire community a hospital serves.

A third and final position attempts to strike a middle ground between patient advocacy and social responsibility. I call this response justly restricted advocacy.

3. Justly Restricted Advocacy: This maintains that providers can ethically ration care provided they can be reasonably certain that their individual measures will contribute to a larger system or plan for health care that is itself just. This approach requires restrictions on patient advocacy conform to standards of justice and fairness.

In support of this view it can be said that it succeeds where the other two views do not. Unrestricted advocacy asks too much: The sky is the limit, and patients are entitled not just to a basic level of care but to anything that stands to benefit them. But restricted advocacy asks too little. It permits limiting care, but does not require that restrictions on care meet justice standards.

It can also be noted that when denials of care are not part of an explicit system or plan, they run the risk of not being thought through, applied consistently, accountable to the public, decided democratically, and insulated from arbitrary and unfair manipulation. By contrast, when rationing is part of an explicit policy or plan, these mistakes are less likely to occur.

Finally, ethical rationing must meet justice standards. As the name suggests, justly restricted advocacy has the advantage of requiring that rationing be held to justice standards, such as ensuring a basic level of care. Rationing that falls short of justice requirements would not be considered justly restricted advocacy.

Following the requirements of justly restricted advocacy clarifies the obligations of Dr. Morris to Mr. Nguyen. It would not be acceptable for Dr. Morris to take boxes of wound dressing or other medical supplies from the hospital and hand them over to Mr. Nguyen free of charge, as unrestricted advocacy would allow. It would also not be ethically defensible for Dr. Morris to tell her patient that he is on his own and the wound dressing belongs to the hospital, as restricted advocacy might suggest. Instead, the model of justly restricted advocacy suggests that Dr. Morris ought to ask the ethics committee to develop an explicit policy giving guidance to physicians about providing care for uninsured and underserved patients – such a policy should enable physicians to serve as just advocates for all their patients. Even if she cannot rob Peter to pay Paul, there is much Dr. Morris can and should do. After all, in this and many cases like it, it helps not only the patient, but also saves money for the hospital and the insurance company, if Mr. Nguyen's postsurgical recovery goes smoothly and further complications are avoided. There is every reason to have a more just policy in place and to direct physicians to abide by it in cases like this.

Understanding Justice: The Role of Healthcare Ethics Committees

There are many advantages to developing an explicit policy for allocating resources within the hospital. In the absence of such a policy, decisions about how to respond to Mr. Nguyen and patients like him will continue to be made, but will be made in an unsystematic and haphazard way. If patients do not receive the care they need, rationing will occur by default, in an implicit manner, without the advantage of open discussion and consideration of the pros and cons of different approaches. This is problematic because such an approach does not even aspire to meet justice standards. Implicit rationing is typically

- not thoroughly considered
- not applied consistently
- not accountable to the public
- not decided democratically
- not insulated from arbitrary and unfair manipulation

These objections suggest the need for a more open and publicly debated set of ethical guidelines.

The HEC can respond to this need on several different levels.

1. **Hospital Policy:** The ethics committee can respond first and foremost by developing hospital policies that aspire to meet justice standards, set out fair procedures for distributing scarce resources, and address the needs of vulnerable populations served by the institution.

For our purposes, justice refers to the ethical problem of distributing scarce resources. While distributive justice traditionally referred to the distribution of income and wealth in a society, we interpret this idea more broadly to include the distribution of other social goods, such as health care. Whenever the problem of distributive justice arises, the background condition is a scarcity of some resource. In health care, for example, there are more patients with end-stage cardiac disease than there are cadaver organs available. Hospitals and patients are also finding it harder to get some medications because drug companies have stopped making them. And there are not always enough hospital beds in ICUs to meet the needs of patients.

The case of Mr. Nguyen does not involve any obvious scarcity of this kind. Yet, it nevertheless raises profound questions of distributive justice. Bandages and wound dressing may not at first blush seem like scarce resources. However, it is important to understand scarcity more broadly. "Scarcity" refers not only to limits in the resources necessary to make a healthcare service available, but also to limits in the money available to spend on health care. Although wound dressings are not scarce in the former sense, they are clearly scarce in the latter sense. Mr. Nguyen cannot afford the prescribed treatment and so he does not receive it. Other examples of fiscal scarcity may include the inability to pay for follow-up care, home health aides, glasses, dental care, asthma medication, or other goods and services that benefit patients. For uninsured and under-insured patients, fiscal scarcity presents as a major obstacle to obtaining needed care.

A variety of solutions to the problem of distributive justice have been proposed, and should be considered by the HEC in the course of developing a hospital policy. It has been proposed, for example, that the ultimate criterion for the distribution of scarce goods should be:

- **Equality:** If interpreted strictly, equality may require that if anyone gets a healthcare resource, it should be available to everyone. Interpreted more moderately, inequality may place certain limits on justified inequalities. For example, no matter how poor surgical patients are, they should have access to bandages and dressings necessary for their surgical incision to heal properly. This is the floor below which no patient should fall.

- **Need:** This requires that we have some basis for rating people's needs for resources and provide a scarce resource first to those whose needs are greatest. For example, in the distribution of influenza vaccine, priority should be given to those who are more vulnerable to getting the flu and are more likely to die from it if they do.

- **Ability to Benefit:** We should provide scarce healthcare resources to those with the greatest quality, length, or likelihood of medical benefit. For example, do not provide a lifesaving surgical procedure to patients who will die soon regardless of our best medical effort.

- **Effort to Maintain Health:** Scarce resources should go first to patients who exert the greatest effort to stay well and make healthy choices. For example, patients with liver cancer should receive liver transplants before patients whose livers fail as a result of abusing alcohol. In the case of Mr. Nguyen, the HEC will need to consider the patient's effort to maintain his health given that he has limited resources to pay for compliance with best medical advice.

- **Social Worth:** Persons who contribute most to the social good should receive scarce resources before those who contribute less, and before those who create positive social harms. For example, police officers, teachers, and nurses should receive priority over citizens who are not contributing vital community services; law-abiding citizens should come before those convicted of violent crimes.

- **Supply and Demand:** Scarce resources should be doled out on the basis of people's ability to pay. For example, surgical patients who can afford dressings should have them, and those who cannot afford them should go without. If this criterion is used, Mr. Nguyen does not have a right to the wound dressings required to properly care for himself postsurgery if he cannot pay for them, and he should look elsewhere, for example to charitable groups or organizations, to obtain the help he needs.

In the final analysis, the HEC will need to evaluate and weigh these kinds of competing values. Its final policy recommendations should make explicit the ethical values at stake that support alternative policy choices.

One policy approach to addressing the needs of uninsured and underinsured patients would be for the ethics committee to propose an institutional policy that sets up a centralized distribution of supplies, including wound care supplies, for needy patients.

Had this been in place when Mr. Nguyen presented for care, Dr. Morris would have a way to justly advocate for her patient, which would be consistently available to all patients based on the same criteria.

This would help in some, but not all, situations. Suppose, for example, that Mr. Nguyen were an undocumented immigrant and the hospital required patients to sign their names to obtain supplies from a centralized distribution source. Mr. Nguyen might reasonably refuse to sign out of fear that he would be found and deported by immigration officials. What recourse would the patient and physician have then?

In the case of undocumented immigrants, policies that are uniformly implemented remain the best way to ensure high-quality care for patients. When the concern is not only financial barriers but risk of deportation, policies must encompass not only charity care, but institutional engagement with the community in the form of networking with social, cultural, and religious leaders and advocates for patients to help them obtain necessary resources (Kuczewski, 2019). The role of Dr. Morris and the ethics committee ought to be to justly advocate and help Mr. Nguyen obtain high-quality care. In tandem with the aid of social work, institutional policies can help patients find community-based nonprofit organizations that offer service to immigrants, even care coordination if these are available in the community (Berlinger and Zacharias, 2019).

The alternative to an institutional-level response is an individual one. For example, Dr. Morris might simply give Mr. Nguyen $30 to pay for bandages (Schiff, 2013). This option is a personal, not a professional response. Even here, just limits must be set, since Dr. Morris presumably cannot afford to pay cash to every needy patient. The problem thus reemerges: How will Dr. Morris set fair limits? The American Medical Association recommends that private and professional efforts alike be systematic and include advocacy for social, economic, educational, and political change to further the dignity of every individual (American Medical Association, Council on Ethical and Judicial Affairs, 2017).

At an institutional level, the ultimate decision about Mr. Nguyen will depend on the hospital's underlying institutional values and mission, for example as a charity hospital, for-profit, or religiously affiliated organization. While such a charge is daunting, the alternative of letting decisions continue to be made by default, and in the absence of any explicitly formulated plan, is ethically unsupportable.

2. **Education:** The ethics committee should also respond by educating its health professionals, patients, and the broader community about the nature and scope of this problem, the hospital's response, and the importance of community involvement.

As noted already, the case of Mr. Nguyen raises a particular kind of ethical problem, which has to do with justice and fairness in the allocation of scarce resources. Justly allocating scarce resources comes into sharp focus in cases involving uninsured and underserved patients. Ethics education should address this topic at all levels. At the most general level, all of the proposed solutions to this problem (discussed above) share certain common features. First, they all purport to tell us what people deserve or what they have a right to possess. For example, some may think that people deserve to have their needs met, while others may hold that people deserve or should rightfully possess the product of their labor. Second, all of the proposed solutions make a distinction between justice and charity. Justice deals with what we ought to do in order to keep from violating the rights of others. Charity addresses what we ought to do if we want to choose what is the most compassionate action or the most responsive to the good of other human beings. One important difference between duties of justice, on the one hand, and duties of charity, on the other hand, is that it is generally thought to be morally blameworthy to fail to do (or allow) what justice requires. By contrast, failing to do what charity requires is often considered to be indecent or inhumane, not wrong. Finally, all solutions to the problem of distributive justice have tended to take either liberty or equality or some particular mix of liberty and equality as a fundamental moral ideal. In general, the more emphasis is placed on equality, the more restrictions on liberty are needed to bring about transfers of wealth. The more emphasis is placed on liberty, the more departures from equality are likely to be tolerated.

3. **Ethics Consultation:** In individual cases, such as Mr. Nguyen's, the HEC can serve as a resource for making recommendations, and can modify and amend hospital policy based on how well or poorly such policies serve in promoting ethical decisions for patients. This supports not only the population of patients who are served by hospital policies, but also providers who may feel caught between a rock and a hard place when uninsured and underserved patients ask for help. It would be irresponsible for Dr. Morris to dismiss Mr. Nguyen as "noncompliant" and move on to the next patient. By unpacking the notion of "noncompliance," and distinguishing between noncompliance based on informed decisions and noncompliance resulting from social and economic barriers, providers can better meet their obligations to justly advocate for all patients.

Conclusion

At the outset of our discussion, Dr. Morris asked the HEC for a recommendation about how she should respond to her patient who cannot afford the wound care she has prescribed. Based on our discussion in this chapter, we can say that Dr. Morris has an obligation to promote Mr. Nguyen's best interests, and help him to obtain needed care. However, this does not mean that Dr. Morris would be justified in stealing hospital supplies and handing them over to the patient. Instead, the HEC should urge Dr. Morris to advocate for her patient in a manner that is just and fair to all patients served by the hospital.

If an institutional policy is in place to guide the response to uninsured and under-served patients, the HEC should point to such a policy in assisting Dr. Morris with this patient. In the absence of such a policy, the committee should use the case consultation as an occasion to reflect on, and develop, a consistent approach that reflects the values of the institution and of the patients it serves. A central advantage of formulating an explicit policy is that we can aspire to justice standards. The substantive justice principles discussed in this chapter can guide the development or refinement of hospital policy.

Finally, the HEC should assume responsibility for educating providers, patients, and the broader community about the plight of uninsured and underserved patients. The goal is not only to raise understanding about the scope of the problem, but also to seek advice and broader community representation in responding in a just and compassionate way to patients.

Questions for Discussion

1. Conceptual: Is caring for Mr. Nguyen required as a matter of justice, or is it instead an act of charity? What are the implications of your answer to this question?

2. Pragmatic: What are the barriers in your institution to responding to uninsured and underserved patients?
3. Strategic: Propose a policy for addressing patients' needs. What substantive justice principles lend support to your proposed policy?

References

American Medical Association, Council on Ethical and Judicial Affairs. (2017). *Declaration of Professional Responsibility: Medicine's Social Contract with Humanity.* https://policysearch.ama-assn.org/policyfinder/detail/medical%20ethic?uri=%2FAMADoc%2FHOD.xml-0-431.xml

American Nursing Association, (2001). Code of Ethics for Nurses with Interpretative Statements. www.princetonhcs.org/-/media/princeton/documentrepository/documentrepository/nurses/code-of-ethics.pdf

Berlinger N, Zacharias RL (2019). Resources for teaching and learning about immigrant health care in health professions education. *AMA Journal of Ethics*, 21(1): E50–E57.

Chen PW (2010, February 5). When the patient can't afford the care. *New York Times.* www.nytimes.com/2010/02/05/health/04chen.html

Jecker, NS (1990). Integrating professional ethics with normative theory: Patient advocacy and social responsibility. *Theoretical Medicine*, 11(2): 125–139.

Jecker NS (2008). A broader view of justice. *American Journal of Bioethics*, 8(10): 2–10.

Kuczewski M (2019). Clinical ethicists awakened: Addressing two generations of clinical ethics issues involving undocumented patients. *American Journal of Bioethics*, 19(4): 51–57.

Schiff GD (2013). Crossing boundaries – violation or obligation? *JAMA*, 310(12): 1233–1234.

Chapter 26

Developing and Implementing Effective Ethics Policy

Sabrina F. Derrington

Objectives

Upon reading and considering the content of this chapter, the reader should be able to:

1. Describe the goal of healthcare ethics committees' (HECs) policy-making activities.
2. Identify tools and strategies supporting HECs' development of effective ethics policies.
3. Explain why it is important for HEC members to engage and educate the broader community in developing and instituting ethics policies.
4. Describe ways that local or institutional-specific ethics policies have broader community implications.

Case 1

A pathologist who oversaw the biorepository at a large, research-oriented hospital asked the HEC chair to develop a policy governing informed consent practices for obtaining biobanked specimens. This request was spurred by a recent change in federal guidelines (the Revised Common Rule) and pressure from the organization's newly endowed Center for Precision Medicine. The Center's director had announced in a recent grand rounds presentation that soon "every patient will be a research subject," and talked about the importance of retaining leftover specimens in order to grow the biorepository. Indeed, the general consent-to-treat form had just been amended (without HEC review) to include a statement that the individual signing the form agreed to allow the hospital to "retain and share their leftover samples, with or without identifying information, in accordance with the law." The pathologist voiced ethical concerns about retention of biospecimens without specific informed consent.

Case 2

A novel coronavirus emerged in late 2019 and quickly became a worldwide pandemic, infecting millions. SARS-CoV2 caused critical illness and respiratory failure in many adults, threatening severe shortages of many key resources including ICU beds, ventilators, dialysis machines, medications, and personal protective equipment. Many HECs across the USA were asked to rapidly develop policies to guide clinicians, hospitals, and regions in the ethical allocation of scarce resources. In one Midwestern metropolis, where medical care is provided by a diverse array of institutions, bioethics representatives from each organization began meeting regularly to discuss the evolving situation and to share their developing policies. In the absence of regional or state-wide guidance, each hospital was writing its own policy for the allocation of critical care resources. It became clear that variability in these policies (whether healthcare providers receive priority, for example, or how comorbidities factored in) created an unjust system wherein the same patient might be able to receive critical care services at one hospital but not at another. The importance of these realizations was highlighted when it became apparent that morbidity and mortality from this pandemic was disproportionately impacting disadvantaged populations, primarily communities of color.

Introduction: Why HEC Policy Work Is Important

Policy work is an important and accepted component of the work of HECs, including both developing new policies for aspects of institutional procedure that have major ethical implications, and reviewing and providing ethics-focused input on drafts of organizational policies created by others (Hester, 2008). This process begins with careful assessment of the institutional environment and history, along with a review of scholarship pertinent to the issue being addressed in the policy. Subsequent steps include engagement of stakeholders within the hospital and in the larger community, and advocacy with hospital leadership. Policy implementation then requires widespread education and careful follow-up to evaluate for unanticipated consequences and barriers to compliance.

While it does not mandate HEC review, the Joint Commission on the Accreditation of Healthcare Organizations does require hospitals to have written policies addressing topics commonly considered to be clinical ethics issues, including informed consent, surrogate decision-making, advance directives, forgoing or withdrawing life-sustaining treatment, and Do Not Attempt Resuscitation orders. However, beyond the typical ethics policies, many organizational procedures have significant moral implications that deserve substantive ethics input. Organ and tissue donation, the evaluation and diagnosis of brain death, triage for mass casualty events or infectious disease outbreaks, conscientious objection by staff, and biorepository data governance are just a few examples.

Healthcare environments can be recognized as moral communities in that they are groups of people united around the common moral ends of promoting the health and well-being of patients and easing their suffering (Austin, 2007). HECs play an important role in cultivating and supporting moral communities through clinical ethics consultations, education, and policy work. These HEC activities provide opportunities to create "open moral spaces" where communities can reflect on concepts such as respect for persons, justice, and confidentiality, deliberating and ultimately applying such moral considerations to patient care, research, and institutional processes (Walker, 1993). And because policies are informed by and contribute to local, regional, and national standards of care, HEC policy work becomes an extension of the moral community that intersects with other communities in significant ways.

First Steps: Identifying the HEC's Goal and Scope of Practice for Policy Development

HECs should conceptualize a clear goal and scope for their policy work. At a basic level, the goal is to produce policies that guide the hospital and those who work within it to ethically optimal decisions, acts, and outcomes. Achieving this goal requires not only ethically sound policy but also widespread buy-in and adherence, without which ethically questionable conduct persists and divergence between policy and practice results in liability for the organization.

The scope of an HEC's policy work depends on that particular HEC's role within its organization: its mission as understood by both the HEC and the hospital leadership. Some HECs might be limited to addressing issues directly impacting patient care, while for others the sphere of influence is more broadly construed. At the most basic level, HECs *could* reasonably participate in development and review of any policy pertaining to practices or procedures where there is potential for disagreement due to different values or diverse perspectives. However, the degree to which HEC involvement is needed and welcomed more broadly will depend on the organization and its leadership. For HEC members and chairs, understanding the implications of their mission and the goal of their policy work, especially as pertains to a particular policy issue, requires thoughtful assessment of both the institutional and community context.

Institutional Context

Important aspects of the institutional context include the HEC's institutional status and the extent of its purview for policy development and revision. Clear and ongoing communication with organizational leadership will help to clarify the HEC's mandate. More importantly, such communication should illuminate institutional priorities and constraints, ensuring the perceived value of the policy work. The structure and tenor of the HEC's relationship with hospital legal counsel and risk management is also relevant. Who has the last word when disagreements arise over policy details? It is also important for the HEC to have as thorough as possible an appreciation of the interests and needs of the entire hospital community, especially the staff most impacted by a new or changing policy. In this regard, knowledge of organizational history, including specific relevant cases, will be helpful. Such information is typically gathered either through individual informal conversations or formal discussions with the HEC. The specific informants will depend on the policy issue.

Community Context

The ethics issues that arise in one hospital, be they from particular patient cases or organizational processes, do not exist in a vacuum. To be most effective, HECs should maintain awareness of regional healthcare interests and ethics concerns. Particularly when attempting to align ethics policy with regional standards and state law, it is helpful to know how neighboring hospitals have interpreted relevant law, as well as the content of their policies. In some cities, regional ethics collaboratives may facilitate such communication whereas in others it may require outreach between individuals.

Beyond the community of local healthcare institutions, HECs should also seek to understand the broader context of the communities in which their patients live. Local history, as well as the current socioeconomic, political, and environmental landscape has relevance to individual patients' health as well as their perceptions of and degree of trust in healthcare institutions. Awareness of local health disparities related to race, ethnicity, socioeconomic status, or geographic location is important to understand any potential justice implications of new or revised policies.

Next Steps: Policy Development and Revision

HECs developing or revising policies will undertake a robust ethical analysis, the content of which is dictated by the subject matter of the policy issue at hand. However, to be ethically both sound *and* effective, their ethics guidance must be accepted and supported by those governed by the policy, and it must be feasible to implement and sustain. This requires a patient, intentional process of stakeholder engagement, iterative discussion and revision, and education and implementation. The following steps are key to the process.

Identify and Engage Key Stakeholders and Advisors

Garnering input and support from stakeholders early on and throughout the policy development process will improve the strength of the policy, help to avoid late discovery of barriers, and increase the likelihood of adoption and adherence. Answering the following questions may assist HECs in identifying as many stakeholders as possible:

- Who participates in the process described in the policy?
- Whose conduct will the policy address?
- Who can inform as to current practice and why it is so?
- Whose buy-in will be needed to implement and obtain adherence to the policy?
- What systems will support the proposed process?
- What coordination is necessary, and who will facilitate?
- Who will need training/education, and who will do that?

One way to ensure meaningful engagement is to include key stakeholders – those who are crucial to the policy's development and/or will be directly affected by the policy – in the working group tasked with developing the policy and shepherding it through to approval and implementation. To keep the working group to a manageable size, other stakeholders and advisors may be invited to contribute expertise to particular questions in a consulting role. Depending on the nature of the policy being worked upon, it may be important to include representatives of the public and of patients/families.

In the first case, the HEC chair should convene a working group including HEC members with expertise in research and clinical ethics, representatives from the patient advisory board, the director and senior staff from the Center for Precision Medicine, clinicians from a variety of specialties, researchers, lab and pathology services, and IRB leadership. During a series of discussions, all working group members would be invited to contribute their perspectives. The relevant ethics literature should be reviewed and policies from peer institutions shared. Additional input can be solicited from hospital legal counsel, patient relations, information technology, and medical records.

Expect an Iterative Process

HEC policy-makers should seek to educate themselves through literature searches and other research into the substantive ethics concern, but also by listening to stakeholders. Members of the working group should expect to learn from each other throughout the process and should intentionally employ empathy and understanding to appreciate the perspectives and responses of others. When differences arise, it may seem as if the opposing parties are speaking completely different languages or are coming from polar opposite perspectives. For example, what if the director of precision medicine told the HEC policy group in the first case that they feel strongly that patients seeking care at an academic institution should be willing to participate in research, and that as long as they are informed ahead of time, specific consent should not be required to retain their biospecimens? They also might argue that the institution has a moral obligation to advance the health of the population through precision medicine research, and that such research cannot be accomplished without a robust biorepository. The HEC chair could argue that some of the patients coming to their hospital do not have a choice to seek care elsewhere because of the complexity of their conditions, and that without a way to opt out of research participation they are being coerced. The committee might agree that the institution has a moral obligation to conduct research that will advance population health but also that there are prima facie duties to provide necessary care and maintain trust with their patients and the community. Through multiple discussions of benefits and burdens, etc., the content of the initial draft policy would be generated and refined through an iterative process, including the ethical analysis and procedures for a standard information form with opt-out consent.

This case can highlight the importance of maintaining the policy working group as an inclusive space for deliberative engagement, framed by a set of substantive values and principles that are recognized by the group as a whole (Kirby, 2012; Kirby and Simpson, 2012). Establishing these values and principles early on is a way for the group to articulate and then focus on "what matters" throughout the deliberative process. There are likely to be times during that process when values conflict or principles are in tension, and the working group must collaboratively consider how best to balance competing obligations.

Anticipate Potential Barriers to Implementation and Adherence

Developing ethically sound, effective policy requires constant evaluation of the potential downstream effects on clinical processes, operational procedures, clinician–patient–family relationships, the organization's identity and public image, and the larger community. An inclusive, diverse working group of stakeholders and advisors will be an advantage in this step, hopefully avoiding blind spots or unanticipated barriers to implementation.

Barriers may come in the form of moral disagreement, pragmatic or operational challenges, or legal and risk management concerns. Of these, moral disagreements are the most vulnerable to being minimized or discouraged in a way that prevents meaningful deliberation because of their sensitive nature. The HEC should be intentional and attentive to enable all stakeholder voices (Kirby, 2012). Moral disagreement may be raised by any member of the working group and should be taken seriously; this may require active compensation for the traditional hierarchies of most healthcare environments (American Society for Bioethics and Humanities, 2010).

Pragmatic and operational challenges may be identified by those with direct knowledge of the practices and processes that will change with the new policy. In Case 1, the laboratory and pathology staff might bring up concerns related to processing of samples and how an "opt-out" decision would reliably prevent leftover biospecimens from being retained. This is a critical operational issue that requires creative problem-solving between laboratory and pathology staff, information technology, and clinician stakeholders.

If unaddressed, legal and risk management concerns can easily destroy an ethics policy initiative. HEC leaders should proactively cultivate effective working relationships with their organization's legal counsel and risk management staff. Representatives from these offices should be engaged in the policy development to greater or lesser degree depending on the issue being addressed; in general, an iterative process is helpful here too, with early consultation and subsequent review and collaborative revision.

Develop a Plan for Education and Feedback

Education is paramount to optimizing adoption and adherence of a new or revised policy, and it starts with the policy itself. A policy should be written with its audience in mind and should provide both compelling ethical reasoning and clear guidance for the employees who will rely upon it in actual practice. The tone should be supportive and respectful, with adequate explanation and justification to support assertions about "the right thing to do." Review by members of the working group and key end-users, prior to final approval, will be helpful in gauging comprehension, gut reactions, and overall response to the wording of the policy.

While email or global announcements are efficient in reaching a large number of people within an organization, the HEC should also design education sessions tailored to the number of employees affected, the degree of change in practice required by the new policy, and the complexity of the procedures involved. These sessions may include grand rounds, organization-wide "town halls," and/or smaller targeted presentations for particular departments or offices.

Even when a policy is well-written and carefully vetted prior to "roll-out," there are likely to be questions and concerns raised. The HEC should develop a method for inviting and responding to questions and feedback from those impacted by the policy.

The Role of Policy Development in Cultivating Moral Community

Hospital policies establish and illustrate the values of an institution, contributing to the creation of a moral community that includes clinicians, other staff and volunteers, as well as the patients and families who receive care there. The field of bioethics addresses topics that raise moral questions; the issues addressed by ethics policies can be expected to generate a range of reactions among various individuals within an organization. These are controversial issues: When and how should parental authority be overridden? How ought medical teams address conflicts with surrogate decision makers about the proper use or discontinuation of life-sustaining treatment? In the context of scarce resources, who should be prioritized for ICU care? Healthcare organizations will have different levels of appreciation and tolerance for the nuances of such issues, depending on organizational culture, risk orientation, and how they hope to be perceived by the larger community. Assessing institutional "readiness" to wrestle with such issues is a critically important step that should begin early in the policy development process. Reluctance or hesitation may be a sign of moral objection, political unease, or merely opposition to change, and thoughtful, respectful discussion is necessary to distinguish those differences and identify collaborative paths forward. The earlier those concerns are elicited, the better the HEC/working group will be able to research, plan, and address those concerns so as to optimize the policy's likelihood of approval.

Successful negotiation with hospital leadership, legal counsel, and other key entities requires appreciation of the different perspectives they have on both the policy issue at hand and the needs and interests of the institution, based on each individual's mandate. For example, the hospital's risk management team will be primarily concerned with protecting the institution from liability. Individual members of the hospital leadership may be focused on financial concerns, academic ranking, employee retention, or a variety of other issues. Each of these perspectives has value to the HEC in developing an effective policy, but when interests conflict, compromise is often necessary. In constructing an ethically acceptable solution that all parties can agree to, the HEC should seek to identify short-term, achievable goals to shift institutional culture, without losing sight of the long-term goal. The common maxim, "Don't let perfect be the enemy of good" is applicable.

Responsible Policy Development within the Larger Community

When hospital policy is created or changed, the surrounding community, which relies on that institution for care, and with whom the institution has a fiduciary relationship, is also affected. Going further, other regional healthcare providers may be impacted by hospital policies that shift the burden of care for certain patient populations, or which influence regional standards of care. Finally, social services agencies, both government and nongovernmental, may be impacted by the way that a hospital chooses to address or manage key issues. HECs have a responsibility to cultivate and maintain awareness of this extended sphere of influence. In Case 2, an unprecedented health crisis resulted in an urgent need for policies to guide allocation of scarce critical care resources. It was not until bioethicists from multiple hospitals within a single region began comparing their policies that the magnitude of potential inequity became apparent. Some of the hospitals prioritized healthcare workers, others did not. Some included chronic medical conditions in the priority scoring system, while others did not. The bioethicists in this group were being pressured by their administrations to develop and finalize policy, while at the same time, public fear of discrimination was growing, exacerbated by preexisting socioeconomic disparities and residential segregation. The group of bioethicists worked to align their policies, advocated for the state and city governments to issue guidance, and developed explanations for popular media that aimed to make the ethical and clinical analysis behind the policy more transparent.

The best way for HECs to avoid negative unanticipated consequences of their policy work is through meaningful community engagement. In the second case, one of the university hospitals had a bioethics center that had already developed a community group; that group provided important feedback that resulted in revisions to their policy to remove any penalty for chronic medical conditions, as this was recognized to disproportionately disadvantage people of color. To be meaningful, engagement activities must include a reasonably representative sample of community members. HECs should identify the communities to be engaged with attention to diversity of attitudes and beliefs, and inclusion of vulnerable and disadvantaged groups (Dresser, 2017). Care should be taken to avoid privileging the professional or expert voice at the expense of meaningful exchange and dialogue, which may contribute to epistemic injustice and deeply flawed policies. Ethical discussion has an integral role in developing trust between the public and healthcare institutions, which requires that people be able to recognize a commitment to understanding, attention, and care (Bowman, 2017).

The policies of a healthcare organization project its (moral) identity. Policies guide hospital procedures and clinical practice – both of which directly impact the health and well-being of patients and their families, their experience of that organization, and the relationships that develop between them and clinicians and staff. When policies enter the public awareness, through media reports, court proceedings, or because of conflict with particular interest groups, those policies, and the ways they play out in particular cases, impact public perception of the entire institution and the individuals who work there. For example, in the second case the resource allocation policy of one institution was widely criticized for its prioritization of younger, healthier patients. As another example, the transfusion refusal policy at one children's hospital resulted in alienation of many members of the Jehovah's Witness community.

Conclusion

HECs play a vital role in cultivating and enriching the moral community of healthcare organizations. The policies that HECs create, critique, or review become tangible representations of the fabric of those moral communities in that they illuminate the values and principles that inform practices and procedures. Policy work is an opportunity to achieve a cultural change in thinking and action regarding an issue, with implications for the institution and the broader community. HECs that understand the goal and scope of their policy work, take time to consider their institutional and community context, and follow an inclusive process of deliberative engagement will be able to develop ethically grounded, contextually appropriate, community responsive policies that can be effectively implemented. After development and implementation, the HEC's responsibility continues, in assessing the impact on the organization and the broader community, eliciting feedback, and revising as necessary.

Given that HECs are often composed of volunteers with many other responsibilities, the amount of work and attention required for high-quality ethics policy work may seem overwhelming. While creation of a new policy or overhaul of an existing policy is a time-intensive effort, these large projects arise infrequently, and may unfold over the course of a year or more. More commonly, HECs review and provide minor updates for existing policies. This type of policy work is less extensive, but deserves the same level of thoughtful preparation, analysis, engagement, and implementation.

Questions for Discussion

1. Conceptual: Consider the potential policy projects that reach your HEC. Are topic areas constrained, explicitly or tacitly, by organizational structure or culture? What implications do these projects have for the broader community beyond your institution?
2. Pragmatic: Has the HEC experienced particular success or failure in policy-making? What were the reasons for the outcome?
3. Strategic: Who, or what offices, within your organization can offer critical insight and advice for your HEC's policy project(s)? Who are key stakeholders in the broader community?

References

American Society for Bioethics and Humanities. (2010). *Core Competencies for Healthcare Ethics Consultation*, 2nd ed. Glenview, IL: ASBH.

Austin W (2007). The ethics of everyday practice: Healthcare environments as moral communities. *Advances in Nursing Science*, 30(1): 81–88.

Bowman D (2017). The moral of the tale: Stories, trust, and public engagement with clinical ethics via radio and theatre. *Bioethical Inquiry*, 14(1): 43–52.

Dresser R (2017). A deep dive into community engagement. *Narrative Inquiry in Bioethics*, 7(1): 41–45.

Hester M (2008). *Ethics by Committee: A Textbook on Consultation, Organization, and Education for Hospital Ethics Committees.* New York: Rowman & Littlefield.

Kirby J (2012). Shifting the emphasis to meaningful ethics engagement in the development of health policies. *American Journal of Bioethics*, 12(11): 18–20.

Kirby J, Simpson C (2012). Deliberative engagement: An inclusive methodology for exploring professionalization. *HealthCare Ethics Committee Forum*, 24(3): 187–201.

Walker MU (1993). Keeping moral space open: New images of ethics consulting. *Hastings Center Report*, 23(2): 33–40.

<table>
<tr><td>Chapter</td></tr>
<tr><td>27</td></tr>
</table>

Ethics In and For the Organization

Margaret Moon

Objectives

Upon reading and considering the content of this chapter, the reader should be able to:

1. Recognize the healthcare ethics committee (HEC) as one contributor to the ethical operation of the healthcare organization (HCO).
2. Identify the ethical implications of the structures, processes, and systems within which the HEC functions.
3. Suggest ways in which the traditional activities of the HEC contribute to the wider ethical enterprise of the HCO.
4. Propose additional tasks suitable for a proactive HEC.

Case 1

At a routine meeting of the ethics committee in an urban quaternary care hospital, committee members express concern about the repetitive nature of several recent consultation requests. These requests all involve patients who are enduring long hospital admissions complicated by recurrent nonadherence to recommended medical care during the current hospitalization and histories of nonadherence to outpatient management. In each case the relationship between patients and staff has become strained, further compounding patient nonadherence, prolonging hospitalization, and increasing staff distress. Providers request ethics consultation as an additional means to resolve frustration and moral distress.

The ethics committee identifies that each of these patients has a history of significant physical or psychosocial trauma. Committee members express concern that the hospital lacks an organized approach to trauma-informed care, and that most providers lack the training and skills necessary to recognize and manage the emotional responses of traumatized patients. The committee concludes that the problem is getting more profound and anticipates increasing distress among patients and providers.

After a robust discussion within the ethics committee, the decision is made to draft a letter to the hospital leadership, describing the problem and recommending several potential approaches to resolution.

Case 2

Ms. N is a pediatric ICU charge nurse and member of the ethics committee at Hospital A. Hospital A is part of a system of eight hospitals with a centralized organizational and policy structure. Ms. N works at Hospital A predominantly, but floats to Hospital B for additional flex shifts. Hospital A is in a densely populated urban center while Hospital B is in a suburban area.

Ms. N is concerned that the system-level policy on pediatric death by neurological criteria (brain death) is not applied consistently between the two hospitals. Specifically, she feels that the ICU providers in Hospital B give parents much more leeway in opting out of brain death exams, while providers in Hospital A offer no options and follow the policy strictly as written. Furthermore, Hospital B does not always follow the established protocol when managing death by neurological criteria, allowing staff providers without the delineated privilege to manage the exam. When she queried the leadership of the ICU, she understood that Hospital B felt itself to be representing the wishes of its community and its medical staff.

Ms. N brings her concerns to the ethics committee at Hospital A, recalling a recent case in which a family objected to the determination of death by neurological criteria but was denied continued ventilatory support due to brain death. The ethics committee members considered the committee's role and whether it had a duty to the system-level organization.

Introduction

HECs exist in almost every hospital in the USA. While their history started with specific conflicts created as advancing medical technology challenged traditional approaches to death, dying, and consent for care, most HECs currently accept three main duties: resolution of conflicts related to clinical care, review of policies related to ethical clinical practice, and education of providers, staff, and patients and families.

This chapter discusses an extension of the traditional role of the HEC as a service focused primarily on clinical ethics consultation and promotes an integrated ethics model for the HEC. The integrated ethics model for an institutional ethics committee "includes the traditional case consultation function with an expanded role in proactive policy development and leadership on organizational ethics" (Moon, 2019, 4). It is based in a focus on "ethics as integral to quality of care" (Schyve, 1996, 18).

Organizational ethics addresses the system within which an organization provides patient care. It addresses not just the policy structure but mission, values, and business considerations central to the institution. Expanding the role of the HECs to include organizational ethics is an extension of its current function, moving beyond the immediate clinical ethics conflicts to incorporate the possible structural causes of the conflicts.

Ethics is a systematic approach to balancing competing moral obligations. Clinical ethics is necessary because conflicting moral obligations are inherent in clinical practice. In parallel fashion, operating a healthcare organization gives rise to numerous moral conflicts such as balancing financial concerns with optimal patient care, avoiding conflicts of interest with industry while embracing new technologies, conducting effective strategic planning while protecting vulnerable communities, and promoting quality and safety while managing cost, among many others. Conflicting moral and professional obligations are inherent to healthcare management.

Clinical ethics typically focuses on moral obligations that affect the care of a patient. Effective management of clinical ethics concerns strengthens the provider–patient relationship. Skill in identifying and managing clinical ethics concerns is a necessary component of competence as a provider. Organizational ethics involves ongoing ethical analysis of the decisions made by the healthcare institution or those acting as agents of the institution. This analysis can help effective leaders balance the competing obligations that affect a healthcare organization. Balance among those obligations is necessary to help a healthcare organization maintain integrity to its mission and values and promote trust within the organization and with its community. An effective and ethically sound organization must have the capacity to identify and manage conflicts in organizational ethics.

While the ethics committee as introduced in the 1970s is reflected in the consultation and conflict resolution dimension of today's HEC, the organizational ethics dimension has been a significant, but less organized, part of the history of healthcare ethics as well. In 1995, the Joint Commission on Healthcare Accreditation (now known as The Joint Commission) changed the name of the standards chapter that supports the need for HECs from "Patient's Rights" to "Patient's Rights and Organization Ethics." The Joint Commission's original discussion of organization ethics focused primarily on the implications of the business of medicine on patient care, calling on healthcare organizations to develop and follow an ethical code to protect the integrity of clinical decision-making from business pressures (Schyve, 1996). An additional component of the organization ethics standard required that hospitals have a code of ethical behavior addressing marketing, admissions, transfer, discharge, and billing practices.

Since the introduction of the "organization ethics" requirement by The Joint Commission, there has been increasing attention paid to the ethical implications of all the operational aspects of the organizations in which we serve.

While there is demand for organization-wide attention to ethical issues, there is little guidance as to the structure of organizational ethics in healthcare systems. Organizational ethics is the purview of the system leadership, but an integrated HEC, combining clinical ethics consultation with proactive assessment and review of the ethics of the organization can support the hospital or system by serving as an avenue for ethical review of the organization's policies, procedures, and practice. Two characteristics of HECs make them prime candidates to support efforts at organizational ethics. An effective HEC is typically a well-organized, multidisciplinary group with experience in systematic analysis of complex situations. As such, the HEC can provide a structure for analysis of organizational dilemmas. Additionally, HECs, in their consultative work, gain a bird's-eye view of many issues that challenge an organization, often before the systematic nature of the issue becomes clear.

Pivoting toward work in organizational ethics requires that the HEC embraces the proactive nature of the organizational ethics perspective. In its clinical ethics consultation function, the ethics committee usually serves as an institutionalized intermediary among healthcare disciplines, professional codes, subspecialties, and institutional departments, as well as among patients and families and caregivers. It mediates disputes and provides ongoing education to help avoid avoidable dilemmas. A commonality is that ethics consultation is usually at the request of the patient, family, or provider(s). The case does not exist until some party feels a challenge or dilemma.

Support for organizational ethics makes the role of an HEC more proactive – it seeks to identify and preempt structural conditions that create avoidable ethical challenges. This chapter recognizes that a fully constituted committee embraces both roles. It mediates between individual cases and the organizational and systemic requirements that structure the context of care.

Identifying Organizational Ethics Issues in an Institution

The consultative role of the ethics committee means that uncertainties, conflicts, or disagreements arising from system-level issues may first be identified as patient-specific dilemmas in clinical care. This puts the committee in a privileged position to become aware of ongoing or emerging system issues that may not yet be obvious to hospital leadership. In settings where hospital leadership is part of the HEC, the framework of ethical analysis can help clarify the meaning of a dilemma as it relates to the organization's values. A committee that seeks to be sensitive to patterns of cases and alert to systemic obstacles to patient care can offer tremendous advantage to an organization whose mission centers on improving health and well-being. These obstacles can present in many ways: as repetitive patterns of clinical ethics dilemmas, as unique cases that highlight unanticipated organizational conflicts, or in the course of policy review.

Patterns of Concern

Repetitions, either in the kind of case that comes to the HEC, or in the source of cases, can suggest the presence of underlying obstacles to excellent care that may be the reason for repeated consults.

For example, in Case 1, the HEC identified, in the repetitive nature of consults about "difficult," nonadherent, and frustrating patients, a concern that traumas, acute, chronic, or complex, were a root cause of the "difficult" patient experience. The HEC members, with a broad range of clinical and nonclinical expertise, reviewed several cases as a set and concluded that the hospital staff was not adequately prepared to manage the level of underlying trauma that was influencing patients' ability to respond to care. While it was not clear whether the level of trauma in the community had increased or the ability of the staff to respond had decreased, the need for a focus on trauma-informed care was evident. The concern did not arise from a single ethics consult, but from a pattern of similar consults in a short period of time. The HEC developed an argument to present to hospital leadership that the pattern of cases identified an ongoing system-level failure to anticipate the impact of trauma on patient care. The HEC suggested a system-wide review of capacity for trauma-informed care as a means to help the institution manage obstacles to successful care of traumatized patients and further its mission of caring.

Awareness of Emerging Issues

Health care involves complex systems and the interplay of technology, science, society, and human nature. Issues that stand to impact the delivery of ethically appropriate care arise from every angle of that interplay. Sensitivity to emerging issues is immensely valuable for the proactive, integrated HEC. Broad interdisciplinary representation on an HEC allows it to identify and evaluate concerns emerging from many components of the organization. The HEC that is willing to entertain discussion of emerging issues and identify avoidable ethical errors can help an organization preempt disaster and further its patient care mission.

In Case 2, the HEC became concerned that significant disparities in care existed between hospitals within the single system. Death by neurological criteria had become a controversial topic in the popular media. Disparities in application of the system-wide policy on death by neurological criteria had the potential to become a flashpoint for the system, reflecting badly on both hospitals and creating distrust in Hospital A's community. The HEC opted to bring the issue to the system-level leadership, requesting that current policy be reviewed for alignment with the organization's mission and values and, at the very least, applied uniformly.

Organizational and Policy Structures as Causal Factors of Ethical Concerns

Integrated HECs can elucidate the organization's structural role in the cases that come to the committee. While most HECs are adept at managing case consultation and conflict resolution in the immediate clinical arena, some issues arise directly from the institution's organizational structure and are most effectively addressed or prevented by interventions at the organizational level. HECs can challenge themselves to look past the specific clinical ethics dilemma and seek structural factors that might serve as root causes of conflict.

Robert Hall, in his *Introduction to Healthcare Organizational Ethics*, describes two operational approaches to analysis of healthcare management decisions. The stakeholder approach focuses on the interests and experiences of various stakeholders including patients, employees, contractors, and the community, to name a few. The analysis is predominantly utilitarian, seeking the balance that offers the most broadly positive consequences to the stakeholders. HECs are likely to be most adept at the "organizational goals" approach. This approach focuses on the identified mission of the organization and challenges policies or practices that do not reflect the mission (Hall, 2000, 16–20).

The mission of a healthcare organization is usually a statement of the intent of the organization, an explanation of why it exists in the community, and where its focus lies. It often includes, or refers to, the core values of the institution such as compassion, fairness, trust, integrity, diversity, stewardship, and respect. Beyond the traditional themes of quality patient care, research, and education, the specific content of the mission and values statements can guide evaluation of policies and practice in an institution (Valsangkar et al., 2014).

Policies that conflict with the institutional mission and values are unfortunately commonplace. Financial, political, or other business efficiencies can easily influence policy, sometimes to the detriment of patient care and in conflict with the stated mission of the organization. An HEC is in an excellent position to consider policies in light of the mission of the organization and raise appropriate challenges.

An "ethics audit" of relevant policies focuses on the accountability of policy structure of the organization. It highlights the shared values, expressed in the mission and values statements or in other key organizational statements and the importance of those values as drivers of policy and practice. In reviewing policy and practice, the ethics audit seeks to make implicit values explicit, identifying unwritten values that might conflict with the stated mission and values (Ells and MacDonald, 2002).

Many clinical ethics dilemmas originate in failed communication. The same is true of organizational ethics concerns. As systems become more complex the opportunities for communication failures expand. Policy changes are not well communicated, growth or expansion of the healthcare system involves new patient populations and unfamiliar patterns of care, and new resource limitations result in unanticipated disparities in care. This is especially true in times of rapid change. As healthcare choices become more constrained, the values of the organization become even more critical for ethical practice.

Institutional policies should articulate and reinforce an organization's mission. When there is conflict between policies and mission, between implicit and explicit values, mistrust can arise. The HEC willing to focus on organizational ethics can support the organization by exploring perceived conflicts between policies and mission.

Cases 1 and 2 both include organizational factors. In Case 1, the HEC asked the hospital leadership to develop a plan to address trauma and develop trauma-informed care education for all providers to prevent further repetition of avoidable distress between clinicians and patients. In Case 2, it appeared that within-system disparities in adherence to important ethics policies had arisen. If left without explanation or resolution, the disparity would lead to mistrust. Resolution of the disparity would have to come from the system-level leadership.

Responding to Organizational Ethics Issues

Communicate, Collaborate, Cooperate

A strength of many HECs is the interprofessional membership. A well-constituted HEC can create space for varied experts, professional and nonprofessional, medical, nursing, social work, psychology, community, legal, clinical and nonclinical, to collaborate respectfully and communicate openly to identify the multiple dimensions of any dilemma. The membership of an integrated HEC should be multidisciplinary with sufficient knowledge and experience to participate in assessment from the organizational level.

The integrated HEC seeking to support the organization in its mission to provide ethical patient care has numerous collaborators and should seek to optimize those collaborations with consistent and reliable reporting structures. Risk management has been a traditional voice at the ethics table in many institutions and responds to many of the same clinical case dilemmas, albeit from a different perspective. Pastoral care, palliative care, and patient advocates are also well represented on most HECs.

Collaboration with quality and safety leadership, while less traditional, can be very valuable for the proactive, organizationally focused HEC. Safety reports, like ethics cases, are often the first hint of deeper system frailties. Quality improvement initiatives can be engaged to respond to structural sources of ethics concerns. Quality and safety planning can benefit from ethics review to ensure that patient rights and organizational mission are reflected in quality improvement programs.

HECs are always at risk of becoming silos in a complex organization. Conscious efforts to further communication and collaboration can better integrate the HEC into the web of interactions that constitutes a functioning organization. HECs should strive for defined and structured collaboration with other system-level functions such as risk management, quality improvement, patient safety, and legal and regulatory compliance.

Report

Ethics committees should have a specific relationship to the professional structure of the hospital and system organization. An ethics committee can be constituted as a medical staff committee, an administrative committee, or a governing board committee. The organizational ethics work of the integrated HEC can be part of the committee as a whole or adopted by a subcommittee, while the HEC retains the authority for coordination, oversight, and approval of activities of the subcommittee. Conflicts of interest should be managed prospectively and openly.

An HEC whose function includes organizational ethics and policy development should establish standards of membership, process, and self-improvement specific to organizational ethics issues and to the organizational structure of its home institution.

It is important that the HEC involved in organizational ethics work has a clear and formal reporting structure, including direction from and access to supportive leadership. Invisibility and isolation inhibit the effectiveness of the integrated HEC as much as would a lack of independence. The integrated HEC should be an identifiable part of the organizational ethics structure of the system or institution.

Except for specific policy development tasks, the output of the HEC engaged in organizational ethics work is recommendations offered to appropriate decision-making leaders. They are not authoritative or binding. Enforcement is the purview of the leadership of the organization.

Healthcare organizations are paying more attention to ethical issues beyond the typical dyadic, individual-level disputes and uncertainties, and will continue to do so. The HEC can be useful because of its diverse membership, its wide representation from the institution, its access to emerging conflicts, and its familiarity with the language and processes of ethical deliberation. If, however, the HEC's founding mandate is restrictive and narrow in focus, the HEC's ability to integrate organizational ethics can suffer. In the present healthcare environment, ethics has a large role to play. HECs may have to work with organizational leadership to redesign themselves for an expanded role. The HEC must have support, collaboration, and specific direction from the leadership of the organization. Additionally, any expansion of the HEC's current role requires resources and support that many committees, staffed primarily or completely by volunteers, do not command. Institutional resources will continue to be devoted to externally imposed regulatory, legal, and business demands with ethical implications. Expansion of the HEC role into organizational ethics may include integration with other programs, but the HEC should maintain independent oversight of its participation.

Conclusion

Ethics is everybody's business, and there is no area of the healthcare enterprise where that is as well-known as in our HECs. That does not mean that everything is the business of our HEC. Our committees have well-defined roles in education, policy formation and review, and case consultation. But, in such a complex, interactive, and fluid system as healthcare organization, clinical actions and decisions tend to have organizational implications and organizational decisions have clinical implications. Careful and systematic expansion of the role of an HEC to integrate participation in organizational ethics work can benefit the HCO. Recognizing this enhances our understanding of what ethics can mean and what it can do.

Questions for Discussion

1. Conceptual: How does the mission and values statement of your organization affect the work of the HEC? How should it?

2. Pragmatic: Would the issue described in Case 1 come to the attention of your HEC? What other organizational departments or functions might be alerted to the problem it represents? Would, or could, they address it? What would you suggest?
3. Strategic: How could your HEC gain organizational support for an effort to compare the implications of specific policies with the mission and values statement of the organization? What policies might you start with?

References

Ells C, MacDonald C (2002). Implications of organizational ethics to healthcare. *Healthcare Management Forum*, 15(3): 32–38.

Hall RT (2000). *Introduction to Healthcare Organizational Ethics*. Oxford University Press.

Moon M (2019). Institutional ethics committees. *Pediatrics*, 143(5): e20190659.

Schyve PM (1996). Patient rights and organizational ethics: The Joint Commission perspective. *Bioethics Forum*, 12(2): 13–20.

Valsangkar B, Chen C, Wohltjen H, Mullan F (2014). Do medical school mission statements align with the nation's health care needs? *Academic Medicine*, 89(6): 892–895.

Chapter

28

The Healthcare Ethics Committee as Educator

Kathy Kinlaw

Objectives

Upon reading and considering the content of this chapter, the reader should be able to:

1. Describe topics in ethics that can be assessed to determine the ethics knowledge level of healthcare ethics committee (HEC) members and the organization at large.
2. Identify at least five strategies for educating physicians and organizational staff about ethics and describe how education can be a "preventive ethics" strategy.
3. Describe mechanisms for tracking and evaluating the HEC's educational efforts.

Case

Metropolitan Care Hospital Ethics Committee received a request for consultation from the ICU regarding whether life-sustaining treatment should be continued for a patient with multiple organ system failure. The patient, Mr. Jansen, had recently been admitted from an area nursing home and had no family or guardian to assist with making healthcare decisions. The ICU physician, who did not believe that continuing treatment would reverse Mr. Jansen's decline and that the treatment might actually be causing Mr. Jansen pain and discomfort, was unsure what decision should be made. The ethics committee consultation tracking system indicated that this was the third case involving medical decision-making for patients without a surrogate decision maker that had been referred to the committee in the last 2 months.

Of all the potential roles of HECs, that of "educator" arguably continues to be the most fundamental and enduring. In addition to traditional training opportunities, every policy examined, every retrospective review of a recurring issue at the institution, every organizational issue studied, and every ethics consult becomes an opportunity for education – not only for committee members but also for patients, families, and healthcare team members. An effective HEC will consider carefully and intentionally how its role as educator will be articulated and implemented and how the institution will evaluate the committee's effectiveness in this role. Though education may not be the role perceived as the primary work of an ethics committee, the task of education by the HEC is essential to the committee's ability to perform its other roles.

Preliminary Questions for Your Institution

In order to target education appropriately, certain foundational assessment questions must be addressed before the HEC can take on the role of educator.

Does the Healthcare Organization's Clinical Team Members Know That an HEC Exists as a Resource?

In the development of or restructuring of an HEC, a survey of physicians, nurses, and other healthcare professionals can provide constructive information. The first question for such a survey might be "Is there an HEC at 'X' hospital?" Responses of "yes," "no," and "unsure" provide quick information about the level of awareness of the HEC. A follow-up question asking "If yes, which of the following are roles of the HEC at 'X'?" will also provide further information both about respondent understanding *and* the effectiveness of the HEC in communicating its roles.

Does the Staff Know What an Ethics Committee Is – and Is Not?

When asked what ethics committees actually "do," many healthcare professionals think first of the role of the HEC in providing consultation in difficult cases. For some professionals the consulting role is misperceived as one of monitoring or oversight of decision-making. This perceived role of "second-guessing" healthcare decision-making along with concerns about the preparedness and effectiveness of committees as consultants raise concerns for some clinicians. In a national sample of US physicians, 11% of respondents reported hesitation in seeking ethics consultation because they believed that ethics consultants were unqualified (DuVal et al., 2004).

Physician-ethicist Mark Siegler warned about the potential for ethics committees to undermine the physician/patient relationship by interrupting the physician's authority in decision-making (Siegler, 1986). A 2006 study confirms that concern, where 72% of physician respondents not using ethics consultation indicated that it was their responsibility to resolve patient or family concerns. Of respondents not using ethics consultation, 28% agreed that using the ethics consult team might lead the patient or family to believe that the physician was not effective in guiding them with these decisions (Orlowski et al., 2006). The demythologizing of ethics committee consultation is being addressed in other chapters of this book, but an early task for ethics committees *as educators* is to recognize this potential for perceived role or responsibility intrusion and to address it proactively and collaboratively throughout the hospital. In addition, some clinicians may gladly turn decision-making over to the HEC in difficult cases, such as that of Mr. Jansen. A survey mechanism developed to assess the prevailing knowledge about and attitudes toward the HEC can aid in addressing the issues, interests, and concerns of the healthcare staff.

HEC Self-Education

In order for the HEC to provide effective ethics education to organizational colleagues, ethics committee members themselves must have an adequate ethics knowledge base. In Mr. Jansen's case, for example, HEC members need to be familiar with ethical issues such as decision-making for patients without decision-making capacity and the issue of withdrawal of life-sustaining treatment. Committees should, therefore, include members with ethics expertise or have ethics resources readily available. Additionally, HEC members must identify effective *mechanisms* for self-education and develop a basic understanding of the field of clinical and organizational ethics themselves.

Self-education of ethics committee members prepares committee members with skills to contribute effectively to all of the functions of the HEC – education, consultation,

Table 28.1 ASBH Core Knowledge Areas for Ethics Consultation

- Moral reasoning and ethical theory
- Bioethical issues and concepts that typically emerge
- Healthcare systems including managed care and governmental systems
- Clinical context, such as medical terminology, common diseases, emerging technologies
- Healthcare institutions in which consultants work, including institutional policies
- Beliefs and perspectives of patient and staff population served by organization
- Relevant codes of ethics, professional conduct, and accrediting organizations' guidelines
- Relevant health law

policy review/formulation, and evaluation. The areas of expertise needed for case consultation as identified in ethics consultation core competency reports by the American Society for Bioethics and Humanities (ASBH, 1998, 2011) remain relevant for HEC self-education (see Table 28.1). This document recognizes that there are some areas in which all HEC members should have basic knowledge or skill and other areas in which advanced knowledge or skill is needed. While all HEC members are not required to have advanced knowledge or skill, at least one member of an HEC should have expertise in each area, or an area expert should be available to the committee (ASBH, 1998). The ASBH 2009 education guide for improving competencies in clinical ethics consultation identifies core ethical issues in caring for adults and for minors and suggests key articles for review (ASBH, 2009). This shared knowledge base is essential for the HEC to participate effectively in educating the broader healthcare staff. In 2017 further in-depth discussion of key patient-centered cases was published in an ASBH study guide (ASBH, 2017) and a resource guide for developing advance ethics consultation skills was also published (Clinical Ethics Consultation Affairs Committee of the ASBH, 2017).

In order to determine how HEC self-education should be focused, it is good practice to survey HEC members routinely about areas in which they desire additional ethics education as well as those areas where their knowledge and comfort is highest. In conjunction with such needs assessments, it is also good practice to survey HEC members in order to identify areas of expertise and/or interest in providing committee or staff education. All HEC members have certain areas of expertise and experience that may provide powerful foundations for education. For example, an HEC member who is a palliative care nurse can bring both patient narratives and questions around the ethics of end-of-life care to educational forums; a transplant surgeon can raise ethical questions about transplant selection criteria and where the patient's ability to comply with post-transplant care intersects with concerns about equity and fairness. Every HEC should look at its own membership for areas of expertise. Pairing these area experts with a clinical ethicist may provide the basis for a highly relevant educational discussion, even early in the HEC member's tenure. When area experts become increasingly informed about ethics as a discipline, the HEC member can effectively provide education alone.

Enabling the HEC and Committee Members as Educators

Several factors facilitate the ability of an ethics committee and each committee member to serve as a resource for the organization. Of paramount importance is support of institutional leadership in communicating the importance of ethics. Further, each member makes a commitment to learning about the field of ethics as well as a significant time commitment, quite distinct from many other organizational committees. In order for committees to effectively bring a body of expertise to education, members must be willing to learn about the normative approaches to ethics in addition to bringing their rich professional experience. Acknowledging the practical moral wisdom that most healthcare professionals possess (Churchill and Schenck, 2005) is important for both HEC members and those colleagues for whom educational programs are focused. Ethical analysis builds upon these strengths and provides additional ways of framing issues and thus should serve as a resource, rather than be viewed as a critique of team competence. HEC education should both support the traditional physician/health team/patient/family relationship as the locus of decision-making and be highly relevant to clinical colleagues on the front line. Helping clinicians examine and clarify their own ethical values, beliefs, and decision-making styles provides a basis for thoughtful, more impartial examination of ethical issues. Supporting members of the clinical team who are struggling with ethical issues may involve equipping team members through coaching that assists clinicians to recognize their moral distress, elicit values among those involved, and discern reasonable options that address ethical concerns (Kockler and Dirksen, 2015).

Perceived Relevance

As mentioned above, relevance of HEC education can be strengthened by utilizing an organization-wide survey mechanism. Clinical colleagues can assess the frequency with which clinical, research, or organizational issues occur and the degree to which these issues are viewed as ethically problematic. Analysis of responses according to demographic information – such as across and within professional disciplines or by affected patient care floors/units – provides important information about what issues may be recurrent and whether issues are discipline- or unit-specific. These indicators provide information that can shape the way in which relevant ethics education proceeds in the institution.

While HEC members will need to develop a foundational level of understanding in a broad array of contemporary ethical topics, educational programming for the broader organizational staff must be more focused. Selecting a recurring issue or a topic surfaced by a recent difficult clinical case or organizational issue (such as decision-making for patients like Mr. Jansen who lack decision-making capacity) ensures a level of interest. Additionally, addressing a cutting-edge issue or one that has had recent national attention may help colleagues stay up-to-date and challenged in their thinking. (Examples of such programming topics are included in Table 28.2.) Engaging formats for education, with moderated discussion of ethical issues, include: detailed case narratives; mock ethics committee meetings where communication skills are key; simulated patient encounters with HEC members role-playing; or viewing a film clip or reading a short story.

The Complexity of Ethical Action

In addition to addressing relevant practice issues, HECs have an opportunity to help clinical and other organizational staff members understand the process of ethical engagement. Case consultation methodologies are only one part of the process of promoting ethical action. Understanding the broader context of how ethical action evolves may be very helpful for HECs. One model for ethical action is derived from the work of educational psychologist James Rest (Rest and Narvaez, 1994, 22–25). This model identifies four components as essential to ethical action:

Table 28.2 Sample Topics for Ethics Education of Healthcare Professionals

- Unrepresented patients: ethical decision-making when there is no decision maker
- Ethical care when healthcare providers feel threatened by patient or family behavior
- Altered medical standards: whether and when emergent conditions justify a different level of treatment
- Legal and ethical perspectives on decision-making near the end of life (multiple program topics: advance directives, do-not-resuscitate decisions, withholding and withdrawal of treatment, artificial hydration and nutrition, medically inappropriate or ineffective treatment, brain death, organ transplantation, assisted suicide)
- Disability perspectives shaping healthcare ethics
- Access to health care for undocumented immigrants
- Addressing moral distress
- Neuroethics in the use of neuroimaging technologies
- Patient confidentiality, privacy, and respect in the Health Insurance Portability and Accountability Act (HIPAA) era
- Respecting difference: How are ethical issues framed and by whom? (a nuanced look at whether and how race, ethnicity, culture, religion, alternative understandings of illness, family systems, and other perspectives unique to those involved in a case make a difference)
- The evolving ethics at the beginning of life (assisted reproductive technologies, neonatal ethics)
- Access, equity of care, and the role of health systems

1. **Ethical sensitivity or attentiveness**: the ability both to recognize that the issue is an ethical one (rather than a legal, cultural, or clinical issue) and to acknowledge one's role responsibility or "agency" in addressing it.
2. **Ethical reasoning**: careful analysis of the situation utilizing various normative approaches and theories.
3. **Ethical commitment**: one's actual willingness to act ethically, rather than to choose other, very real, competing commitments, often of a nonmoral nature (e.g., time, self-preservation, conflict avoidance, etc.)
4. **Ethical character/implementation**, which includes an assessment of whether one will actually take the next steps, and whether one knows what resources and practical options are needed to act

Rest indicates that all four of these components must be present for ethical action to occur. This model acknowledges that ethical issues are situated in complex contexts and that awareness of these layers and practice competencies may be powerful for clinical teams and HEC members. Before one can analyze a situation, one must be able to recognize and name what ethical issues are at stake. Then one must decide whether one will actually speak up or act in the complex situation and if one has the knowledge and skills to do so.

Acknowledging Existing Educational Pathways

Logistics also matter in constructing educational opportunities, and existing forums provide important venues for ethics education. For example, each hospital unit has existing administrative and educational meetings. If the ICU staff meetings at Metropolitan Hospital occur at a regular weekly time, working with meeting conveners to address the issues in Mr. Jansen's case at this existing meeting may best respect staff time and result in well-attended discussions. The ethics session may need to be repeated during other shifts; asynchronous (online) learning modalities may also facilitate delivering education to multiple audiences at multiple times. HEC members can work with unit leaders to determine a topic of current interest or concern (Is a new ethics-related policy being implemented in the hospital or unit? Did unit staff struggle with a difficult patient case recently? Are there recurring ethical issues in the unit [as in Mr. Jansen's case] that staff would like to address?).

Each meeting provides a chance to demonstrate the relevance of ethics to the everyday life of staff and patients/families. Some issues can best be addressed in a discussion format in which procedural ethics is modeled as unit staff are able to voice their concerns, and questions that help frame the ethical issues are asked. Because limited time is available in standing meetings, especially when other agenda items are also addressed, HEC members' initial discussions may lead to an invitation to return for a more in-depth dialogue. Simply the presence of the HEC members and their method of approaching the discussion will convey important information about the overall role and effectiveness of the HEC.

Further, choosing the "right" HEC members to lead the educational forum is important. An HEC member who is knowledgeable about the practices of a particular unit may be especially helpful in the discussion, but only if staff in that unit can acknowledge that in this discussion the individual has a separate role as a member of the HEC and possesses a level of expertise in ethics. Additionally, the HEC member leading the discussion must be able to follow up and support the unit in addressing concerns arising in these discussions.

Other Opportunities for Ethics Education

Beyond existing unit meetings, there are other opportunities for education organization-wide. Medical staff meetings or grand rounds formats provide collaborative opportunities to address large groups who are already accustomed to attending the forum. Ethics grand rounds, with a committed, interdisciplinary planning group and ideally a budget to occasionally bring in outside speakers, may provide an effective venue in many organizational settings. The ability to offer continuing education credits encourages participation.

Additionally, bringing ethical discussions to leadership groups (such as the clinical practice committee or conflict of interest committee or the health system or organizational board) can provide an important resource for these groups and will demonstrate the importance of the work of the HEC as a resource to the organization. Having members of these leadership groups also serve on the membership of the HEC provides an ongoing mechanism for information exchange and assists in the identification of issues about which the HEC might provide further education. Where other committees at the organization have responsibilities that clearly intersect with ethical concerns in the organization (e.g., risk management, compliance, palliative care, institutional research boards), HECs should establish regular mechanisms for discussion and information sharing. Finally, nontraditional strategies for education can also be important for HECs to consider. For example:

- Every note that an HEC team or member writes in the chart becomes an educational tool for anyone accessing the chart. HEC members need training on how to structure notes and effectively utilize ethics language in writing notes.

- Some HECs have instituted nurse liaison programs or rounding in those units in which ethical issues are frequently encountered. These mechanisms can be effective in identifying patient care concerns early and may help to clarify patient preferences or resolve decision-making conflict, thus preventing conflict from becoming intractable. The HEC process must be carefully constructed so that committee liaisons and regular ethics rounding are not viewed as oversight mechanisms looking for problems in patient care, but rather as resources to the team. These mechanisms provide excellent opportunities for staff and patient/family education.
- The practice of including ethics as a part of new staff orientation – whether in person or via online techniques – recognizes the importance of ethics as an integral part of organizational structure. At this level, basic information with relevant examples may be most helpful to address: what is meant by "ethics" and why ethics is important; respect for differing values and perspectives; recurring ethical issues for which the HEC is a resource; and information on the role of the HEC.
- Social media, brochures, and posted announcements that describe the purpose of the HEC and how to access it as a resource may help colleagues (and patients and visitors) understand the role of the HEC. Having an online ethics presence can establish a recognized resource for clinical teams and organizational leadership as well as patients and families.
- Inclusion of timely ethical articles/discussions in print or online newsletters, on websites, on internal cable TV channels, or via other established communication routes provides an opportunity for more in-depth coverage of issues.

Education as Preventive Ethics

Many of the educational approaches previously discussed are also "preventive" in nature, addressing organizational issues or practices in ways that may avoid ethical controversies later – both in caring for particular patients and within the unit or organization as a whole.

- HEC members committed to developing knowledge and skills in ethics become adept at early recognition of ethical issues, allowing for discussion and responses that may keep issues from escalating. As ethics-related policies are developed, HEC members can help extend information about new policies throughout the organization, both at educational events and in specific care units. For example, HECs may lead efforts to develop guidelines and communication techniques regarding working with families who wish to continue treatments that the team has determined are clinically ineffective or potentially inappropriate for the patient. HEC members might facilitate education and discussions around these guidelines, particularly in those critical care units where these patients frequently receive care. Providing discussions in or rounding with teams in a variety of units demonstrates deep interest in clinical teams and builds awareness of issues in each unit as well as trust relationships for future work.
- As educational activities are extended throughout the organization, the HEC will find clinical staff alerting the HEC to recurrent issues, such as the lack of a pathway for decision-making for "unrepresented patients" like Mr. Jansen. This provides an opportunity for the HEC to be a resource across the organization to facilitate development of preventive strategies to identify unrepresented patients at admission

and to address pathways for decision-making for these patients. This might involve collaborative work with other key groups at the organization, as well as with other community organizations who can assist with public education and possible public policy initiatives.

• Each of these programs may be one part of a strategic effort to work with organizational leadership to build a culture of ethics. In such a culture, the disciplinary and experiential knowledge of all staff is recognized, ethics is better understood as a discipline and a resource, and potentially difficult issues are recognized and addressed early so that patient care is improved and moral distress is decreased.

Accountability and Effectiveness

Evaluation of the effectiveness of the HEC in achieving each of its stated roles and responsibilities is essential. HECs should utilize outcomes research resources at the organization in determining a methodology for assessing effectiveness of educational efforts. Utilizing the survey tool discussed earlier would provide a baseline about knowledge level and areas of interest. HECs can track their educational activities throughout the year, describing meeting information such as number, frequency, format, topic, and attendees. In addition, brief evaluations can assess attendee satisfaction, knowledge gained, effectiveness of presenters and formats, and identification of future topics of interest. In some settings, pre- and post-tests can be utilized to better assess the knowledge and skills gained. It would also be helpful to initiate periodic follow-up assessments with clinicians who have participated in educational programming to determine whether and how the information gained had impacted their practice. Similarly, soliciting feedback from individuals involved in more informal educational formats (e.g., occasional meetings with the risk management committee) may provide valuable evaluative information. Because each consultation is an opportunity for education, follow-up questionnaires with those involved in case consultation also provide significant information about knowledge gained. A year-end, organization-wide survey covering those knowledge and skill areas that were the focus of that year's educational programming would provide an assessment of community understanding along with direction for future programming opportunities.

HEC as Educator and the Broader Community

HECs often report limited success in providing educational events for the public community the organization serves. Because HEC members most often do not receive specific release time or compensation for their work on the HEC, formal educational efforts focused on the community are limited unless there is will and investment at the organizational level. Historically, HECs have had some success with community education on end-of-life planning and advance directives or joining with civic organizations or religious organizations/worship sites to host such programs. Primary education of the public community often occurs at the bedside, with particular patients and families who are receiving care. Each encounter can, of course, have far-reaching impact in the community as these care narratives are communicated by patients and families.

HECs are not alone in serving as ethics educators in their communities. Many regions have an ethics consortium or collaborative that provides educational programming for interested healthcare professionals and the public and can supplement and support HECs in their role as educators. Educational programming is available through university-based bioethics centers, professional associations, and national associations like the ASBH. HECs can make information about these broader programs available to staff members. Hosting speakers and educational opportunities "at home," within the organization, is also an effective way for ethical reflection to permeate organizational culture. HECs may work with local bioethics programs to assess the ethical environment at the institution and bring educational opportunities and consultation training to the institution. HEC leadership and members should remain keenly aware that all HEC actions and responsibilities become "ethics teaching moments" for colleagues. Tracking educational activity and impact provides important information about the effectiveness of the HEC for organizational leadership and the organization as a whole.

Questions for Discussion

1. Conceptual: What are the primary ethical issues that are currently relevant at your organization and that, if creatively addressed, would support patient care and institutional staff?
2. Pragmatic: What measures for continually assessing ethics knowledge and tracking ethical activity can be instituted at your organization this year and how can these data be used to educate key constituents?
3. Strategic: What individuals at your organization or in your local area possess ethics expertise, including the ability to put the theory and language of ethics into practice?

References

American Society for Bioethics and Humanities. (1998). *Core Competencies for Health Care Ethics Consultation*. Glenview, IL: ASBH.

American Society for Bioethics and Humanities. (2009). *Improving Competencies in Clinical Ethics Consultation: An Education Guide*. Glenview, IL: ASBH.

American Society for Bioethics and Humanities. (2011). *Core Competencies for Health Care Ethics Consultation*, 2nd ed. Glenview, IL: ASBH.

American Society for Bioethics and Humanities. (2017). *Addressing Patient-Centered Ethical Issues in Health Care: A Case-Based Study Guide*. Chicago: ASBH.

Churchill LR, Schenck D (2005). One cheer for bioethics: Engaging the moral experiences of patients and practitioners beyond the big decisions. *Cambridge Quarterly of Healthcare Ethics*, 14(4): 389–403.

Clinical Ethics Consultation Affairs Committee of the American Society for Bioethics and Humanities. (2017). *Resources for Developing Advanced Skills in Ethics Consultation*. Chicago: ASBH.

DuVal G, Clarridge B, Gensler G, Danis, M (2004). A national survey of U.S. internists' experiences with ethical dilemmas and ethics consultation. *Journal of General Internal Medicine*, 19(3): 251–258.

Kockler NJ, Dirksen KM (2015). Competencies required for clinical ethics consultation as coaching. *Healthcare Ethics USA*, 23(4): 25–33.

Orlowski J, Hein S, Christensen J, et al. (2006). Why doctors use or do not use ethics consultation. *Journal of Medical Ethics*, 32(9): 499–502.

Rest JR, Narvaez D, eds. (1994). *Moral Development in the Professions: Psychology and Applied Ethics*. Hillsdale, NJ: Lawrence Erlbaum Associates, Inc.

Siegler M (1986). Ethics committees: Decisions by bureaucracy. *Hastings Center Report*, 16(3): 22–24.

Chapter

29

Understanding Ethics Pedagogy

Felicia Cohn

Objectives

Upon reading and considering the content of this chapter, the reader should be able to:

1. Identify the ways instruction about ethics is different from instruction about other clinical or scientific topics.
2. Describe important educational objectives for ethics and the teaching strategies that facilitate them.
3. Describe common barriers in teaching about ethics to a broad audience.

Case

Mary Rivera, 82, was admitted to the hospital with shortness of breath, diarrhea, weakness, and near syncope. She has a history of Alzheimer's Disease, diabetes, hypertension, chronic aspiration, and multiple episodes of pneumonia. She is again diagnosed with aspiration pneumonia. On admission, she is awake and oriented, requests treatment to "help her breathe," and notes she has an advance directive on file. Subsequently, her cognition declines. Her kidneys begin to fail and recovery is considered unlikely.

Mary was widowed years before and has seven adult children, all of whom regularly visit her in the hospital. Her youngest son, Jimmy, 43, has continued to live with her since childhood. Jimmy is a large man who previously worked part-time as a bouncer at a local nightclub, but states he quit his job to stay home to care for his mother. His demeanor is intimidating and the unit nurses often call security when he visits. He presents an advance directive Mary prepared 8 years prior that names him as durable power of attorney (DPOA) and expresses a preference for continued treatment. He states Mary had told him repeatedly to fight for her. The advance healthcare directive in the chart is more recent, dated 3 years ago, and names Mary's eldest daughter, Emily, as DPOA, and states a preference to forgo life-sustaining treatment in the event that her condition is irreversible and incurable. Emily is a quiet woman, married with four children, and works as an accountant. Brother and sister have been at odds regarding their mother's treatment and the other siblings have taken sides. At issue medically is Mary's code status and use of hemodialysis. Socially, the siblings report that Jimmy is living on Mary's social security and wants to continue treatment to maintain his source of income. Emily believes their mother is suffering and that treatment is contrary to Mary's wishes.

The healthcare ethics committee (HEC) consultant discovers legal issues that raise questions about the validity of both advance directives. The consultant reviews hospital policy regarding the selection of a surrogate decision maker, advance directives, and nonbeneficial treatment; consults other intensivists and palliative care physicians; and contacts hospital legal counsel. After several contentious family meetings and further deterioration in Mary's condition, Jimmy is persuaded that Mary is unlikely to recover, and all agree to a plan to withdraw life-sustaining treatment.

This ongoing saga has garnered a lot of interest throughout the hospital. The HEC chair requests that the ethics consultant present the case at the next HEC meeting and at an upcoming community lecture. The medical director asks for a presentation at the next physician group meeting.

Introduction

Ethics case consultations often highlight ethical issues within an organization that may be best addressed with education. Ethics education is an integral and essential role for HECs, yet HEC members are often not prepared to support this challenging role. To teach ethics, the HEC member should understand and be able to convey what ethics is and what makes it unique, be prepared to overcome common barriers to ethics education, define goals of the education efforts, and utilize vital and clinically relevant educational methods. Some key insights can help guide educational efforts.

What the Educator Needs to Know about Teaching Medical Ethics

The Focus of Ethics Education Is Values, Not Character, Opinions, or Law

Teaching ethics must necessarily begin with a determination of what ethics is. The term "ethics" may be used in various ways, to refer to evaluations of right and wrong, better and worse with regard to our actions, goals, and roles (Chapter 2). Defining ethics by delimiting what ethics is not can further help clarify its meaning. Ethics is not a personal or religious belief system, a professional code, or law. It is not an opinion, an abstract principle, or a legal requirement. It is not what one feels might be done, what might be expected, or what one must do. Ethics education is neither like Sunday school nor a court of law. No heaven and hell, no threat of incarceration – the intent is not to impugn an individual's moral compass, but to help calibrate it to particular circumstances. Since Aristotle, ethics has been recognized as a practical discipline that provides individuals "with the intellectual tools and interactional skills to give that moral character its best behavioral expression" (Culver et al., 1985, 253). Ethics is a well-reasoned response to difficult questions or conflicts. Ethics suggests what one should do in a specific situation, and so a case provides useful context for applying these tools and skills in a manner that is relevant and interesting to the audience. Using Mary's case, for example, the HEC member may focus other committee members on the relevant policies, principles, and practices; focus the physicians on ethics consultation as a useful tool; and focus the community audience on the value of proper advance care planning and family discussion.

Ethics Education Is Different

Teaching clinical ethics is different from other topics, like reading or chemistry, in which there are clear rules and exceptions, a clear content to be mastered and practiced, and a clear goal to attain. Teaching ethics is more like teaching someone how to cook. With cooking, there are many concepts, terms, principles, and theories to learn, most of which can be conveyed through textbooks and instruction. The key content can be taught, but with the ever-changing environment, the applications vary widely.

Clinical ethics is similar. The content and application evolve with new situations and technologies, which create new and revisit old questions. Effective case presentation offers something useful and interesting for the audience. While each presentation will start with Mary's case, each will vary significantly in the objectives to achieve, the details provided, and the topics raised.

Responding to Ethical Questions Requires Evaluation of the Options Available

Ethics education is not about right and wrong in any absolute sense; rather, it is concerned with the systematic and critical reflection on the right and wrong or the good and bad of human acts and human character. Ethics education involves nuanced clarification of questions, attention to process, and decision analysis in order to determine the options available and which appears best in a given situation.

Each audience will respond to the case based on their experiences and worldviews. An effective presentation can help audience members reason beyond their "gut" reactions and emotional responses. The presentation may begin with an examination of the situation to identify the questions it raises and proceed with consideration of goals, judgments, and reasons. Both a challenge and opportunity for ethics education are the lack of clear guidelines, easy rules to follow, and simple learning objectives. A review of relevant literature, including religious, philosophical, historical, legal, and literary references, may inform ethical analysis, but may not provide answers. There is no algorithm, or textbook with the answers at the back, just the opportunity for critical reflection, open communication, and moral reasoning. In Mary's case, like most, several options for resolution were possible. The various audiences and members within each might argue for different outcomes. For example, some might suggest that Jimmy not be allowed to participate, that a judge determine who should make the decision, that the family work it out among themselves, or that the physicians act on the treatment preferences expressed in Mary's most recent advance directive. The HEC member may explore such options to demonstrate how to build arguments and justify decisions.

Goals of Ethics Education

Ethics education can offer the tools necessary to consider enduring conflicts and questions. For most audiences, ethics education can help the learner build a knowledge base (e.g., relevant laws, policies, and paradigms); recognize diverse moral viewpoints; increase self-awareness; identify ethical questions and dilemmas; reflect critically; communicate effectively; build relationships; and tolerate ambiguity, uncertainty, complexity, and discord. Ethics education supports the development of critical thinking skills, the ability to discern the best response to real and complex situations, and the expression of recommended courses of action. Trained and experienced HEC members can share their content expertise, skill set, and wisdom, enabling others to engage in ethics consultation, and in turn, empowering their constituents to address the questions and conflicts they regularly face on their own.

In Mary's case, identifying and assessing the conflicting perspectives among the family members and between the family and clinicians was important in understanding ethical conflicts, highlighted the complexity of the case, and suggested lessons for communication, relationship development, and options for resolution. These content areas may be refined into more specific objectives relevant to the particular audience. The lessons learned may then be applied to similar situations in the future. When comparable cases arise repeatedly, these lessons can inform ethics policies, which, in turn, may guide clinical ethics practice. Education can then reflect this practical guidance and the policies developed.

Methods of Ethics Pedagogy

What and How to Teach Ethics

Determining what and how to teach is an exercise in maximizing opportunity. Planning starts with consideration of the reasons the HEC member is offering or was invited to teach. Every clinical case consultation or question raised is an opportunity for "just in time" education for those involved that should focus on the knowledge, skills, and attitudes essential for addressing that situation, for example guidance from paradigm cases, the use of reasoning tools, or acceptance of a policy. Formal presentations may build on these immediate needs so that the presentation is relevant and interesting.

For further guidance, some common course objectives have emerged from medical ethics education programs. Among these are important skills such as the recognition of ethics issues, ethical reasoning and problem-solving skills, understanding ethical frameworks, familiarity with relevant law and medicine, personal values clarification, communication, and identification of ethics resources (DuBois and Burkemper, 2002). Some core topic areas from the bioethics literature include ethical theories, issues in reproduction, end-of-life care, privacy and confidentiality, professionalism, shared decision-making, research, patient safety, and resource allocation. The American Society for Bioethics and Humanities (ASBH) has offered a curricular guide that identifies competencies for those engaged in clinical ethics consultation services. Their thoughtful report offers an array of content domains and further specifies basic and advanced skill levels as appropriate for different roles (ASBH, 2011). The domains identified form the basis of the Healthcare Ethics Consultant-Certified (HEC-C) program, launched in 2018, to promote excellence and professionalism within the field of healthcare ethics consultation (ASBH, 2019). ASBH also offers an education guide that offers strategies for teaching core knowledge about clinical ethics generally and specific ethical issues, ethics consultation skills, and responsibilities of healthcare ethics consultants. In addition to identifying key resources, this guide also suggests educational approaches to engaging ethics committee members, such as group discussions, literature reviews, values clarification exercises, case analysis, and policy comparisons. These frameworks may be useful starting points when developing ethics education for a variety of audiences.

Helpful Teaching Methods

The teaching methods are as important as the content and will also vary with the audience, as well as the time available and the setting. Medical ethics has been described as a self-consciously multidisciplinary field that borrows from the humanities, social sciences, health professions, law, and business, among others (Sugarman and Sulmasy, 2001). The methods may be qualitative or quantitative, abstract or concrete, deductive or inductive, normative or descriptive. The educator may choose the most comfortable or appropriate approach. Common techniques include lecture with question/answer sessions, discussion and debate, writing exercises, the use of movies or program clips, role-playing, computer simulations, and clinical rounds or field visits. Regardless of the specific approach selected, ethics education may benefit from incorporating self-reflection, dialogue, narrative, and role-modeling. Students may benefit further from consideration of their learning styles and the instructor's efforts to match those styles with various pedagogical methods (Dunn, 2000).

Know Thyself

Ethics education requires self-reflection. It is imperative that one understands one's own beliefs and the premises from which they arise, biases, strengths and weaknesses, and limits. As human beings, it is impossible to separate personal and professional beliefs completely, and consciously or subconsciously those personal beliefs will affect one's judgment. Self-knowledge is wisdom, without which it is impossible to recognize when and the extent to which personal beliefs influence behavior and decisions. The HEC member must assess and address their own beliefs and biases, and their impact on the evaluation of a case. Ethics education allows such development of the self as moral agent, for the educator and learners.

In Mary's case, the ethics committee member may have strong feelings about the best course of treatment for Mary, or about which family member should be making decisions on her behalf. It was easy, for example, to dislike Jimmy and sympathize with Emily, and these feelings affected the perspectives of many involved. It is important to acknowledge those beliefs and feelings, and to recognize their effect on the consultation and education about the case. These beliefs can be useful in teaching many audiences to acknowledge and work with their own biases and emotional responses.

Talk With, Not At

There is a place for lecture, PowerPoint presentation, and textbook review in ethics education, but after offering fundamental definitions and citing critical references, the HEC member may help the audience apply them in the context of a real ethical dilemma. This may be accomplished through a process of discovery using the concepts described to identify and respond to ethical questions. Discussion is useful for facilitating awareness of an ethical issue, identifying differing points of view, discerning underlying premises, assessing points of commonality, and promoting active reasoning. The Socratic method, for example, involves a dialogue among people with different positions or perspectives on a subject, who challenge and examine contrary viewpoints and work toward agreement by reasoned argument. Engaging the learner in any audience in this process rather than dictating to the student facilitates understanding and skill development and may enhance positive attitudes about the role and value of ethics in the clinical setting.

Role Models

Consider the best teacher you had in elementary school or college. It was probably not the teacher's selection of textbook, assignments, or even the syllabus that you most remember. The classroom materials were important to what you learned, but it was likely the teacher themself that was most significant. What did that teacher do? Usually good teachers are passionate about their subject, know the material well, and demonstrate how the material impacts the student or the community. Students recall the content because of its presentation and its relevance. A teacher, as a role model, does more than impart knowledge; they also demonstrate competent practice and positive attitudes, ultimately habituating students into their roles. Research suggests that students are more influenced by what they see than what they are taught; the hidden curriculum is more powerful than the formal (Lehmann et al., 2018). Observing ethical practice will normalize that behavior, create expectations, and sensitize learners to contrary behaviors. With regard to Mary's case, the HEC member must do more than extol the value of good communication; they must demonstrate it. A controversial case provides an opportunity to show how other HEC members or clinicians might facilitate difficult discussions or how community members can ask questions they otherwise might hesitate to raise.

Narrative

Every patient, every question, every conflict has a story. These stories are informative and transformative, and can be instructive (Charon, 2006). Most people learn and have learned from stories, from the fairytales of their childhoods, the biblical stories of their religious education, to the news stories of the day. The educator must convey and help the learner interpret the complex narratives of patient cases and societal conundrums, to help discern the ethical questions and determine ethical options. Weaving together the story enriches understanding of the ethical question and provides insights into addressing it. Mary's case offers a rich narrative. The HEC member can tease out the details to support the educational objectives designed for the particular audience. HEC members, for example, may benefit from details about specific problems with Mary's advance directives; physicians from discussion about the various decision points; and the lay community from a better understanding of the family dynamic. The details build the big picture and allow the educator to guide the audience in discerning the moral of the story or the take-home messages.

Online Pedagogy

Ethics education is not limited to the classroom or the clinic and may increasingly move online. Web-based education with its unique possibilities for engaging information and extending communication offers opportunities to broaden the audience, reaching beyond usual educational settings and providing ongoing learning and review (Broadhurst et al., 2012). Webinars, social media platforms, blogs, educational websites, and recorded lectures and case simulations offer interactive forums or resources for HEC members that may afford time for reflection not available in a traditional classroom. Online offerings can provide specific content education, training, values clarification exercises, knowledge or performance evaluation, mentorship, and networking. The opportunities may be live, instructor-led meetings, or asynchronous passive learning resources. Mary's case may offer several options for further learning, as long as care is taken to avoid any breaches of patient privacy and confidentiality. The HEC may record a deidentified case review, detailing case-based analysis skills and relevant literature, posted to a website for future use. The HEC could develop a secure chat forum or blog to discuss such cases, building critical thinking skills and identifying lessons for application to future cases. The case may be the basis for an interactive online case simulation or webinar on cases involving similar issues to enhance content knowledge and develop case analysis skills.

Obstacles to Ethics Education

When offering ethics education, the HEC member may face a number of obstacles beyond logistical difficulties. While the HEC will likely be predisposed to appreciating the educational presentation, clinician audiences may be disinterested or resistant, and even those from the community who elected to attend might not understand what ethics is. A prepared presenter will be ready to address some common objections.

"I Don't Need Ethics"

Some audience members may submit that "I am a good person," "I learned at my mother's knee/my preacher's pulpit/my kindergarten desk," "I know right from wrong; I don't need ethics." Morality is appropriately understood as a matter of personal values or individual character but being good does not necessarily result in doing good. Ethics attends to the varied worldviews and experiences that can produce conflict, conflict resolution tools, and ongoing moral development. Every time someone asks, "What should I do?" they are asking an ethical question, which ethics education can help address. The goal of a case presentation is not to suggest that anyone did anything wrong, or that anyone involved is a bad person, but to derive lessons from the case. All involved in Mary's case were trying to do what they thought best for Mary, but the persistent conflict required detailed analysis and skilled facilitation.

"Ethics Cannot Be Taught"

Edmund Pellegrino famously asked, "Can ethics be taught?" He responded in the affirmative, but explained: "Critics assert that a course in ethics does not make one necessarily more ethical or more virtuous. This is true. One may have knowledge of ethics, a cognitive grasp, but lack the motivation to do the right thing. No course could automatically close the gap between knowing what is right and doing it" (Pellegrino, 1989, 492).

Yet, he continues: "there is unwarranted pessimism in concluding that one's students are beyond our influence" (Pellegrino, 1989, 493). The difficulties with teaching ethics do not mean "that ethics cannot be taught at all, nor that virtue is entirely unteachable" (Pellegrino, 1989, 492). Rather, the "criticisms leveled against the possibility or utility of teaching stem from a misunderstanding of what ethics is, what it can teach and what it cannot, and the illusory nature of substitutes for teaching. Ethics decisions are intrinsic to every important clinical decision" (Pellegrino, 1989, 494).

Responding to the claim that ethics cannot be taught requires recourse to the goals of education, which must be realistic. Education is intended to have a formative effect on thinking, physical skills, or character, but these may be separate categories that require distinct objectives and methods, but that are interdependent (Giubilini et al., 2016, 130). Ethics education may target the knowledge and skills necessary for successful work in ethics consultation or with an ethics committee. Objectives may include increasing understanding of ethical conflicts, identifying potential areas of disagreement, developing communication skills, facilitating compromise, and/or motivating thoughtful reflection. Ethics education may also aim to address the attitudes that affect virtue and character, with objectives such as enhancing awareness of personal beliefs, understanding conflicts between self-interest and the interests of others, and developing sensitivity to diverse individuals. As cases arise, they will offer specific teaching opportunities and can serve as real and relatable examples in a more comprehensive curriculum that employs teaching techniques such as case review, role play, and exercises in applying ethical theory. Goals in Mary's case may be general and appropriate to multiple audiences such as identifying the source(s) of conflict, illustrating helpful communication processes, and sensitivity to alternate perspectives of stakeholders in a case, or more specific such as writing valid advance directives for the lay audience, or understanding hospital policy and law on the process of selecting a surrogate decision maker for the clinician and HEC member audiences. These educational efforts should be coordinated with intention, expressing explicit objectives that address both cognition and character. While taking advantage of the teachable moments in specific cases, the education should be offered regularly demonstrating the ethical issues embedded in health care and the opportunities for learning.

"Don't Tell Me What to Do"

A goal of education is often to inform action, and students expect to be told what to do to compute a chemical equation or to write a clear essay. Students of ethics, whether in a lecture or the clinical setting, may similarly expect that they will be told what to do – what the "right" answer to an ethical question is – especially if they believe that ethics is about right/wrong in some absolute sense. This misplaced expectation may result in resentment, either if one is told what to do or if an answer is not forthcoming. Neither in the classroom nor in the hospital room are ethics educators or clinical ethicists likely to tell someone what to do or believe (even if they really want to). Instead, the HEC member will help others clarify their values, identify the questions they face, and reason about those questions in a manner that is consistent with their values. Ethics provides methods for decision-making and processes, not specific answers. The HEC member's role is not to decide whether Jimmy or Emily should make the decision, or to decide what decision should be made, but instead to help the family determine what course of action best reflects Mary's values. Understanding this process will be helpful to all audiences, as each may engage in it from their distinct positions.

The HEC member may also encounter the opposite complaint. Ethics may prove to be frustrating for those who do simply want to be told what to do. While the HEC member may be tempted to make pronouncements about right and wrong, case-based teaching provides an occasion to assist others with that determination.

Conclusion

HECs are responsible for ethics education, in addition to clinical ethics consultation and policy review and development. Every case consultation provides opportunities for education. Determining educational objectives or goals related to developing knowledge, skills, and attitudes must begin with a consideration of the audience. The case may shape the objectives or may be used to support specific objectives. Because medical ethics is a living discipline with real impact on day-to-day lives and individual actions, ethics education must draw on its relevance to the real world and clinical setting. Effective pedagogy should engage, enlighten, and encourage. As American scholar and educator William Arthur Ward once said, "The mediocre teacher tells. The good teacher explains. The superior teacher demonstrates. The great teacher inspires."

Questions for Discussion

1. Conceptual: Consider the objections and obstacles to ethics education. How might you respond in your institution?
2. Practical: Reflect on a recent case. Consider the three most important educational objectives for the HEC, clinicians, and community members, and the most effective method for teaching those objectives.
3. Strategic: Consider a case in which you have been tempted to dictate action. What did you learn from that experience and how can you teach about that learning?

References

American Society for Bioethics and Humanities. (2011). *Core Competencies for Healthcare Ethics Consultation*, 2nd ed. Glenview, IL: ASBH.

American Society for Bioethics and Humanities. (2019). *Healthcare Ethics Consulting Certification Candidate Handbook.* https://asbh.org/hec-c-candidate-handbook (accessed September 30, 2019).

Broadhurst J, Gormley S, Haywood J (2012). Are MOOCs a game-changer for higher education? The Observatory on Borderless Higher Education, Borderless Report, October. www.obhe.ac.uk/newsletters/borderless_report_october_2012/are_moocs_a_game_changer_for_higher_education (accessed August 18, 2020).

Charon R (2006). *Narrative Medicine: Honoring the Stories of Illness.* New York: Oxford University Press.

Culver CM, Clouser KD, Gert B, et al. (1985). Basic curricular goals in medical ethics. *New England Journal of Medicine*, 312(4): 253–256.

DuBois JM, Burkemper J (2002). Ethics education in US medical schools: A study essay. *Mount Sinai Journal of Medicine*, 77(5): 432–437.

Dunn, R. (2000). Learning styles: Theory, research, and practice. *National Forum of Applied Educational Research Journal*, 13(1): 3–22.

Giubilini A, Milnes S, Savulescu J (2016). The medical ethics curriculum in medical schools: Present and future. *Journal of Clinical Ethics*, 27(2): 129–145.

Lehmann LS, Snyder Sulmasy L, Desai S, ACP Ethics, Professionalism and Human Rights Committee. (2018). Hidden curricula, ethics, and professionalism: Optimizing clinical learning environments in becoming and being a physician: A position paper of the American College of Physicians. *Annals of Internal Medicine*, 168(7): 506–508.

Pellegrino EP (1989). Can ethics be taught? An essay. *Mount Sinai Journal of Medicine*, 56(6): 490–494.

Sugarman J, Sulmasy D, eds. (2001). *Medical Ethics*. Washington, DC: Georgetown University Press.

Chapter

30

Quality Assessment of Healthcare Ethics Committees

Katherine Wasson

Objectives

Upon reading and considering the content of this chapter, the reader should be able to:

1. Defend the ethical imperative to perform quality assessment (QA) and quality improvement (QI) strategies for all of the work of the healthcare ethics committee (HEC).
2. Implement effective strategies to assess the ethics committee's consultation, education, and policy functions.
3. Recommend QI processes for the committee's functions.

Case 1

A 72-year-old patient with advanced lung cancer is admitted to the hospital and tells the medical team he does not want to be resuscitated. His condition deteriorates, he is placed on a ventilator and loses capacity, and his wife and son then demand the do-not-resuscitate (DNR) order be rescinded. The hospital policy supports maintaining the DNR order in the chart without the wife's "consent." The team is distressed but unsure how strongly to push back against her wishes at such a difficult time. Additionally, the adult son adamantly opposes the DNR order and is a physician himself. An ethics consult is requested. During the consultation, the ethics consultant elicits the team's desire to respect the patient's wishes, explains the hospital policy, and explores why the wife and son disagree. The patient's wife expresses her reservations about her husband's decision, as it was a change from prior discussions, and anticipatory grief about losing him. The son remains convinced that his father would not "give up," that a DNR order is not in his best interests, and that the medical team's recommendations are dissatisfactory. The ethics consultant attempts to clarify the ethical issues and options, explore the values of each person, and facilitate a decision upon which all can agree.

Case 2

In undertaking QA efforts, the HEC chair requests that a retrospective review of ethics consultations be done for the past 2 years. A subcommittee is formed to conduct the review and examine the data. The subcommittee notices that there has been an upward trend in consult requests from the medical ICU (MICU) by 30% in the past year and a 25% decrease in requests from the neonatal ICU (NICU). Further investigation ensues and the subcommittee reports back that one reason for these trends is that the MICU has a new nurse manager and multiple new and less experienced nurses on the unit. Therefore, it concludes that quality improvement strategies are needed to help educate these new health professionals. In contrast, the HEC and clinical ethics consultation (CEC) service have been providing monthly ethics "brown bag" sessions on the NICU for all staff. The new medical director and a nurse manager have stressed the importance of attending and participating. These sessions seem to have been a factor in decreasing the need for ethics consultation as clinicians have become more comfortable addressing the issues themselves and when to request an ethics consult for more in-depth help.

Why Healthcare Professionals Ought to Care about Quality in Relation to Healthcare Ethics Committees

The duties of an HEC consists of policy development and review, ethics education, and CEC. All three domains impact patients, families, staff, clinicians, and the institution as a whole. These domains are integral to the mission and function of the hospital or healthcare system as they embody the values of the organization and provide practical guidance.

The moral imperative underlying the duty to provide and assess quality in the HEC's functions rests on two ethical principles: the duty to care and nonmaleficence. Members of the HEC are part of a hospital or healthcare setting that provides care for patients. They have a duty to care for these patients and part of that care is providing services that are at minimum competent and, ideally, high quality, both in direct patient care and those that indirectly support it. For the HEC, that includes having ethically sound and effective policies, educational efforts, and ethics consultation services. Poor-quality ethics services (e.g., those that give inaccurate information) may cause harm to stakeholders. Part of assessing the quality of these functions is to examine whether the three domains, at minimum, do no harm or help avoid harm to stakeholders.

On another level, QA includes at least basic competence in each domain. For ethics consultants, the American Society for Bioethics and Humanities (ASBH) has established clear quality standards and expectations in its *Core Competencies for Healthcare Ethics Consultation*; these standards also include the obligation to evaluate the consultation service (ASBH, 2011). Additionally, The Joint Commission requires each facility to provide access to ethics services, and it evaluates those services for quality during accreditation. The professional standards help to set the stage for QA of the work of HECs.

Policy: While the HEC is not responsible for developing and reviewing all institutional policies, ethical policy development and review impacts all levels of the hospital. Policies provide guidelines, standards, and processes on specific issues. There are organizational policies, such as conflicts of interest, and those that deal with specific patient care situations, such as cardiopulmonary resuscitation (CPR), which contain ethical components or concerns. HEC policies also may include information on moral frameworks, principles, and rationales that support the policy to help stakeholders understand the context in which the policy was developed. QA of policies examines whether a policy meets its aims and objectives, addresses relevant issues and needs identified, and provides and communicates the guidance effectively to stakeholders.

Ethics Education: The quality of ethics education for the HEC is important because its members are charged with overseeing a significant proportion of the ethics work in a hospital. At minimum, HEC members need a basic knowledge and understanding of ethical principles, theories, and approaches to moral decision-making. Assessing this knowledge and any educational efforts is a first step in QA.

Clinical Ethics Consultation: The quality of the ethics consultation service is important because it directly impacts patients, families, staff, and clinicians often at a vulnerable moment dealing with highly sensitive issues. The HEC may provide QA for the ethics consultation service it provides itself or it may serve as the QA body for an independent ethics consultation service. An ethics consultation is requested precisely when those involved in the case or issue are uncertain about what to do and, thus, seek moral guidance. An ethics consultant attempts to identify and clarify ethical issues and resolve conflict when possible. The ASBH recognizes that ethics consultation is part of providing quality health care (ASBH, 2011), therefore, it needs to be a quality service too. The first standard in the *Code of Ethics and Professional Responsibilities for Healthcare Ethics Consultants* is "Be competent" (ASBH, 2014).

For all three domains, caring about quality is a necessary first step. While quality may be low or high, the first level of quality is defined as competence. Assessing quality at a basic level must take place before striving for excellence, and it highlights areas for QI.

Strategies for Quality Assessment and Quality Improvement for HECs

Policy: Sound practices in policy development include articulating a clear rationale or need for the new policy or revision, agreeing on the aims and scope, identifying key stakeholders and experts from across the institution, especially those affected by it in practice, surveying current guidelines in the field, and seeking feedback on drafts (Flamm, 2012). QA ought to include drawing up clear process steps for every policy and assuring they are followed, similar to a checklist in the operating room. Policy implementation includes education on multiple levels of the institution and should be part of the specified or required process steps and assessed.

QA can be triggered by the normal review cycle in an institution, for example all policies are reviewed on a 3- to 5-year cycle, a change in national or specialty-specific guidelines, or institutional mergers may mean policies need to be reviewed and aligned. If the aims or scope of an existing policy must change significantly to meet current needs, then it can either be revised or a new policy written. A new policy might need to be developed to address a recurring issue or consideration that is not covered by existing policies or not in sufficient detail. Ideally, the HEC and larger organization will have processes to trigger a policy review or development that are known and accessible to stakeholders. To help identify which policies are appropriate for the HEC, Frolic and colleagues (2013) developed a "Notice of Intent Form" for requestors: Does the policy involve a potentially controversial moral or social issue? Could this policy conflict with the health system's mission, vision, values, or code of conduct? Could this policy negatively impact patient/family/staff interests or rights? Consistency in this QA approach is inherently important to establish and maintain the quality of policies and will help maintain standards even among institutional changes.

As policies are reviewed, issues for QI will emerge. Frolic and colleagues (2013) have published the most detailed framework for policy QI: (1) identify ethical issues raised by the policy; (2) study the facts; (3) seek possible recommendations; (4) understand values and duties; (5) evaluate and justify recommendations; and (6) sustain and review the policy. To engage QI efforts regarding policy development and implementation, the HEC should pilot test the policy once drafted and obtain feedback from a range of key stakeholders to anticipate barriers (Flamm, 2012). Specifically, Frolic et al. (2013) recommend seeking feedback from the requestor and HEC about the process of the policy review and how much of the HEC's input was adopted in the final policy as part of QA. The HEC can also create evaluations to assess needs before a policy roll-out and then evaluate once it is implemented. Eliciting formal and informal feedback over time to evaluate the implementation efforts and effectiveness of the policy is also important for QA. A policy subgroup can be formed and meet to discuss the feedback and conduct QI projects, for example necessary changes to the electronic medical record (EHR) or additional education. Policy education should include multiple levels in the institution, such as department chairs, managers, and frontline staff, and different media, for example written information, formal education sessions, grand rounds, and webinars.

Ethics Education: The HEC is responsible for educating its membership, ideally when the members join as well as afterward (Zaidi and Kesselheim, 2018). It also has a duty to educate staff about ethics policies, the ethics consultation service, and ethical issues that arise. Such efforts may include unit-based brown bag sessions, case consultations, grand rounds, or a series of sessions on a given topic or unit. QA should be done to evaluate those efforts for quality and effectiveness, specifically increased knowledge of participants, and also identify future topics of interest to stakeholders. QA might include short quizzes before and after the education offering or soliciting narrative feedback from participants. While common, satisfaction surveys are of limited usefulness because of inherent biases of the participants and the fact that satisfaction and increased knowledge are not equivalent.

While ethics education is viewed as necessary in a healthcare institution, there is no agreed-upon effective method to deliver and evaluate education. Carlin et al. (2011) developed the Health Professional Ethics Rubric for assessing ethics education in health professional schools. Bardon (2004) challenges the assumption that ethics education is beneficial for an HEC, stating there is a dearth of evidence linking such education with improved moral development, reasoning, confidence, or performance. He also claims the potential content of ethics education for HECs is not clear. Given these gaps in the literature, the HEC will need to determine its focus, set clear objectives, and evaluate its efforts using appropriate methods. Tools for evaluating changes in knowledge can be developed through pre- and post-tests or existing scales, while moral reasoning can be assessed using case vignettes or simulations. More research is needed on QA in ethics education for HECs specifically.

ASBH sets clear standards for knowledge in ethics and articulates whether one or all members of the HEC should possess it (ASBH, 2011). QI educational needs can be addressed using ASBH *Core Competencies* and other related case-based resources. As of 2018, there is a formal certification for healthcare ethics consultants (HEC-C) via eligibility criteria and a multiple-choice examination developed by ASBH. Passing the examination demonstrates minimum competence and attests to basic quality for someone doing ethics consultation and is a vital element of QA in the field. To educate its members, an HEC could break down the relevant content areas from ASBH and address them via case-based discussion, presentations by members or guest speakers, and webinars.

Clinical Ethics Consultation Services: A key responsibility of the HEC is to do QA via retrospective case review regularly (e.g., monthly or quarterly), including the nature of the consultation request, requestor, unit, processes followed, and ethical issues and reasoning for recommendations. The HEC should assess whether any steps were omitted or additional input is needed. Are there recurring ethical challenges or organizational ethics issues that should be communicated to administration? The retrospective review also provides an educational opportunity for committee members who do not provide consultation.

A desirable outcome of QA is to examine patterns, for example to see which units request ethics consults most frequently, what ethical issues arise, and whether there have been changes in the requests over time. Important questions for tailoring such efforts include: Who are the "frequent flyers" of this service? Do they remain the same or change over time? Which services underutilize the service? What are the most common ethical issues and questions? What are some appropriate responses to the needs raised and patterns observed? Any service should examine how it "counts" or captures ethics consults, related efforts, and time spent. In Case 2, a review of the ethics consults identified a sharp rise in requests from the MICU. The HEC chair and ethics consultants were able to evaluate the data, identify this rise, and develop a strategy to investigate the reasons behind it. Once it was known that the nurse manager had changed and multiple new and less experienced nurses were hired, the CEC service developed a strategy to provide ethics education and identify champions on the unit. The QA naturally led to QI. HECs are also responsible for ensuring that a more comprehensive review is done at regular intervals, for example 1–5 years depending on consult volume, and to examine patterns, gaps, and needs and formulate appropriate responses. Services should publish these results, especially larger services with more resources, to contribute to knowledge about QA and QI in the field more widely.

Determining appropriate measures for evaluating the quality of CEC services is a challenge with little consensus and limited data on what approaches are most effective. Needs assessments, satisfaction surveys, and data analyses from ethics consults have all been used. Satisfaction surveys are limited in their usefulness depending on how the different participants viewed the process and outcomes (Repenshek, 2018). When ethics consultations are called in the midst of conflict, they have the potential to be unsatisfactory to one or more parties. For example, in Case 1 the son remained dissatisfied that his wishes for his father were not followed even though his mother is the appropriate surrogate decision maker and the patient's wishes were respected by upholding the DNR order. He might not complete this type of evaluation or is likely to express his dissatisfaction because he disagrees with the decision. Even though an ethically justifiable resolution was reached, the satisfaction score will be lowered because of one participant's experience and views. Surveys also pose practical challenges about response rates and how to locate those outside the hospital to gather feedback. Responses are likely to be skewed toward hospital staff who, again, may or may not be "happy" with the recommendations or outcomes of the ethics consultation.

Other potential empirical measures for QA and effectiveness, such as length of stay and potential cost savings, have been used and their benefits and detriments evaluated

(Schneiderman et al., 2003; Repenshek, 2018). Whether the ethical recommendations in the case have been followed is another potential outcome measure. However, this is time-consuming to assess, and other factors, such as the patient's death, may take place before implementation, thus skewing the results.

There is a range of approaches to QI for CEC (Volpe, 2017). At a basic level, the annual retrospective review of all cases provides an opportunity to identify changes, needs, and areas for growth. Ethics consultants should meet regularly outside of the HEC meetings to discuss ongoing concerns, patterns, and processes for the service. Having each consultant review their own cases and write-ups for a given period (a year or a specific number of consults) and present that assessment to colleagues may prove useful both in self-reflection and gathering input from the group in a more systematic manner than the HEC meetings. Over time, it will also highlight differences in style and content and allow the group to clarify processes and best practices.

Many hospitals have or are shifting to an EHR. Developing a template for CEC notes is an important QI project. Providing a consistent structure and format that is easy to identify allows the ethics consultant to focus on the content. It also allows other users of the EHR to elicit quickly the key information and recommendations in the chart and provides data for QA, QI, and research.

As for clinical ethics skills, the ASBH identifies standards in this arena (ASBH, 2011). However, there are few opportunities to learn and assess those skills, much less practice and improve them in a standardized manner. While individuals can now complete degrees in bioethics and concentrate on clinical ethics, fellowships with practical training remain limited in number and may not be feasible or realistic for the many mid-career professionals who volunteer their time for the HEC.

The Assessing Clinical Ethics Skills (ACES) tool focuses on the interpersonal skills and knowledge of CECs (Wasson et al., 2016). The ACES tool can be used as part of educational efforts within an HEC or CEC service. The ACES website includes clinical ethics cases and teaches the user to evaluate the ethics consultant in the video case. Individuals can complete a case before the HEC meeting and compare responses or the committee can view scenes from the case and discuss the correct responses together. Another goal could be to use the ACES tool to rate a CEC colleague in "real time" as they conduct an ethics consultation providing structured feedback for improvement.

Other tools include the Ethics Consultation Quality Assessment Tool that trains raters to review ethics consultation written records as a means of QA. Raters assess the Ethics Question; Consultation-Specific Information; Ethical Analysis; Conclusions/Recommendations (Pearlman et al., 2016). The United States Department of Veterans Affairs National Center for Ethics in Health Care provides multiple ethics consultation resources on its website, including proficiency tools that may be useful to an HEC (National Center for Ethics in Health Care, US Department of Veterans Affairs, 2020).

Live role-play or formal simulations are other valuable QI approaches to hone ethics consultation skills. The ethics team can select a case and then each play a role while observers use the ACES tool or other evaluation tool to provide structured feedback. Then, participants can switch and play other roles or observe. Cases can be drawn from real life or texts. If a formal simulation center is used, the participants will be video recorded and be able to review their performance as well as receiving "real time" feedback. Sensitive and balanced feedback is vital and using an outside expert may aid this process with colleagues. The range of QI efforts may seem overwhelming, and those carrying out this responsibility need to assess their institutional context and constraints, identify what is most important and/or practical, and start somewhere, even if the effort is modest.

Broader Quality Improvement for HECs

Stepping back for a broader view of QI, another approach is to identify champions on specific units who are either part of the HEC or brought in to contribute to a specific policy, educational effort, or ethical issue. The champions should receive education and training and can become frontline persons who answer questions on the unit or direct colleagues to further resources as needed. They can be trained to address more straightforward ethical questions, such as identifying the appropriate surrogate decision maker, examining advance directives, or obtaining valid informed consent. Individuals may be motivated to be a champion by a particular interest or concern, for example withholding/withdrawing life-sustaining treatment, and can be offered professional recognition for their service and efforts, such as clinical ladder points or promotion. Residents and nurses may be able to develop QI projects more formally or a related research project. Finding projects where all stakeholders benefit is a savvy approach and builds commitment to the efforts in the longer term.

QA often should begin with a needs assessment or feedback from an "intervention." This naturally leads to QI ideas. Different institutions may have ways of fostering QI initiatives from separate departments, for example Quality and Patient Safety, to specific individuals who take ownership of the initiative. HECs should partner with these key resources to maximize their efforts and learn what is most effective when trying to communicate across the institution. Finding QI initiatives that involve people from different levels of the institution, that is, from bedside staff to managers to leadership, creates a greater likelihood the initiatives will be implemented and maintained.

Questions for Discussion

1. Conceptual: What are the purposes/objectives of QA and QI practices for HECs, and are there any that particularly resonate with your HEC?
2. Pragmatic: How might your HEC implement QA in one of the three domains, namely policy, education, or ethics consultation?
3. Strategic: Which individuals are vital to ensuring the long-term quality and health of your HEC and its roles in the institution? What opportunities do you have to communicate the outcomes of your QA and QI initiatives?

References

American Society for Bioethics and Humanities. (2011). *Core Competencies for Health Care Ethics Consultants*, 2nd ed. Glenview, IL: ASBH.

American Society for Bioethics and Humanities. (2014). *Code of Ethics and Professional Responsibilities for Healthcare*

Ethics Consultants. https://asbh.org/resources/guidelines-standards

Bardon A (2004). Ethics education and value prioritization among members of U.S. hospital ethics committees. *Kennedy Institute of Ethics Journal*, 14(4): 395–406.

Carlin N, Rozmus C, Spike J, et al. (2011). The Health Professional Ethics Rubric: Practical assessment in ethics education for health professional schools. *Journal of Academic Ethics*, 9(4): 277–290.

Flamm AL (2012). Developing effective ethics policy. In Hester DM, Schonfeld T, eds., *Guidance for Healthcare Ethics Committees*. Cambridge University Press, 130–138.

Frolic AN, Drolet K, HHS Policy Working Group. (2013). Ethics policy review: A case study in quality improvement. *Journal of Medical Ethics*, 39(2): 96–103.

National Center for Ethics in Health Care, US Department of Veterans Affairs. (2020). IntegratedEthics™ resources. www.ethics.va .gov/integratedethics/IE_Resources .asp#Ethics%20Consultation (accessed July 18, 2020).

Pearlman RA, Foglia MB, Fox E, Cohen JH, Chanko BL, Berkowitz KA (2016). Ethics Consultation Quality Assessment Tool: A novel method for assessing the quality of ethics case consultations based on written records. *American Journal of Bioethics*, 16(3): 3–14.

Repenshek M (2018). Examining quality and value in ethics consultation services. *The National Catholic Bioethics Quarterly*, 18(1): 59–68.

Schneiderman LJ, Gilmer T, Teetzel HD, et al. (2003). Effects of ethics consultations on nonbeneficial life-sustaining treatments in the intensive care setting: A randomized controlled trial. *JAMA*, 290(9): 1166–1172.

Volpe RL (2017). Ongoing evaluation of clinical ethics consultations as a form of continuous quality improvement. *The Journal of Clinical Ethics*, 28(4): 314–317.

Wasson K, Parsi K, McCarthy M, Siddall VJ, Kuczewski M (2016). Developing an evaluation tool for assessing clinical ethics consultation skills in simulation based education: The ACES project. *HEC Forum*, 28(2): 103–113.

Zaidi D, Kesselheim JC (2018). Assessment of orientation practices for ethics consultation at Harvard Medical School-affiliated hospitals. *The Journal of Medical Ethics*, 44(2): 91–96.

Index

Printed in the United States
by Baker & Taylor Publisher Services

Printed in the United States
by Baker & Taylor Publisher Services